CAMBRIDGE LIBRARY COLLECTION

Books of enduring scholarly value

History of Medicine

It is sobering to realise that as recently as the year in which On the Origin of Species was published, learned opinion was that diseases such as typhus and cholera were spread by a 'miasma', and suggestions that doctors should wash their hands before examining patients were greeted with mockery by the profession. The Cambridge Library Collection reissues milestone publications in the history of Western medicine as well as studies of other medical traditions. Its coverage ranges from Galen on anatomical procedures to Florence Nightingale's common-sense advice to nurses, and includes early research into genetics and mental health, colonial reports on tropical diseases, documents on public health and military medicine, and publications on spa culture and medicinal plants.

The Works, Literary, Moral, and Medical, of Thomas Percival, M.D.

A physician and medical reformer enthused by the scientific and cultural progress of the Enlightenment as it took hold in Britain, Thomas Percival (1740–1804) wrote on many topics, including public health and demography. His influential publication on medical ethics is considered the first modern formulation. In 1807, his son Edward published this four-volume collection of his father's diverse work. Some of the items here had never been published before, including a selection of Percival's private correspondence and a biographical account written by Edward. Volume 3 contains the first two parts of *Essays Medical and Experimental*, the revised edition of which has been reissued separately in this series in one volume in addition to his *Medical Ethics* (1803). The essays reflect Percival's wide range of interests, such as the application of philosophical methods to medical questions, the importance of accurate record keeping, and the risks of inoculating very young children against smallpox.

Cambridge University Press has long been a pioneer in the reissuing of out-of-print titles from its own backlist, producing digital reprints of books that are still sought after by scholars and students but could not be reprinted economically using traditional technology. The Cambridge Library Collection extends this activity to a wider range of books which are still of importance to researchers and professionals, either for the source material they contain, or as landmarks in the history of their academic discipline.

Drawing from the world-renowned collections in the Cambridge University Library and other partner libraries, and guided by the advice of experts in each subject area, Cambridge University Press is using state-of-the-art scanning machines in its own Printing House to capture the content of each book selected for inclusion. The files are processed to give a consistently clear, crisp image, and the books finished to the high quality standard for which the Press is recognised around the world. The latest print-on-demand technology ensures that the books will remain available indefinitely, and that orders for single or multiple copies can quickly be supplied.

The Cambridge Library Collection brings back to life books of enduring scholarly value (including out-of-copyright works originally issued by other publishers) across a wide range of disciplines in the humanities and social sciences and in science and technology.

The Works,
Literary, Moral, and Medical,
of Thomas Percival, M.D.

To which are Prefixed,
Memoirs of His Life and Writings,
and a Selection from
His Literary Correspondence

VOLUME 3

THOMAS PERCIVAL

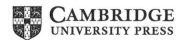

CAMBRIDGE
UNIVERSITY PRESS

CAMBRIDGE
UNIVERSITY PRESS

University Printing House, Cambridge, CB2 8BS, United Kingdom

Published in the United States of America by Cambridge University Press, New York

Cambridge University Press is part of the University of Cambridge.
It furthers the University's mission by disseminating knowledge in the pursuit of
education, learning and research at the highest international levels of excellence.

www.cambridge.org
Information on this title: www.cambridge.org/9781108067355

© in this compilation Cambridge University Press 2014

This edition first published 1807
This digitally printed version 2014

ISBN 978-1-108-06735-5 Paperback

THE

WORKS

OF

THOMAS PERCIVAL, M.D.

IN FOUR VOLUMES.

THE

WORKS,

LITERARY, MORAL,

AND

MEDICAL,

OF

THOMAS PERCIVAL, M.D.

F. R. S. AND A. S.—F. R. S. AND R. M. S. EDIN.

LATE PRES. OF THE LIT. AND PHIL. SOC. AT MANCHESTER; MEMBER OF
THE ROYAL SOCIETIES OF PARIS AND OF LYONS, OF THE MEDICAL
SOCIETIES OF LONDON, AND OF AIX EN PROVENCE, OF THE
AMERIC. ACAD. OF ARTS, &c. AND OF THE AMERIC.
PHIL. SOC. AT PHILADELPHIA.

TO WHICH ARE PREFIXED,

MEMOIRS of his LIFE and WRITINGS,

AND A SELECTION FROM HIS

LITERARY CORRESPONDENCE.

A NEW EDITION.

VOL. III.

PRINTED BY RICHARD CRUTTWELL, ST. JAMES's-STREET, BATH;
FOR J. JOHNSON, ST. PAUL's CHURCH-YARD, LONDON.

1807.

ESSAYS,

LITERARY, MORAL,

AND

MEDICAL.

ADVERTISEMENT.

THE present Edition of this Work comprehends not only the author's former volumes, of Medical, Philosophical, and Experimental Essays; but also many detached pieces, written at distant times, and on various occasions, that have been inserted either in the Transactions of some of the learned Societies, of which he is a member, or in other Periodical Journals. He has attentively revised the whole; has made numerous practical additions; and corrected or expunged whatever appeared to be inconsistent with his later experience, and better informed judgment. On certain philosophical subjects, of which he has treated, much light has been thrown by subsequent inquirers. He has not, however, attempted to model such Essays anew; or to weave into their texture discoveries and improvements, made since the period when they were written. For he deems anachronism, of this kind, to be a violation of literary property; and unfavourable to the interests of science, by creating perplexity in the view of its progressive advancement.

Manchester, February 11, 1788.

B O O K S

PUBLISHED BY THE AUTHOR.

I. A FATHER's INSTRUCTIONS, confisting of MORAL TALES, FABLES, and REFLECTIONS; defigned to promote the LOVE OF VIRTUE; and an early acquaintance with the WORKS OF NATURE. Sixth edit. crown 8vo. price 3 s. 6 d. fewed.

II. MORAL and LITERARY DISSERTATIONS, on the following fubjects: 1. On Truth and Faithful- nefs. 2. On Habit and Affociation. 3. On Incon- fiftency of Expectation in Literary Purfuits. 4. On a Tafte for the general Beauties of Nature. 5. On a Tafte for the Fine Arts. 6. On the Alliance of Natural Hiftory and Philofophy with Poetry. Crown 8vo. price 4 s. fewed.

TABLE

THE

CONTENTS.

PART I.

Vol. I. b *Experiments*

ESSAYS

E S S A Y S

MEDICAL, PHILOSOPHICAL,

AND

EXPERIMENTAL.

P A R T I.

Quantacunque fuerint aliorum conamina, semper existimavi mihi vitalis auræ usum frustra datum fore, nisi et ipse, in hoc studio versatus, symbolum aliquod, utcunque exiguum, in commune medicinæ ærarium contribuerem.

SYDENHAM.

T H E

P R E F A C E.

THE Author of the following
Eſſays, preſuming on the candour with which they have
been received, commits to the ſame
indulgence, the preſent enlarged and improved edition of them. The firſt and
ſecond Diſſertations are the productions
of his youth, and illuſtrate both the in-
ſufficiency of THEORY, and the danger
of truſting to EXPERIENCE alone in the
practice of phyſic. The annals of medicine abound with inſtances of the fatal
effects of empiricifm, and hypothetical
reaſoning, founded on fictitious principles.
But theſe examples, painful as they are
to a feeling mind, impeach not the honour

or

or ufefulnefs of the healing art; and
are chargeable only on the ignorance of a
few of its profeffors, and on the credulity
of mankind. The Hiftory of the Chriftian Church prefents us with a picture
ftill more fhocking to humanity: But
who difputes the influence of religion,
to promote the peace, order, and happi-
nefs of fociety, becaufe fuperftition hath
occafioned fo much confufion, mifery,
and devaftation? It is ferioufly to be
lamented that jufter ideas are not formed
of the nature, extent, and objects of
medicine in general; and of the feveral
branches, into which, as a practical fcience
too comprehenfive for any individual to
profefs, it is now divided. This would
prevent the encouragement of illiterate
pretenders; would conciliate harmony,
and excite a generous emulation amongft
the different orders of the faculty; and by
confining the exertions of each, within
the fphere adapted to their genius and
education, would powerfully promote the
improvement of Phyfic, Surgery, and
Pharmacy. No profeffion requires a more
enlarged

enlarged and cultivated underftanding, or
comprehends a wider circle of knowledge
than that of phyfic. And to the honour
of the phyficians of this age and country,
it may with truth be afferted, that they
are peculiarly diftinguifhed as men of
liberal education, and extenfive learning.

THE third Effay confifts of Experiments and Obfervations on BITTERS and
ASTRINGENTS in general, and on the
PERUVIAN BARK in particular *(a)*. The
utility

(a) Of this Effay, which was firft publifhed in 1767,
large portions have been copied into feveral Cyclopædias,
and Treatifes on the Materia Medica, both foreign and
domeftic. The author has reafon to believe that the
practical and pharmaceutical doctrines it contains have
been generally adopted. Two very ingenious writers,
however, have lately controverted the refults of fome of
the experiments which he has related. He acknowledges
with fatisfaction the candour of thefe Gentlemen ; and
thinks himfelf honoured by their approbation of his
works. But the points in difpute, he muft leave to the
decifion of others ; having *now* no leifure for fuch
inveftigations. He is fenfible that, in the courfe of his
inquiries, he muft have been liable to many fources of
fallacy : But the fame obfervation, he prefumes, is not
more applicable to him than to others engaged in
experimental refearches. And he trufts the reader will
perceive,

utility of this method of inquiry is
univerſally acknowledged ; and nothing
can tend more to the advancement of
real ſcience, than the ſteady purſuit of
it. The improvements made in the
art of medicine for this century paſt,
are more than equal to thoſe of a thou-
ſand preceding years. And theſe improvements may be juſtly aſcribed to
that taſte for experiment, which hath of
late ſo generally prevailed. But though
much hath been done in this way of inveſtigation, there are ſtill numberleſs un-
trodden paths in phyſic which remain to
be explored. And every perſon of tolerable abilities, who has patience, aſſi-
duity, and a ſufficient minuteneſs of
attention, may almoſt aſſure himſelf that

perceive, in the following pages, that he has endeavoured with cautious ſolicitude, to guard againſt the
undue influence of preconceptions ; that he has faithfully related faĉts and appearances as they occurred,
whether favourable or unfavourable to his opinions ;
that his experiments are numerous, diverſified, and
frequently repeated in the purſuit of different truths ;
and that they were made at a period when the Peruvian bark was eaſily obtained unadulterated, and of
a good quality.

MARCH 7, 1788.

his

his labours will be rewarded with fuccefs,
and that he cannot fail of adding fome
new and ufeful difcoveries to the common
ftock of medical knowledge. *Multum
egerunt qui ante nos fuerunt, fed non pere-
gerunt ; multum adhuc reftat operæ, mul-
tumq; reftabit, neque ulli nato poft mille
fecula præcidetur occafio aliquid adhuc ad-
jiciendi (b).* The author might have confirmed many of the obfervations contained
in this Effay by a variety of experiments,
which he has lately made on the Columbo
Root; a medicine, which from its efficacy,
deferves to be more generally known in
practice. But his papers on that fubject
are laid before the Royal Society, and
will probably be publifhed in the next
volume of Philofophical Tranfactions.

THE title of the fourth Effay fully
explains the purport of it. An attempt
to afcertain the ufe and operation of a
remedy fo well known as BLISTERS, may
at firft view appear to be unneceffary.
But a more attentive examination will

(b) Seneca.

convince us of our miſtake. The trite-
neſs of the ſubject is the reaſon that it has
been ſo much overlooked and neglected;
and though veſicatories are employed and
recommended by almoſt every medical
practitioner, yet few have attended to their
real action, or to the general principles
which ought to direct their application.

THE ſubject of the fifth Eſſay, the
author confeſſes, is rather curious than
uſeful; of more importance to the in-
quiſitive phyſiologiſt, than to the practical phyſician. But as all reſearches into
the operations of nature merit our notice
and regard, an inquiry into the reſem-
blance between the CHYLE and MILK
hath certainly ſome claim to attention. And if it appear probable, as he
preſumes it will, that milk is the chyle
unaſſimilated, or at leaſt very little
changed, it may lead to ſome uſeful inferences concerning the proper diet for
nurſes.

THE tracts on WATER, and on early
INOCULATION, were publiſhed, ſeparately,
a few

a few years ago; and as no copies of the former impreffions now remain, they are reprinted and annexed to this volume of Effays.

THE Obfervations on the efficacy of External Applications in the ULCEROUS SORE THROAT were written in the fummer of 1770, a period when that difeafe was epidemical in the town and neighbourhood of Manchefter. The Meafles alfo prevailed very generally at the fame time; but though thefe diforders have been often obferved to affociate together, and may feem to bear fome analogy to each other, from the efflorefcence on the fkin, and inflammation of the eyes, with which they are both accompanied, no inftance then occurred to the author of their union.

MANCHESTER,
JANUARY 1, 1772.

E S S A Y

E S S A Y I.

T H E

E M P I R I C

O R

M A N OF E X P E R I E N C E,

BEING ARGUMENTS AGAINST THE USE OF

THEORY AND REASONING IN PHYSIC. *(a)*

Sufficit fi quid fiat intelligamus, etiamfi quomodo quidque
fiat ignoremus. CICERO.

IN this polifhed age, when every art is ad-
vancing towards perfection, and every fcience
enlarging its boundaries, it is a melancholy
confideration that MEDICINE fhould alone be
left behind, in the general career of improvement.
The

(a) THIS and the following differtation contain a dif-
cuffion of the arguments for and againft the ufe of theory
and reafoning in medicine. They are not intended as
an explanation of the tenets of thofe two ancient and
celebrated fects of phyficians, the Empirics and Ration-
alifts, of which Celfus hath given us fo elegant an ac-
VOL. I.   B   count;

The mifts of ignorance and error are now vanifh-
ing before the lights of genuine philofophy; and
knowledge, practical and fpeculative, extends its
influence even to the meaneft mechanic. But the
Hippocratic art, amidft this rapid and almoft univerfal revolution, is at leaft ftationary, if it move
not in a retrograde courfe. And what is fingular
in its fate, the fame caufes which have promoted
the advancement of the fifter fciences, have, by a
wrong direction, checked the growth, and retarded
the progrefs of one, which is

—— fairly worth the feven.

POPE.

THE induftry of its profeffors, by an injudicious
application, hath ferved only to darken and perplex
it. Inftead of patiently treading in the fure fteps
of EXPERIENCE, they have followed the falfe clue of

count; but to point out opinions which now prevail in
the world, and which naturally arife from the different
lights, in which the fame fubject is viewed by different
minds. The author hath endeavoured to fuppofe himfelf
firft of the one party, and then of the other; in order
more fully to enter into the fentiments of each, and by
that means to do juftice to both fides of the queftion. In
this kind of writing it is not eafy to avoid declamation;
and he hopes to be excufed, if he has indulged fome degree of that enthufiafm, with which two antagonifts may
be fuppofed to be actuated, when pleading againft each
other, in fupport of a favourite caufe.

THEORY;

THEORY; and whilft, with infinite pains and labour, they endeavour to penetrate into the receffes of phyfic, they have loft themfelves in the labyrinths of error. Unhappily for the healing art, their miftakes have coincided with the common propenfities of mankind, who are more inclined to fearch after hidden and undifcoverable caufes, than to attend to the obvious phænomena of nature. Blinded with their own fictions, thefe wanton theorifts conceal their ignorance from themfelves and the world, by unmeaning terms and pompous phrafes.

" *Omnia enim ftolidi magis admirantur amantque*
" *Inverfis quæ fub verbis latitantia cernunt.*"
                                    LUCRETIUS.

BUT defcending from the flights of declamation, let us point out the folly, detect the fallacy, and trace the dangerous confequences of theory and reafoning in medicine.

WHOEVER fearches into the annals of phyfic, cannot fail of being aftonifhed at the almoft infinite variety of fyftems and hypothefes, which at different times have been obtruded on the world. The amazing fertility of the imagination is there difplayed in its full extent; and perhaps fo ample an exhibition of the powers of human invention might gratify the vanity of man, if the agreeable effect were not more than counterbalanced by the

B 2   humbling

humbling view of fo much abfurdity, contradiction, and falfehood. The idleft opinions have had their abettors; the moft groundlefs fictions have been fwallowed with credulity. A lift of all the follies which, at different periods, have been eftablifhed as articles of faith in medicine, would form the fevereft fatire on the healing art. Who can withhold his laughter when he reads of expelling, attracting, and concocting faculties; of energies, fympathies, antipathies, idiofyncrafies, and occult caufes; of the body being nothing but falt, fulphur, and mercury; of man being a microcofm, and uniting in his frame the motion of the ftars, the nature of the earth, of water, air, all vegetables and minerals, the conftellations, and the four winds. Yet ridiculous as thefe feveral tenets may appear, they have given rife to fects, have been efpoufed with warmth, and defended with acrimony. But the excentric genius of the theorifts hath not been confined within the limits of phyfiology, and the laws of the animal œconomy: the hidden caufes of difeafes, the elements or firft principles of medicines, and their fecret mode of action on the body, have afforded another no lefs extenfive field for the exercife of their creative imaginations. The bare recital of their fictions, would fufficiently demonftrate their abfurdity. But to enumerate them would be an almoft endlefs tafk. Erafiftratus defines difeafe to be a tranflation of blood from

the

the veins to the arteries; whereas Galen afferts
that, as health confifts in the equilibrium between
drynefs and moifture, heat and cold, ficknefs muft
depend upon the fubverfion of that equilibrium.
One fect adopts *plethora* as the caufe of all difeafes;
another denies the poffibility of its exiftence in
the body.   Sylvius exults in the difcovery that an
acid is the fole morbid principle; his antagonifts
afcribe that honour to their alkali.   Salt, fulphur,
acrimonies, cauftics, volatiles, ferments, &c. &c.
have each, at different times and by different fyftematics, been received as the undoubted *principia
morborum.*   No lefs abfurd are the fictions of the
theorifts, concerning the elements and qualities of
medicines, and their operation on the body.   The
fame drug is reprefented as hot in one degree and
cold in another, or as dry in one proportion and
moift in another.   Certain remedies are whimfi-
cally affigned to particular parts of the body, on
which they are fuppofed to exert their effects by a
peculiar predilection.   Hence the claffes of pectorals, ftomachics, hepatics, cephalics, cordials, &c.
One medicine attracts and eliminates the bile,
another the *pituita,* and a third the *atra bilis* or
melancholy.   Some preparations *irradiate* the animal fpirits, others *darken* and *obfcure* them.   But
enough of thefe idle conceits, the offspring of
theory, and the difgrace of phyfic!

PERHAPS it may be objected, that though many vain and groundlefs hypothefes have been advanced, there are two which will bear the teft of ridicule, and which have had the fuffrages of the wifeft and moft learned men in their favour. Let us briefly examine their pretenfions to credibility.

1. GEORGE ERNEST STAHL, a German phyfician, of a fubtil and metaphyfical genius, fuppofes two oppofite principles or propenfities in the human frame; one conftantly and uniformly tending to corruption and decay, the other to life and health. The former is founded on the elementary compofition of the body, the latter depends on the power and energy of the mind. By means of the nerves, the influence of the mind is extended to every part of the fyftem, and if their action be impeded, difeafe is the unavoidable confequence. A fuperabundance and fpiffitude of the blood is therefore the proximate caufe of ficknefs, as the energy of the mind is thereby diminifhed, and its action on the body obftructed. Hence to leffen the quantity, and break down the *lentor* of the blood, the foul exerts all its powers and excites hemorrhages, fweats, diarrhœas, fevers, and the like. Dr. Porterfield and Dr. Nichols have carried this theory ftill further. The latter, in his prælection *de anima medica*, affirms without referve, that the foul at firft forms the body, and afterwards governs

governs it; that she regulates and conducts all its vital and natural motions; circulates the fluids and distributes them to the different parts of the system, with such velocity and in such proportion as she judges right; and that whenever the body is disordered, she excites those conflicts and commotions, which are best adapted to restore it to health and soundness.

Such are the principles of the Stahlians.—Let the unprejudiced judge whether they need a serious refutation. Could a mariner plan and construct a ship, launch it into the wide ocean, govern it in storms, direct it from shoals and rocks, and steer it safe into the destined harbour, without being conscious of the skill he exerts, and the labour he employs? The analogy is obvious; and it would be equally absurd to suppose that the mind could form the body, regulate all its motions, superintend its health, rescue it from disease, and be perpetually occupied in planning and executing the wisest designs, without the least knowledge or consciousness of the power and energy she every moment exerts.

But the first proposition of the Stahlians confutes itself. For if the body and mind, with equal force, be constantly and uniformly tending different ways, no change can possibly ensue; agree-

ably

ably to the well known axiom in phyfics, that action and reaction are equal, and deſtroy each other's effect. Not to inſiſt however on this error in philoſophy, the doctrine of the Stahlians in confining all diſeaſes to *lentor* and *plethora* is falſe and abſurd. The dropſy, ſcurvy, *cacochymia,* jaundice, putrid fevers, and many of the nervous claſs of ailments, are accompanied for the moſt part with a thin and colliquated ſtate of the fluids. Nor is there more truth in the aſſertion, that every diſtemper is an effort of the mind to relieve the body. The ſlighteſt laceration of a tendon has been ſucceeded by the locked jaw, convulſions, and death. An indolent glandular tumour terminates not unfrequently in a cancer. A neglect to evacuate the bladder in due time hath occaſioned a ſuppreſſion of urine; and the palſy has been the conſequence of a profuſe he-morrhage. Are theſe then the wiſe conflicts of the ſoul, to reſcue her ſuffering partner from im-pending evil! And muſt we view in the ſame light the *angina maligna,* the *tuſſis convulſiva,* the ſpaſ-modic colic, the *tetanus, catalepſis,* worms, rickets, &c. &c. No one but a theoriſt, blinded with the miſts of his own brain, would anſwer in the affir-mative.

2. THE important diſcovery of the circulation of the blood, in the beginning of the laſt century, by

by the ever memorable Dr. Harvey, gave rife to
the introduction of MECHANICS into medicine.
And as that fyftem of philofophy was founded on
the general laws of nature, it was obvious to infer
its application to the human body; which was
fuppofed to differ only from the univerfe of things,
in the wonderful variety and complication of its
machinery. Bellini, Borelli, Pitcairn, Keil and
Boerhaave are the great fupporters of this theory.
According to the defcription of the latter, the body
is chiefly compofed of a conic, elaftic, inflected
canal, divided into fimilar leffer ones proceeding
from the fame trunk, which being at laft collected into a retiform contexture, mutually open
into each other, and fend off two orders of veffels,
lymphatics and veins, the one terminating in different cavities of the body, the other in the heart.
Thefe tubes are deftined for the conveyance of the
animal fluids; in the circulation of which life
confifts, and on whofe free and undifturbed motion health depends. *Obftruction* therefore is the
proximate caufe of moft difeafes. And as it is
produced either by a conftriction of the veffels, or
by a *lentor* in the blood, thefe are confidered as
the remote caufes.

However plaufible this theory may appear to
be at firft fight, it will be found, on a ftricter examination, to be fallacious and defective. The
mathematician

mathematician, who calculates the projectile force of the heart, the velocity of the blood in the arteries, and the various secretions of the glands, from the known laws of fluids in motion, and the nature of tubes of different shapes and sizes, must unavoidably be exposed to a thousand mistakes. The vessels of the body are too numerous and minute to admit of an accurate mensuration; and they are perhaps every moment undergoing changes, from the diversified action of that vital power which animates our wonderful system. Hence arises the contrariety in the computations of philosophers on this subject. Borelli reckons the resistance which the heart overcomes, in propelling the blood through the arteries and veins, to be equal to 180,000 pounds weight: Dr. Hales makes it amount to no more than 51 pounds; and Keil, though he computes the fluids of the human body to be five times more in quantity than Borelli supposes, hath reduced the sum to a single pound. One asserts that the pressure of air, overcome in ordinary respiration, is equivalent to the weight of 14000 pounds; a second proves it to be equal only to a 100 pounds; and a third makes it so inconsiderable, as to be almost below comparison; whilst all the three appeal to mathematical demonstration. A similar diversity appears in the conclusions of the mathematicians, concerning the quantity of bile separated by the liver.

liver. To determine this point, Borelli firſt mea-
ſures the diameter of the *duƈtus communis choledo-
chus*, which he finds to be the 225th part of the
diameter of the *vena cava*, juſt before it enters
the right auricle of the heart. Hence he infers
that if 7680 pounds of blood (ſuppoſing the whole
maſs to be twenty pounds, and to circulate ſixteen
times every hour) paſſes through the *vena cava*
in twenty-four hours, the 225th part of this quantity, i. e. thirty-four pounds of bile muſt, in the
ſame ſpace of time, be tranſmitted through the
hepatic duƈts: a concluſion altogether repugnant
to faƈt and experience. And it will appear to be
much more ſo, if we admit, with the latter mathematicians, that the veſſels of the human body
contain at a medium thirty pounds of blood ; for
then the quantity of bile, according to Borelli's
method of reaſoning, muſt amount to eighty-five
pounds in one day. But in this, as in the former
inſtance, Keil widely differs from Borelli, and
with greater probability concludes that two
drachms of bile and no more, are hourly ſeparated
from the liver. In theſe calculations no attention
is paid to the peculiar nature of the animal fluids.
Water and wine, a poiſonous and wholeſome
liquid, are governed by the ſame hydraulic laws,
but their effeƈts when circulating in the body
would certainly be very different. We know,
from experience, that the velocity of the pulſe is
                                              influenced

influenced by the ftate of the blood. Even the
acceffion of new chyle, after each meal, quickens
the action of the heart and arteries. The human
body therefore is not to be confidered as a mere
machine; and that theory which is built on this
foundation is evidently fallacious. *(b)*

But the mechanic hypothefis is alfo inadequate
and defective; for the animal frame is incident to
numberlefs difeafes which have no dependence on
obftruction. The *morbi fibræ debilis et laxæ* are
not, even by Boerhaave himfelf, afcribed to this
caufe. The dropfy, fcurvy, putrid fevers, fmall-
pox, meafles, and *lues venerea* are inexplicable on
mechanical principles. The *hydrophobia* feems to
be entirely a nervous affection, and cannot with
the leaft propriety be fuppofed to arife from obftruction. No inflammation is obfervable on diffection in the fauces or gullet; nor is there any
palfy in the mufcles fubfervient to deglutition. A
numerous clafs of difeafes depend upon that fympathetic connexion, which fubfifts between different

(b) In the Philofophical Tranfactions there is a table,
in which the feveral purgatives and emetics, commonly
in ufe, are enumerated and adjufted by mathematical rules
to all ages, fexes, and conftitutions. The dofes of the medicines are as the fquares of the conftitutions. And in
the Edinburgh Medical Effays there is a formal attempt
to correct the errors of this table.

parts of the body. When the ftomach is out of order, languor, debility, watchfulnefs, the night mare, and fometimes a *cephalæa, vertigo,* or *hemi-crania* are the confequences. A rough bone fti-mulating the nerves of the great toe, hath pro-duced epileptic fits. And it is well known that children, from the irritation of the gums in denti-tion, are liable to vomiting, purging, fever, and convulfions. Thefe few inftances are fufficient to fhew that the body is unhappily fubject to many diforders, befides thofe which proceed from ob-ftruction. And perhaps the conclufion may be carried ftill further, when we confider that in the operation for the aneurifm a large artery is tied up, and the circulation of the blood for fome time almoft totally fuppreffed in the part, without any material injury to health. Morgagni relates that Valfalva affixed two ligatures to the carotids of a dog, who lived above twenty days after the ope-ration, and might have continued longer, if he had not been killed for the purpofe of diffection. Is it then to be fuppofed that the obftruction of a few capillaries, which are united together by an infinite number of anaftomofing branches, can be pro-ductive of fuch fatal confequences, whilft the courfe of the blood is ftopped in large veffels with impunity? Equally falfe and abfurd is the mecha-nical hypothefis, concerning the operation of me-dicines, which is fuppofed to depend upon the fize,

figure,

figure, and gravity of their conftituent particles. Thus chalybeates, for example, are recommended in obftructions of the *catamenia*, on account of the *momentum* which they communicate to the blood. And on the fame principles, mercury is faid to break down the texture, and produce a colliquation of the animal fluids. But both thefe explanations, however elegant in theory, are falfe in fact. From the experiments of the late Dr. Wright *(c)* it is evident that fteel never enters the lacteals, and that it exerts its effects folely on the ftomach and bowels. And it is furely beyond the bounds of credibility to fuppofe, that a few grains of corrofive fublimate, which are light enough to be fufpended and diffolved in brandy, are capable, by their extraordinary weight, of diffolving the *craffamentum* of the blood. But it is the genius of theory to dignify trifles, and to afcribe the moft wonderful effects to the moft infignificant caufes.

Happy however had it been for the world, if the medical fyftems, which have been obtruded on it, were only chargeable with inutility, abfurdity, or falfehood. But alas! they have mifled the underftanding, perverted the judgment, and given rife to the moft dangerous and fatal errors in practice. A fhort view of the hiftory of phyfic

(c) Phil. Tranf. vol. L. part II. p. 595.

will

will convince us of this melancholy truth. The divine Hippocrates knew how to diftinguifh between theory and experience; and he fuffered not his doctrines of fire and water, his elements with their powers, nature with its inclinations, averfions, attractions, repulfions, and ratiocinations, to influence his treatment of difeafes. But the conduct of his fucceffors was widely different.

ERASISTRATUS reafoning on falfe and precarious principles, and neglecting experience, the fole teft of utility, profcribes the ufe of venæfection and purgatives, and condemns them as remedies equally infamous and dangerous.

ASCLEPIADES, from whom the modern fect of mechanics have borrowed many of their doctrines, fuppofing that health depends on the juft proportion between the pores of the body and certain corpufcles, which they are deftined to receive and tranfmit, and that it is impaired whenever thefe corpufcles are obftructed in their paffage, orders exercife on horfeback in the moft ardent fevers. He advances it as a maxim, that one fever is to be cured by raifing another; and that the ftrength of the patient is to be exhaufted by watching, and the endurance of thirft. And his practice was ftrictly and feverely conformable to his principles; for he would not allow the fick to cool their mouths with a drop of water, during the two firft days of

the

the diforder.   But he indulged his phrenitic patients in the ufe of wine, even to intoxication.

THEMISON, the difciple of Afclepiades, re-
jeéted fome of the opinions of his mafter, and
founded a new feét, called the Methodics.   But
his praétice did not materially differ from that of
Afclepiades, and his fuccefs is recorded by Juvenal in the following line:

Quot Themifon ægros autumno occiderit uno.

GALEN for the moft part followed the plan of
Hippocrates, in the treatment of difeafes.   But as
the *materia medica* in the courfe of five hundred
years had been much augmented, the prefcrip-
tions of Galen were devoid of the Hippocratic
fimplicity.   And it is more than probable that
his falfe and ridiculous theory, concerning the
primary qualities of hot and cold, dry and moift,
led him into dangerous errors in the compofition
of medicines.

ORIBASIUS, Ætius, Alexander, Trallianus,
Paulus Ægineta, and their fucceffors the Arabian
phyficians, attempted no material innovations, but
humbly trod in the footfteps of Galen.   The Arabians indeed introduced feveral new and valuable
medicines into praétice, fuch as manna, fenna, ta-
marinds, caffia, and rhubarb.   And by the culti-
vation of chemiftry, they laid a foundation for the
greateft

greateft and moft important revolutions in the art of medicine. I omit the mention of Albertus Magnus, Arnoldus de Villa Nova, Raymund Lully, Johannes de Rupefciffa, Ifaac and John Hollandus, and Bafil Valentine, who were all che-mifts, many of them inventors of *panaceas*, and probably the authors of much mifchief. In the beginning of the fixteenth century, Paracelfus, a native of Switzerland, ftood forth, and with match-lefs arrogance, and the moft fupercilious contempt of others, proclaimed his opinions to the world. Seated in his Profefforial chair at Bafil, he fo-lemnly burnt the writings of Galen and Avicenna, intending to become himfelf the fole oracle in phyfic. But his theory is wild, romantic, ab-furd, and dangerous; a ridiculous mixture of ma-gic, aftrology, and chemiftry. The body, he fays, is compofed of falt, fulphur, and mercury; and in thefe three firft fubftances, as he terms them, health and difeafes confift. The mercury, in pro-portion to its degree of volatility, produces tre-mors, mortifications in the ligaments, madnefs, phrenfy, and delirium. Fevers, phlegmons, im-pofthumations, and the jaundice, are the offspring of the fulphureous principle; and the colic, ftone, gravel, gout, and fciatica derive their origin from falt. What fatal errors, in the treatment of difeafes, muft fuch idle notions of their caufes unavoidably produce? The medicines which Paracelfus and his followers employed, were generally metallic preparations, which, in such rash and presumptuous hands, were doubtless frequently pernicious, and always dangerous. Their common purge, in every disorder, was *mercurius præcipitatus,* reduced to pills, and made up with the *theriaca* or *mithridate.* About a century after Paracelsus, Van Helmont took the lead in physic; a man of such indefatigable industry, that he spent fifty years in torturing, by every chemical experiment the animal, vegetable, and mineral kingdoms. He was a person of learning and ability, but, like his predecessor, had the folly of pretending to an universal remedy *(d).* By his writings he defended, enlarged, and promoted the chemical theory; and as Sylvius de la Boe, and Otho Tachenius soon after adopted his system, it became almost universal. All the operations of nature, in the world at large, as well as in the animal œconomy, were reduced to the laws of chemistry; and every phænomenon was accounted for, on the principles of fermentation, putrefaction, corrosion, effervescence, solution, or mixture. The functions of the body

(d) Veteres chemici, quorum interpres est Helmontius, dixerunt, in cuprum insitum esse genium metallicum, qui vix mole corporea, sed tantum irradiatione sanat omnes ferè morbos; et Helmontius dixit, hoc fieri solo attactu tincturæ cupri ad linguam.

Boerhaave de morb. Nervor. p. 764.

were

were explained by analogies, drawn from chemical experiments. Thus the folution of the aliments in the ftomach was afcribed to an acid, becaufe acids were obferved to diffolve metals, and other fubftances of the firmeft texture. Mufcular motion was accounted for, by an effervefcence and explofion, in the imaginary rhomboidal receptacles, refembling the tumults raifed by the mixture of an acid and an alkali. The generation of animal heat was imputed to the combination of the acid chyle, with a fuppofed balfam of the blood, becaufe a fimilar effect is produced by uniting acids with diftilled oils. If the acid of the chyle happen to be highly concentrated, and the juices very acrimonious, according to this theory, an ardent fever is excited. The cold fit of an intermittent was afcribed to the action of nitre, fea falt, or fal ammoniac in the blood, becaufe thefe fubftances were found to refrigerate water, in a remarkable degree.

FROM this abfurd and groundlefs theory, the practice of the chemical fect was deduced; of which I fhall give one memorable and fatal inftance. In the year 1669, an epidemic fever raged at Leyden, and carried off more than two thirds of the principal inhabitants of that city. The fymptoms which accompanied it were a difordered ftomach, vomitings, anxiety, quotidian or tertian paroxyfms, fpots, oozing of blood from

different

different parts of the body, dyfenteric ftools, fœtid urine, great debility, apthæ, and other appearances, which indicated a very high degree of putrefaction. But Sylvius de la Boe, who was at that time a Profeffor in the Univerfity of Leyden, afcribed the diftemper to a prevailing acid, and attempted the cure of it by abforbents, and other medicines of a feptic nature; to which injudicious practice, we may juftly impute a confiderable fhare of that uncommon fatality, which attended the progrefs of this fever. And is it not more than probable that the prefent practice, of giving the *tef-tacea* in accute diftempers, hath a dangerous and pernicious tendency? If acidities prevail in the *primæ viæ*, they will indeed correct them; but with this inconvenience, that they generally occafion coftivenefs. And if they remain unneutralized in the firft paffages, they will powerfully promote putrefaction, and by concreting with the mucus of the ftomach and bowels, prove highly oppreffive and injurious.

I HAD almoft omitted to mention a theory, of the moft dangerous tendency, which the chemifts adopted from Galen, and enriched with many abfurd additions of their own invention. They fuppofed the body to be endued with certain *animal fpirits*, as they were called, generated in a manner, fimilar to that of obtaining brandy from wine by diftillation. Thefe fpirits were confidered

fidered as the feat of various difeafes, particularly
of inflammations; and were thought capable of
being infected with *fomething* of a peculiarly
deleterious nature. Hence it became a *defideratum*,
to expel this unknown enemy out of the fyftem;
and as it was obferved, that acute diftempers are
fometimes terminated by a critical fweat, it was
concluded, that the moft powerful fudorifics were
the beft means of accomplifhing this defirable end.
This gave rife to the deftructive and fatal practice,
which foon became univerfal, of adminiftering
heating remedies, in difeafes of an inflammatory nature; a practice productive of great devaftation
amongft the inhabitants of Europe. Sydenham,
the Englifh Hippocrates, was the firft phyfician
who had underftanding and courage enough, to
ftem the rapid and overwhelming torrent: and we
are now at laft taught, by fad experience, founded
on the deftruction of numbers of our fellow creatures, that the cooling regimen is alone to be employed, in fuch diftempers. The fmall-pox affords us a remarkable example of the oppofite
effects of the two different methods of treatment.
And the amazing fuccefs which hath attended the
new mode of inoculation, is a proof, undeniably
convincing, of the excellence and fafety of the
one, and of the danger and frequent fatality of the
other. So powerful is the action of heating remedies, in this diforder, that a fingle glafs of

mountain

mountain wine, given even after the eruption is completed, is faid to have produced an additional number of puftules.

The fyftem of Stahl, which fucceeded that of the chemifts, though falfe and abfurd, is not chargeable with any pernicious tendency. As it chiefly relates to the influence of the mind over the body, the doctrine of difeafes which it inculcates is fimple, and the indications of cure which it furnifhes are few, and at leaft harmlefs. Thus when the foul, in her efforts to relieve the body, runs into excefs, and excites an immoderate hæmorrhage, *diarrhæa*, or fever, fhe is to be checked and reftrained. On the contrary, when fhe acts negligently, or too feebly, fhe is to be roufed and ftimulated to an exertion of her powers. In thefe inftances, the conclufions of the Stahlians, though deduced from groundlefs principles, are certainly juft, and their practice is fupported by experience, the true ftandard of fitnefs and propriety in phyfic.

The Mechanic Theory, though better fupported than the Stahlian, hath a more dangerous influence on the treatment of difeafes. Thus for example, in the management of the fmall-pox, a phyfician, who is ftrongly attached to the fyftem of obftruction, and regardlefs of experience, might commit the moft

fatal

fatal errors. As the diftemper, according to
the mechanical hypothefis, confifts in a certain
matter thrown off from the blood, and locked
up in the capillaries of the fkin, where being
gradually accumulated, it forms puftules; he
would probably attempt, either to difperfe it
by repeated purging and venæfection, or to
promote its paffage through the fmall cutaneous veffels, by the moft powerful fudorifics.
The firft method of cure would occafion a
fudden finking of the pocks; the fecond would
render them putrid, confluent, and malignant.
And thus the unfortunate patient would fall a
facrifice to reafoning and theory. I mean not,
by this illuftration, to charge the mechanic fect,
with having adopted fo dangerous a method of
treating the difeafe under confideration. The
plan of cure, prefcribed by Boerhaave, is judicious and fuccefsful; but it is a deviation from
his favourite hypothefis of obftruction, and is
founded on experience and obfervation. There
are however fome fatal inftances, in which the
mechanical fyftematics have regulated their
practice by their theory. How many unhappy
wretches fell by the lancet, or funk under the
operation of cathartics, in the ulcerated fore
throat, till the fagacious Fothergill pointed
out the true nature and right management of
that difeafe? It is not long fince crude mer-

cury was confidered as a *panacea*, and taken univerfally, by the healthy, as well as the fick, to prevent obftructions in the one, and to break down by its gravity thofe which were already formed in the other. On the fame principle, the fpirit and falt of hartfhorn were exhibited indifcriminately, in almoft every ailment; for as they colliquate the blood, when taken out of the body, it was not doubted but they would diffolve that lentor of the fluids, which was, and is ftill by many, regarded as the moft general caufe of difeafes.

It is evident then, that THEORY is abfurd and fallacious, always ufelefs, and often in the higheft degree pernicious. The annals of medicine afford the moft ftriking proof, that it hath, in all ages, been the bane and difgrace of the healing art. And as it favours the indolence, flatters the vanity, and gratifies the curiofity of man, ever inquifitive after caufes, I fear the paffion for it will not be eafily fuppreffed, amongft the profeffors of medicine. The invention of an hypothefis is a work of no difficulty to a lively imagination; and the fiction, by its tinfel glitter, never fails to dazzle the ignorant and vulgar. But to watch with clofe attention the operations of nature, to treafure up a ftore of ufeful facts, to learn, by accurate obfervation, the diagnoftics of difeafes,

and

and by unbiaffed experience, the true method
of cure, requires unwearied labour, affiduity,
and patience, at the fame time that it admits
of no pompous difplay of wit or knowledge.
The wife, however, value not genuine fcience
lefs, for her unaffuming deportment and fimplicity of attire; and the opinion of the ignorant would be unworthy the confideration of a
jndicious phyfician, if humanity did not intereft him in the concerns of fuch numbers of
his fellow creatures, as unhappily fall under
that denomination.

ESSAY

E S S A Y II.

T H E

DOGMATIC, or RATIONALIST;

BEING ARGUMENTS FOR THE USE OF

THEORY AND REASONING IN PHYSIC.

Medicina, in philosophia non fundata, res infirma est.

BACON.

THOUGH reason is the most exalted
faculty of man, and the source of that
high rank which he holds, in the universe of
God, there is a set of groveling spirits in the
world, who vilify the powers of the understanding, and with inverted pride, glory in sink-
ing themselves to a level with the brute crea-
tion. Of this class are the EMPIRICS, who have
laboured with infinite pains, to banish all
theory and reasoning from the art of medicine.
Experience, they affirm, is the sole guide to
safe and successful practice; and fatal is the
temerity of those, who deviate from the beaten

path,

this implies the exercife of reafon, and, befides
experience, requires a knowledge of the ftructure and functions of the animal frame, of the
changes produced in it by difeafe, and of the
powers and qualities of medicines; all which
the empiric rejects as vifionary and ufelefs.
" In a watch every one obferves when the
" finger deviates; but the artift alone, who is
" acquainted with the exquifite ftructure of the
" machine, can correct and amend its move-
" ments." A conftant and diligent atten-
dance on the fick may inftruct us in the external face of difeafes, and enable us, with fome
degree of certainty, to prognofticate their iffue.
But without theory, and an exertion of our rational faculties, it will never furnifh any other
than the mere fortuitous means of relieving
them. The favage Indian, by his accurate obfervation of natural figns, can frequently foretel
thofe tremendous ftorms, to which America, at
certain feafons, is expofed: But of what avail
would this have been, in preventing the im-
pending ruin, if philofophy had not accomplifhed what was impoffible to rude experience?
To the ingenious Franklin, our colonies owe
the warmeft gratitude; who by inveftigating
the nature and caufes of thunder and lightning,
hath pointed out the method of warding off
their deftructive effects. How blind and dangerous

gerous would be all attempts to cure the diforders of the eye, without a knowledge of its
ftructure, and an acquaintance with the theory
of vifion! And yet the empiric is, profeffedly,
ignorant of both. Suppofe him to be confulted by a patient labouring under the *gutta
ferena:* No external defect appears, no pain is
complained of, and the health of the body, in
every other refpect, is perhaps unimpaired.
By what figns will he be able to determine the
feat of the difeafe; or upon what principles
will he proceed, in the treatment of it ? Confufion, uncertainty, and danger muft neceffarily attend his random practice. By the laws
of the animal œconomy, there fubfifts a certain
fympathy between different parts of the body;
by which the difordered ftate of one organ
impairs the functions of another. The head
and ftomach, for inftance, have an almoft univerfal confent with the reft of the fyftem, and,
of confequence, are fubject to various, and fometimes oppofite caufes of indifpofition, each in-
dicating a different and peculiar method of
cure. Thus watching, flatulency, indigeftion,
the gout, rheumatifm, or inflammation may
produce the head-ach; and ficknefs or vomit-
ting may arife from furfeiting, from a load of
mucus, from putrid bile, from an affection of
the kidneys, and from many other fources.

In

In all thefe cafes the empiric, if he act confif-
tently with his principles, will attend only to the
leading fymptom, and will indifcriminately apply
his ftomachic cordial, or cephalic plaifter, without
any regard to the origin or nature of the malady.

MAY we not therefore juftly conclude, that
mere experience, whether derived from books, or
acquired by perfonal obfervation, is infufficient of
itfelf to qualify us for judicious and fuccefsful
practice. " I look upon a good phyfician," fays
the amiable Mr. Boyle, " not properly as a fervant
" to nature, but as a counfellor and friendly affift-
" ant, who in his patient's body furthers every
" thing, which he judges to be conducive to the
" welfare and recovery of it." To this end, a
knowledge of the animal œconomy, of the influence of external caufes on the human frame, of the
ftate of health, and the changes induced by difeafe,
is abfolutely neceffary. And this is the foundation, on which the Rationalift erects the fuperftruc-
ture of medicine. He explores the writings of
the ancients and moderns, he attends diligently to
nature in her operations, he felects and arranges
facts, and deduces general conclufions, and thus
forms a confiftent, rational, and ufeful theory, on
which his practice is built (e). He neither indulges

(e) ALTHOUGH the arguing from experiments and
obfervations, by induction, be no demonftration of ge-

neral

dulges a warm and creative imagination, nor yet
confines himfelf within the limits of one narrow
hypothefis, well knowing the abfurdity of either
extreme.   With the Stahlians he believes that the
foul, or nature, as it is now called, frequently
exerts herfelf in the cure of difeafes, or in expelling
from the body whatever is offenfive and hurtful.
Thus a *crapula* occafions a *diarrhœa*, and a crumb
of bread, in the wind-pipe, excites a fit of coughing.
But he is aware likewife, that the efforts of nature
in fuch cafes may be too powerful ; that a falutary *diarrhœa* may terminate in a dyfentery, and a
fit of coughing in univerfal convulfions.   He
adopts alfo, with reftrictions, the mechanical and
chemical hypothefes, and admits that obftruction
is often a caufe of difeafe, and that many changes
in the body are reducible to chemical and mechanical principles, of which he deems inflammation
and acrimony to be fufficient proofs.   But he is
not wedded to fyftems, nor anxioufly bent upon
explaining every phænomenon, which occurs in
the animal frame.   He diligently avails himfelf
indeed of all the affiftances, with which philofophy
furnifhes the healing art ; but fenfible of its im-

neral conclufions, yet it is the beft way of arguing which
the nature of things admits of ; and may be looked upon
as fo much the ftronger, by how much the induction is
more general.   NEWTON.

perfection.

perfection, he ingenuously acknowledges, that in
diseases there are numberless anomalous symptoms,
that the operation of medicines is often irregular
and uncertain, and that even in the healthy body,
there are many appearances, which are inexplicable to the wisest and most experienced of the
faculty.   But where his theory is deficient, his
practice is proportionably more cautious and re-
served.   If experience fail him, he calls in analogy to his aid *(f)*; and judges it better to pursue
a doubtful path, than to stand still in uncertainty
and suspense.   In the most intricate cases, however, he is not totally without a clue : Reason and
philosophy are his guides; and under such direction, there is at least a probability that he will not
mistake his course.   And by thus treading occasionally in unbeaten tracks, he enlarges the boundaries of general science, and adds new discoveries to the art of medicine.   In a word, the Ra-
tionalist has every advantage which the Empiric
can boast, from reading, observation, and practice,
accompanied with superior knowledge, understanding, and judgment.

(f) Ejus (analogiæ) hæc vis est, ut id quod dubium
est, ad aliquod simile, de quo non quæritur, referat; ut
incerta certis probet.

Quint. Inst. Orat. l. 1. c. 6.

E S S A Y III.

EXPERIMENTS AND OBSERVATIONS

O N

ASTRINGENTS AND BITTERS.

S E C T I O N I.

EXPERIMENT I. AN ounce of PERUVIAN BARK, coarsely powdered, was divided into two equal parts, one of which was infused forty-eight hours, in six ounces of cold spring water; the other was boiled over a slow fire forty minutes, in nine ounces of water, till about a third part of the water was evaporated. The infusion and decoction were each filtered through linen rags doubled, and of the same fineness.

FOUR grains of *sal martis* were dissolved in an ounce of spring water, and one drachm of this solution was added to equal quantities (viz. half an ounce) of the turbid decoction and infusion. Each assumed a deep purple colour, scarce perceptibly different in degree, though I thought the

infusion

infufion, after ftanding a while, acquired rather a more dufky purple than the decoction. The infufion had a deeper tinge, and more of the tafte and fmell of the bark in fubftance than the decoction: Its tafte indeed exactly refembled the bark, after it has been broken down, and chewed for fome time, in the mouth.

EXPERIMENT II. Equal quantities of each *rifiduum* were boiled over a flow fire, in three ounces of fpring water, for the fpace of twenty minutes. The decoctions were equally turbid, exactly fimilar in tafte, and on the addition of the chalybeate folution, in the proportion of one drachm to half an ounce, they affumed precifely the fame colour, viz. a dufky brown, like chocolate, but inclining fomewhat to purple.

EXPERIMENT III. Five drachms of each *refiduum* were infufed, for the fpace of forty hours, in an ounce and an half of Jamaica rum, which was fufficiently pure, and unimpregnated with any aftringent matter from the cafk. The tinctures were exactly alike in tafte and colour; and, on the addition of one drachm of the chalybeate folution, they were inftantly changed from a deep red, to a dark and dirty brown, which was precifely the fame in both tinctures.

EXPERIMENT IV. To half an ounce of powdered bark, was added an ounce of cold fpring water. The mixture was well triturated in a

D 3   marble

marble mortar, after which it was suffered to remain at rest, till the gross powder subsided. The clear liquor was then carefully poured off, and fresh water, to the quantity of half an ounce, was added; the trituration was renewed, and afterwards part of the *menstruum* poured off again, as before. This method was pursued for the space of thirty-four hours, in which time six ounces of water were combined with the bark. The mixture was then infused fourteen hours, without heat, and strained off. This infusion was found to have the smell and taste of the bark, in a considerably greater degree, than either the decoction, or the infusion without trituration, [Exper. I.] and it assumed a much blacker colour, on mixing with it one drachm of the chalybeate solution, than either of the two former preparations.

EXPERIMENT V. It was attempted to determine the comparative strength, or rather astringency, of five preparations of the bark, viz. the extract, decoction, cold infusion, tincture, and triturated infusion.

TEN grains of the extract, carefully made, and as free from *empyreuma* as this officinal preparation is generally found to be, were mixed with an ounce of hot water. But so imperfect was the solution, or to speak more
properly,

properly, the fufpenfion of the bark, that in
a few minutes, a large powder was depofited
at the bottom of the glafs. This however
was fhaken up, and one drachm of the chalybeate folution was added to the mixture.
The fame quantity was added to half an
ounce of the decoction, infufion, tincture of
the London Difpenfatory, and triturated
infufion. The laft affumed by far the deepeft
black, the extract approached neareft to it,
and the tincture appeared to be the leaft
tinged. The decoction and infufion were
precifely alike in colour.

EXPERIMENT VI. The *refiduum* of the triturated infufion, [Exper. IV.] was boiled over
a flow fire, in three ounces of water, for the
fpace of twenty minutes. The decoction,
when cold, was ftrained off. It was of a
paler colour than the decoctions mentioned
in Exper. II. although there was a portion
of powdered bark fufpended in it, which,
by the trituration, had been rendered fine
enough to pafs through the filter. This
powder, on ftanding, fubfided to the bottom
of the veffel, and left the decoction much
more limpid than it was before.

To equal quantities of this, and of the two
decoctions mentioned above, one drachm of
the chalybeate folution was added. The

black

black tinge was manifeſtly weakeſt in this decoction, though the difference was not ſo great, as might have been expected, from the diverſity in their ſenſible qualities of taſte and ſmell ; owing perhaps to the fine powder of the bark, which floated in it, and retained ſome degree of its original aſtringency.

EXPERIMENT VII. Equal quantities of the ſimple, and of the triturated infuſion, were boiled for the ſpace of ſeven minutes, over a quick fire. Both loſt their tranſparency, when cool ; but the latter aſſumed a much more turbid appearance than the former, exceeding even that of the decoction from freſh bark, [Exper. I.] and after ſtanding twenty-four hours, it depoſited a very copious ſediment.

EXPERIMENT VIII. Half an ounce of pow-dered bark was infuſed forty-eight hours, in five ounces of ſpring water, and one ounce of white wine vinegar. The mixture was placed near a warm fire, and at certain intervals was ſmartly ſhaken. It was then filtered through a linen rag doubled. The taſte of the vinegar was in a good meaſure covered, though the ſmell was not ; but the *menſtruum* was not ſo fully impregnated with the flavour of the bark, as the infuſion [Exper. I.]. One drachm of the chalybeate ſolution was added

to

to half an ounce of this acid infufion ; at firft, no change of colour took place, but in a few hours a flight black tinge appeared.

EXPERIMENT IX. Half an ounce of powdered bark was well triturated, in the manner defcribed in Exper. IV. with fix ounces of warm water; after which the mixture was poured into a bottle, placed near the fire, and frequently fhaken. This procefs lafted forty-eight hours. The infufion, when ftrained off, was found to be more perfectly impregnated with the bark, than the triturated infufion with cold water, [Exper. IV.] as appeared by comparing their colour, tafte and fmell, and by the deeper black, which it inftantly affumed on the mixture of one drachm of the folution of *fal martis.*

EXPERIMENT X. Half an ounce of powdered bark, and two drachms of ftone quick lime, warm from the kiln, were rubbed together until they were thoroughly united; then fix ounces of fpring water were gradually poured on, the powder and water were well incorporated by triture, and the mixture was fet by, to infufe for twelve hours. Two ounces of it were then filtered through a double linen cloth: the remainder ftood thirty-fix hours longer, and was often agitated; after which, it was ftrained off. The fmell of the bark was
almoft

almoſt entirely covered in both the infuſions, which were ſtrongly impregnated with the lime, and had an extremely diſagreeable flavour. The firſt was of a pale colour, and poſſeſſed but a ſlight degree of bitternefs; the latter had a deeper tinge, and was equally bitter and nauſeous. Neither of them ſtruck a black colour with the chalybeate ſolution, which, as ſoon as it was added, occaſioned the ſeparation of a yellow ſediment, that ſubſided, in a few hours, to the bottom of the glaſs. Compared with the triturated infuſion, [Exper. IV.] theſe preparations appeared to be much weaker, both in colour and taſte. The *reſiduum* did not ſenſibly effervefce with oil of vitriol.

EXPERIMENT XI. The decoction and in-fuſion were found to be impaired in ſtrength, afrer ſtanding ſix or ſeven days; although it was the winter ſeaſon, and the weather was ſeverely cold. The infuſion became paler coloured, and at the ſame time depoſited a ſlimy ſediment. The decoction, at the end of ſeven days, aſſumed an almoſt milky hue, and ſtruck but a faint black with the chaly-beate ſolution. The ſimple infuſion alſo had loſt much of its aſtringency; but the two triturated infuſions were very little altered in that reſpect.

EXPERIMENT

EXPERIMENT XII. To determine the time, requifite for obtaining a fufficiently ftrong impregnation of the Peruvian bark, in cold water; four infufions were prepared, by macerating equal quantities (two drachms) of the fine powder of the *cortex*, in four ounces of rain water *(g)*. After two hours infufion, the firft was filtered; the fecond after feven hours; the third after nineteen hours; and the fourth after forty-eight hours. The fecond infufion, which had been prepared by feven hours maceration, appeared by its tafte, fmell, colour, and by the hue, which it affumed on droping into it a faturated folution of green vitriol, to be confiderably more impregnated with the bark than the firft, and to be equal in ftrength to the other two preparations. This experiment feems to evince that the *cortex* yields its virtues, in a fhort time, to cold water, and that it is unneceffary to continue the infufion longer than feven or eight hours.

PHYSICIANS in general agree, that the PERUVIAN BARK is moft powerful in its effects, when taken in fubftance. But as the ftomach is frequently

---

(g) The foregoing infufions of the bark would have been ftronger, had they been made with the fine powder of the cortex; and they would have ftruck a deeper black with green vitriol, had a lefs quantity of the chalybeate been employed.

unable

unable to bear it, and as many patients have an almoſt invincible averſion to it in that form, it is of importance to determine, in what preparations the virtues of this valuable drug are leaſt impaired, and whether it may not be adminiſtered under a form, that is elegant, palatable, and at the ſame time ſufficiently efficacious. The decoction of the bark hath always appeared to me, to be an injudicious preparation: For though the *cortex* is not a ſubſtance of much volatility *(h)*, yet there is a certain *aroma* accompanying it, which the heat of boiling water cannot fail to diſſipate *(i)*; and conſequently the medicine is deprived of one of its component parts, in which probably ſome

---

(h) Astringency is perhaps not ſo fixed a quality in vegetables, as is commonly ſuppoſed; for I am well informed that artichoke ſtalks, by being gently dried in an oven, loſe their property of ſtriking a black colour with chalybeates.

(i) The vapour, which exhales in the firſt coction, being caught in proper veſſels, condenſes into a limpid liquor, which ſmells ſtrongly of the bark.

Lewis's Mat. Med. p. 431.

Genuinus cortex, ſapore ſatis grato, et aromatice-amaro eſt; odorem ſpirat peculiari modo mucidum, attamen ſuavem, gratum, et *aromaticum*; atque huic ſenſui, in corticis ſinceritate deprehendenda, præ cæteris omnibus credere ſoleo.

Morton. lib. I. p. 66.

ſhare

fhare of its virtues refides. The bark likewife undergoes a decompofition by boiling; the refin is feparated from the gum, and remains fufpended in the watery *menftruum*. This renders its appearance inelegant, its tafte naufeous, and, I fhould apprehend, muft confiderably diminifh its efficacy. For as the virtues of the bark are ftrongeft in its native ftate, they depend, in all probability, on its compofition as a *mixt*; and muft of courfe be impaired by the difuniting of its conftituent principles. Intermittents have been cured by oak bark and gentian combined, when neither aftringents nor bitters feparately, had any effect. By the firft, fecond, and third experiments it appears, that the *cortex* yields its virtues at leaft, as perfectly to cold, as to boiling water: And the fimple infufion hath certainly many advantages over the decoction. It is a much more agreeable and elegant preparation, and the principles of the bark remain perfectly unaltered in it, retaining the fame proportions to each other, as in the fubftance of the drug itfelf. Nature hath fo accurately combined, and blended together the gummy and refinous parts of the *cortex*, that by their union, they become foluble in *menftrua*, with which, when feparated, they refufe to unite. Thus they reciprocally promote the folution of each other in water and ardent fpirits; and both the tincture and infufion are found, by experiment, to

be

be ftrongly impregnated with thefe two conftituent principles of the bark. The tincture is, without doubt, an elegant and palatable medicine; but it is liable to this objection, which indeed holds equally true againft fpirituous tinctures in general, that a fufficient dofe of the medicine cannot be given, on account of the heating nature of its vehicle. This preparation, however, might be rendered much ftronger, if a larger proportion of bark, than is prefcribed by the college of phyficians, were to be employed.

EXPERIMENT XIII. Equal quantities, viz. fix ounces by meafure, of two tinctures of the bark, the one made after the *formula* of the London Difpenfatory, the other with double the ufual quantity of bark, were weighed with great exact-nefs, in a nice pair of fcales; and the latter was found to be eighteen grains heavier than the former, and to exceed in gravity the fimple proof fpirit thirty-feven grains. The ftronger tincture had alfo a confiderably deeper hue, and when mixed with water, became much more turbid.

IN nervous fevers, hyfterical diforders, and other low cafes, where it is neceffary to join cordials to the bark, an infufion of it, in red port wine, may be prefcribed with advantage. Under this form the famous empiric Talbot ufed to adminifter the *cortex*, in the paroxyfms of intermittents; and fo fuccefsful was his practice, that LOUIS XIV.

was

was induced to purchafe, at a large price, the fecret of his fpecific. Orange peel is an ufeful ingredient in preparations of the bark; it gives a grateful warmth to the infufion, and adds, I think, confiderably to its efficacy. The following *formula* is agreeable to the tafte, and well adapted to a weak and delicate ftomach.

R. *Pulv. cort. peruv.* ʒj. *cort. aurant.* ʒfs. *aq. cinnamom. ten.* ℔j. *aq. cinnamom. fp.* ℥ij. *m. et infunde, fine calore, per horas octo, vel duodecim, deinde filtra.*

THE ufe of trituration, in promoting the powers of folution, is evident, from Experiments IV. VI. and VII; and would have been ftill more fo, if a proper apparatus had been employed. The Count de la Garaye, a French nobleman, who is diftinguifhed for his affiduity in applying the different branches of philofophy to the improvement of medicine, hath defcribed a very convenient machine, and pointed out an admirable procefs, for obtaining from vegetables, by triture with water, the matters in which their virtues chiefly refide. The contrivance is extremely fimple, confifting only of a veffel to which a churning ftaff is fitted, which, by means of a cord and a wheel, is perpetually whirled with a rotatory motion. By this conftant agitation, the moft accurate diffufion is produced, and different portions of the *menftruum*

are

are, in quick fucceffion, applied to every particle of the folvend.

From the fifth experiment no certain con-clufions can be deduced; except that the extract is a much weaker preparation, than is commonly fuppofed. It is liable to all the objections which have been advanced againft the decoction, with this additional one, that it is hardly poffible to make it according to the procefs of the London Difpenfatory, without giving it fome degree of *empyreuma.* The extract, employed in my experi-ment, was prepared by a very diligent and careful apothecary, yet a confiderable portion of it pre-fently fubfided, in a powdery form, to the bottom of the glafs, which on examination appeared to be the burnt parts of the bark. How little then is this officinal medicine to be depended upon, when we confider the careleffnefs and inaccuracy of many of our druggifts, and apothecaries *(k).*

It

(k) It were to be wifhed, that the college of phyfi-cians would direct all extracts to be made, by means of a water bath. The following fimple contrivance will fully, commodioufly, and with very little trouble to the operator, anfwer this purpofe. Let a pan be made of fuitable dimenfions, with a large circular hole in the cover of it, adapted to receive a china or glafs bafon, and with a curved pipe, two inches high, and half an inch in diameter, on one fide: The cover fhould be clofely cemented to the pan. Fill the veffel with a fufficient

quantity

IT is the practice of the most eminent physicians to join acids with the bark, in the cure of
putrid diseases; and Sir John Pringle hath observed, that in bilious fevers, the *cortex* answered
best in Rhenish wine, after standing a night in
infusion *(l)*. This suggested to me the eighth experiment; and I flattered myself that, by macerating the bark in a mixture of vinegar and water,
these two antiseptic medicines would be more accurately combined, and that perhaps the acid
might promote the dissolvent power of the aqueous *menstruum*. In the latter expectation, it appears that I was disappointed; and whether the
former was better founded must be left to abler
judges to determine *(m)*.

quantity of water; then place the bason in the cavity
designed to receive it, and lute it well to the cover.
The pan may now be set over a kitchen fire, and the
liquor, intended for evaporation, poured into the china
bason. From the closeness of the vessel, the heat which
the water acquires, will exceed the common boiling
point; and the evaporation will be proportionably expe-
dited, without the least danger of producing an *empyreuma*. The pipe will serve the double purpose of conveying a fresh supply of water into the pan, when it is
wanted, and of carrying off some part of the steam. If
a greater degree of heat be required, the pipe may be
closed with a cork.

(l) Diseases of the Army, edit. 4, p. 213.

(m) Vide Experiments, XIX. XXVI.

THAT moderate heat promotes and affifts the action of water, as a *menftruum*, on the bark, is evident from experiment the ninth; and it would be of advantage to determine, what degree of heat this drug will admit, without fuffering a decompofition. It fhould however be remarked, that this infufion, though ftronger, had neither fo agreeable a flavour, nor was fo fenfibly impregnated with the *aroma* of the bark, as the two made with cold water.

IN an effay on the DISSOLVENT POWER OF QUICK LIME, a very ingenious chemift hath obferved, that all refinous bodies become foluble in water, when the cohefion of their particles is deftroyed, by withdrawing the fixed air which they contain. This method of folution he endeavours to apply to many valuable purpofes in medicine; and hath defcribed feveral ufeful and curious proceffes, for obtaining ftrong and elegant tinctures of the moft active drugs by means of quick lime. The firft part of the tenth experiment, *mutatis mutandis*, was borrowed from him; and it was hoped that an efficacious and palatable infufion might, with tolerable expedition, be made by the procefs, which he has laid down. But the fuccefs of my experiment was not anfwerable to the plaufibility and ingenuity of the theory, which induced me to attempt it. The infufion, after ftanding twelve hours, the time prefcribed

fcribed by Dr. Macbride, was but weakly impregnated with the bark: And when the maceration had been continued forty-eight hours, it by
no means equalled, in ftrength, the preparation
defcribed, Exper. IV. It appears therefore, that
quick lime, whatever its effect may be upon
other medicines, neither quickens nor increafes
the folubility of bark in water: And it communicates to the infufion a tafte, which is intolerably
naufeous and difagreeable. That the chalybeate
folution fhould produce no change, in the colour
of thefe preparations, is agreeable to the laws of
elective attraction. For the acid of the vitriol,
having a ftronger affinity with abforbent earths,
than with metallic fubftances, forfakes the iron,
with which it was combined, and unites itfelf to
the quick lime. Hence arofe the yellow, ochery
fediment, taken notice of in the experiment. As
the *refiduum*, after filtration, did not effervefce with
oil of vitriol, it is evident that quick lime is not
endued with the power of abftracting, from bark,
the fixed air which it contains.

EXPERIMENT XI. furnifhes no other inference
than this obvious one, that the decoction and
infufion of the bark are calculated only for immediate ufe. The *cortex* is a fubftance of a very
fermentable nature, as appears from the experiments of Dr. Macbride; and when its active
parts are diffufed in water, and feparated from

fuch

such as are merely ligneous and inert, it is not to be wondered at, that it undergoes those changes, to which all vegetables, when favourably circumstanced, are liable.

As it is to be feared, that decoctions of the bark, from the facility with which they are prepared, will still continue in use, it may be necessary to suggest, that they should be poured upon the filter as soon as they are taken from the fire. Whilst the water is hot, the resinous part of the *cortex* will continue dissolved in it, and will readily pass through a coarse strainer; but if the *menstruum* be suffered to cool, it will separate, concrete together, and a considerable portion of it will remain in the filter: And thus the efficacy of the medicine will be greatly diminished.

SECTION II.

IT appears from the preceding section, that the PERUVIAN BARK yields its virtues as perfectly to cold, as to boiling water; and that the simple infusion, in point of elegance and efficacy, is preferable to the decoction. But the latter preparation hath this advantage, that it is made with great expedition: For it is a fundamental

mental principle in chemiſtry, that heat quickens
the action of almoſt every *menſtruum*. To avail
myſelf therefore of this aſſiſtance, without decom-
poſing the bark, I made the following experiment,
in the iſſue of which it will appear that I was diſ-
appointed.

EXPERIMENT XIV. A glaſs phial, lightly
ſtopped, containing two drachms of powdered
bark well incorporated with three ounces of ſpring
water, was placed in a half-pint cup of cold
water.   The cup was ſet in a pan of boiling
water, and kept in the boiling heat, for the ſpace
of an hour and a half. The phial was then taken
out of the veſſel, and the heat of it meaſured by
Sir Iſaac Newton's thermometer, when it was
found to be about eight degrees below the boiling
point, which is nearly equal to forty degrees in
Farenheit's ſcale. The infuſion whilſt hot was
clear, and of a deep red, but when cold it aſſumed
a brown colour, and had a turbid appearance.

SEVERAL other experiments were tried, in order
to determine what degree of heat the bark will
bear, without decompoſition; but I was unable
to hit upon the preciſe point. And when I
conſidered, that if it could be aſcertained, few
apothecaries in extemporaneous preſcriptions
would pay an exact attention to it, I dropt all
further attempts towards the diſcovery of it.
But the following experiment, which I have

made

made since the first edition of these essays, obviates the necessity of using heat, and points out a method of making, with sufficient ease and expedition, a saturated infusion of the bark.

EXPERIMENT XV. Two drachms of the *cortex*, finely powdered, were diligently triturated, fifteen minutes, in a marble mortar, with four ounces of rain water; and afterwards macerated without heat, three quarters of an hour. The infusion was then filtered through paper, and appeared, by all the tests used in the preceding experiments, to be considerably stronger than another preparation, which had been macerated twenty-four hours. Three ounces of it, by measure, weighed a grain and a half more than the infusion, prepared, according to the same proportions, without attrition.

A SIMILAR preparation was made by triturating the *cortex* ten minutes only, and then filtering without digestion. But the *menstruum* was by this method less impregnated with the bark, as its taste, colour, specific gravity, and the diminished effect of the chalybeate solution, clearly evinced. The elegance and strength of this preparation are increased, by the addition of a small quantity of French brandy, during the triture.

EXPERIMENT XVI. It is evident from the seventh experiment, that a considerable quantity of the resin of the bark is soluble in cold water; but

but I was defirous of trying, whether the whole of it might not be diffolved, by repeated affufions of the fame *menftruum*. For this purpofe I macerated half an ounce of powdered bark, for the fpace of three days, in fix ounces of fpring water: The *menftruum* was then decanted off, and frefh water added in the fame quantity as before. This affufion was repeated at equal intervals thirty times, till the water was infipid, colourlefs, and unalterable by the addition of green vitriol. The *refiduum* alfo, when chewed in the mouth, had no fenfible bitternefs or aftringency. Two drachms of this *refiduum*, carefully dried by a very gentle heat, were infufed in an ounce of rectified fpirit of wine; and in two days, a tincture was produced of an orange colour, and bitter tafte.

EXPERIMENT XVII. Half an ounce of pow-dered bark, loofely tied up in a linen rag, was boiled over a quick fire twenty-five times, in fo many different pints of fpring water. Each coction was continued twenty minutes, and re-peated till the *menftruum* received no fenfible im-pregnation from the bark. After the twenty-fifth boiling, it was perfectly taftelefs, ftruck no black with *fal martis*, and the powder, when chewed in the mouth, was equally infipid with the liquor. Two drachms of the *refiduum*, cautioufly dried, were digefted forty-eight hours, in an ounce of *fp. vin. rectificat*. The fpirits acquired a deeper colour, and were more ftrongly impregnated with the bitternefs of the *cortex*, than in the preceding experiment. But neither this nor the former tincture ftruck a black with green vitriol, owing probably to the infolubility of that metallic falt in rectified fpirit of wine.

EXPERIMENT XVIII. A drachm of powdered bark was digefted, without heat, forty-eight hours, in two ounces of rectified fpirit of wine. The clear tincture was then poured off, and frefh fpirit, in the fame quantity as before, was added to the *refiduum*. The digeftion was thus repeated fix times, until the *menftruum* acquired neither tafte nor colour from the bark. The powder was then carefully dried, and afterwards fucceffively macerated without heat, in two feveral portions of fpring water; to each of which it communicated the property of ftriking a purple colour with green vitriol. Both thefe infufions were infipid; fo that rectified fpirit feems to have the power of extracting all the bitternefs of the *cortex*, though not all its aftringency. Is not this fact repugnant to what Dr. Lewis hath obferved of this drug, " that " its aftringency refides wholly in its refin, which " does not appear to be in any degree foluble in " watery liquors ?" (*n*) The fame ingenious writer is likewife miftaken, when he afferts that

(*n*) Neumann's Chem. by Lewis, p. 339, note (*x*).

the

the refin of the bark melts out in the firft boilings,
and that the fubfequent decoctions are tranfparent
and bitter, without the leaft turbidnefs or aftringency *(o)*. For in making the feventeenth experiment, I found the decoction, after the twen-
tieth boiling, ftruck a purple colour with *fal
martis*. The three laft trials furnifh a clear
proof of the flow and difficult folubility of the
bark. Fuller fays, with fome degree of admi-
ration, *Cum olim experimenti caufa ejufdem (corticis)
pulverem fæpius decoxiffem, non eo ufque vires ejus
exhaurire valui, quin vel octavum decoctum adhuc
amaricaret (p).* If his patience had permitted
him to extend his experiment, what would have
been his furprize to find, that even twenty-five
coctions, and thirty cold macerations, are infufficient to exhauft the virtues of the *cinchona!*
An ingenious friend of mine informs mc, that
he reduced the bark, by extraction and decoction, to an infipid powder, which was given in
the dofe of two drachms to a patient labouring
under a quotidian fever, an hour or two before
the acceffion of the paroxyfm. It mitigated the
fits by degrees, changed the quotidian into a tertian, and then entirely removed it.

EXPERIMENT XIX. To determine, with
more accuracy, the relation which different

(o) Ibid.   *(p)* Fuller. Pharm. Extemp. p. 5.

menftrua

menftrua bear to the bark, I digefted a drachm
of the *cortex* weighed with great exactnefs, in
equal quantities, viz. three ounces, of each of the
following liquors. 1. Spirit of wine rectified.
2. French brandy. 3. Rhenifh wine. 4. Cold
water. 5. Cold water, with the addition of a
drachm and a half of white wine vinegar. After
feven days infufion, the clear part of each
menftruum was carefully poured off, and the
refiduum evaporated to drynefs. The weight,
which the bark loft by digeftion, is expreffed in
the following table, which fhews the comparative
powers of folution of the feveral liquors, men
tioned above.

Cort. Peruv. ʒj. infufed feven days in

		Grains.
Sp. vin. rectificat.	loft	6
Sp. vin. gallic.	—	$8\frac{1}{4}$
Rhenifh wine	—	9
Water	—	8
Water and vinegar	—	8

RHENISH wine, from this experiment, appears
to be the moft active *menftruum* for the bark.
Whether it owes any part of its fuperior folvent
power to the acid, with which it is replete, cannot
with certainty be determined; but I am inclined
to think it doth not, becaufe the folution of the
cortex is not in the leaft promoted, by the addition
of

of vinegar to water. Dr. Lewis fays, that proof fpirit extracts lefs from bark than rectified fpirit *(q)*; but from the preceding trial, which was made with all poffible exactnefs, it is evident he is miftaken. This experiment likewife affords the moft fatisfactory proof, that cold water is a powerful *menftruum* for the *cinchona.* It is confiderably more active than rectified fpirit of wine, and is very little inferior to brandy. Perhaps the *refiduum* of the watery infufion would have weighed lefs, if the maceration had been continued only two days: For water, after extracting from bark all that it is capable of diffolving, precipitates fome part of it again.

EXPERIMENT XX. Two drachms of gentian root were macerated forty-eight hours, in three ounces of cold fpring water: The fame quantity was boiled over a quick fire, in four ounces of water, till a fourth part was confumed. The infufion had a more intenfely bitter, and at the fame time a much lefs difagreeable tafte than the decoction, which was mucilaginous, and highly naufeous. Six grains of *fal martis* were added to each; but neither of them changed colour. The fame experiment was repeated with Aleppo galls. The decoction manifefted more roughnefs and aftringency to the tafte, than

(q) Mat. Medica, p. 432.

the

the infusion, but did not strike so black a colour with green vitriol. Dr. Lewis informs us, that by steeping the *carduus benedictus* for a few hours in cold water, a very agreeable bitter is procured; but if heat be employed, the more ungrateful parts of the plant are taken up, and the infusion becomes so nauseous, as to provoke vomiting. If sena be infused in cold or, for a little time, in warm water, the liquor will purge far more mildly, than an infusion made in hot water for a longer time, though both infusions be reduced to the same degree of strength, by a suitable evaporation(r). Camomile flowers, as I have long experienced, have their bitterness very perfectly extracted by cold maceration; and in this way they are much more grateful, than when infused in boiling water. An ounce of flowers, and half an ounce of orange peel, macerated in three pints of water, for twenty-four hours, make a light, cheap, and agreeable stomachic medicine. Green and bohea tea yield a finer flavour to a cold than hot infusion, and they strike as deep a black by the former, as by the latter method of preparation. Oak bark, it is well known, is always steeped in cold water, for the purpose of tanning: And I suppose the artists, in that branch of trade, find that the

(r) Vide Neumann's Chem. p. 267.

application

application of heat is not neceffary to extract its aftringency. May we not therefore juftly conclude, from the preceding experiments and obfervations, that cold water is a more univerfal and powerful *menftruum*, than hath hitherto been apprehended; and that its ufe in pharmacy is at prefent too much neglected.

THE refult of the eighth experiment was fo contrary to my expectations, that I determined to make further trials of the effects of acids, in deftroying that property in certain vegetable fubftances, by which they ftrike a black colour with chalybeates, which hath been long regarded as an indubitable teft of aftringency.

EXPERIMENT XXI. An ounce of the infufion of camomile flowers was divided into two equal portions; to one was added a drachm of white wine vinegar, to the other an equal quantity of fpring water. Thus, with refpect to dilution, they were precifely in the fame circumftances. A tea fpoonful of the folution of *fal martis* was then mixed with each of them. The portion, which contained the vinegar, fuffered no change of colour; the other inftantly affumed a dufky hue. The fame experiment was repeated, with a very ftrong triturated infufion of the bark, and the refult was nearly the fame. As foon as a drachm of the vinegar was added to half an ounce of the infufion, it changed the colour of it, from a

deep

deep and reddish brown to a bright yellow; whilst the same quantity of water had no sensible diluting effect on the other portion, with which it was mixed. The chalybeate solution, as in the former experiment, was then added. It produced no alteration in the portion with vinegar, but the other it changed into a perfect ink.

EXPERIMENT XXII. To half an ounce of a strong infusion of galls, were added two drachms of the solution of *sal martis*. It presently assumed the appearance of ink. Forty drops of the acid of vitriol restored it to its original colour. Thirty drops of the *sp. c. c. vol.* renewed the inky blackness.

IN these experiments, it is obvious that an affinity subsists between acids, astringents, and bitters; and this suggested to me that they may possibly neutralize each other, and when combined together in due proportion, form what the chemists term a *tertium quid*. This important point, from which many useful inferences may be deduced, I attempted to ascertain in the following manner.

EXPERIMENT XXIII. To half an ounce of a light infusion of the bark, I added twenty drops of white wine vinegar. The acid and the bitter entirely corrected each other, and a new taste was induced: After standing twelve hours, the

mixture

mixture changed from a light yellow to a deep chocolate, and depofited a large brown fediment.

Experiment XXIV. The fame quantity of vinegar was added to half an ounce of an infufion of Aleppo galls. The mixture was more auftere and aftringent to the tafte, than the infufion. After ftanding twelve hours, it depofited a flocculent, whitifh fediment, and the liquor above became lefs auftere to the tafte, than the fimple infufion itfelf.

Experiment XXV. To equal quantities of fpring water, and of a ftrong infufion of gentian root, in feparate glaffes, was added one drachm of white wine vinegar. The acid was entirely covered by the infufion, but the fpring water was manifeftly four to the tafte. Sixty drops of the fyrup of violets were then added to each. The infufion fuffered no change of colour; but the water affumed a light red, inclining fomewhat to purple. Imagining that the deep colour of the infufion prevented me from perceiving the action of the acid on the vegetable blue, I took the fame quantity of old mountain wine, which was precifely of the colour of the infufion of gentian, and adding to it a drachm of vinegar, and fixty drops of fyrup of violets, I found a flight purple rednefs manifeft itfelf, about an hour after the mixture. The fame experiment was repeated, with a ftrong infufion of galls and

diftilled

diftilled vinegar; but the refult was not fo obvious as in the former one, probably on account
of the weaker powers of the acid employed.

EXPERIMENT XXVI. Sir John Pringle hath
proved, that neutral falts refift putrefaction with
confiderably lefs force, than the acids and alkalis
of which they are compofed. *Spiritus mindereri,*
for inftance, is not half fo aptifeptic as the *fal.
c. c. vol:* And the common faline mixture of *fal
abfinth.* and *fucc. limon.* is only three fourths as
antiputrefcent, as falt of wormwood feparately
taken *(s)*. Dr. Macbride alfo hath fhewn,
that acids and alkalis have the power of reftoring
fweetnefs to putrid fubftances, but that, when
mixed together to the point of faturation, they
lofe this property *(t)*. As there feems therefore,
by the three foregoing experiments, to be an
analogy between the combination of acids, aftringents, or bitters, and acids and alkalis, curiofity
induced me to purfue it; and I flattered myfelf
that, though my attempts fhould prove unfuccefsful, fome ufeful facts might offer themfelves
to my notice, and that my labour would not be
without reward.

AN ounce and a half of mutton, chopped very
fmall, was divided into five equal parts, and put

(s) Difeafes of the Army, Append. Exp. v. IX.
(t) Macbride's Effays, p. 129.

into

into fo many different phials. To the firft, which was defigned for a ftandard, were added twelve drachms of fpring water; to the fecond, ten drachms of water, and two drachms of white wine vinegar; to the third, ten drachms of the decoction of the bark, and two drachms of vinegar; to the fourth, ten drachms of the decoction of the bark; to the fifth, ten drachms of water, and one fcruple of bark finely powdered. The bottles were lightly ftopped, and fet in a fand bath, the heat of which was regulated by a thermometer, and kept up to the hundredth degree of Farenheit's fcale. In the night, the lamp was fuffered to go out. The changes, as they occurred in the mixtures, were carefully noted down, and were as follows:

The ftandard phial, in feven hours, emitted many air bubbles, and was frothy at top; but had acquired no fetor; No. 4. the decoction of the bark, was alfo a little frothy. The next day the ftandard fmelled offenfively, and No. 4. was juft perceptibly tainted. The third day, the ftandard was very fetid; No. 4. was evidently putrid. The fourth day, the ftandard was fo extremely offenfive, that I removed it. No. 2. the vinegar and water, was not quite fweet. No. 3. the decoction of the bark and vinegar, was unchanged. No. 4. the decoction of the bark, was very fetid. No. 5. the powder of bark and water, was quite sweet, but a little mouldy. The fifth day, No. 2. the vinegar and water, was more offensive than before. No. 4. the decoction of bark, was so putrid that I removed it. No. 3. and 5. were quite sweet.

THE sixth day. The phials were removed from the sand bath yesterday, on account of an accident which happened to the lamp; and they remained in the cold for twenty hours. This morning, they were set by a warm fire. They were not much changed, since the last examination.

THE seventh day. No. 2. the vinegar and water, was very offensive, but had a peculiar fetor, totally different from the putrid smell of No. 1. and No. 4. It was therefore removed. No. 3. and No. 5. were sweet.

THE eighth day. No. 3. the decoction of bark and vinegar, was a little tainted. No. 5. the powder of bark and water, was perfectly sweet, and did not become sensibly putrid, till the thirteenth day from the time of mixture.

EXPERIMENT XXVII. To an ounce of putrid ox-gall, were added, an ounce and a half of the decoction of bark, one drachm of the powder of bark, and three drachms of white wine vinegar. The putrid smell of the gall was entirely corrected; and the mixture continued sweet fourteen days, though it was placed near a warm fire.

In

In the event of the two laſt experiments, I was very much deceived. Before I undertook them, I was almoſt fully perſuaded, that there ſubſiſted a complete analogy between the combination of acids and aſtringents or bitters, and acids and al-kalis; and that the neutrals, formed by the mixture of the former, like thoſe of the latter, would prove leſs antiſeptic than the ſubſtances, ſeparately taken, of which they are compoſed. This preconceived hypotheſis led me to ſuſpect the preſent practice of joining acids and the bark, in the cure of putrid diſeaſes, to be very improper, as I imagined they would counteract each other's effect. To aſcertain this important point, I made the two preceding experiments, with the moſt minute exactneſs; and though the reſult of them was the very re-verſe of what I had ſuppoſed, I was neither mortified with my diſappointment, at that time, nor am I now aſhamed to acknowledge it. In a long courſe of experiments, which are undertaken with ſome particular view, and not made at ran-dom, inſtances of ſelf-deception frequently and unavoidably occur; and in general they happily ſerve as a ſpur to induſtry. We firſt conceive a fact, and then ſet about the demonſtration of it. If the trial ſucceed, our end is obtained, and for the moſt part we reſt ſatisfied. But if the proof fail, ſome unexpected phænomena oftentimes occur, which awaken our attention, and excite us

to

to new purfuits. But whether this be the cafe or not, fuccefs or difappointment are equally ufeful, in experimental inquiries; becaufe a negative truth may be of as much importance as a pofitive one.

THE five laft experiments furnifh, at leaft, a prefumptive proof, that acids and aftringents or bitters, neutralize each other. By mixture, it appears their tafte and fmell are altered; the acids lofe their property of ftriking a red colour with fyrup of violets; and their antifeptic powers, in combination, are double the fum of them, when feparately employed. The bark likewife, with vinegar, [Exper. XXVII.] hath the power of reftoring fweetnefs to putrid fubftances, which it hath not alone, as Dr. Macbride affirms (t). Sir John Pringle hath indeed afferted the contrary; but, in his experiment, the putrid alkali feems to have been wafhed off, not corrected, by repeated affufions of the decoction of the bark.

EXPERIMENT XXVIII. Four pieces of calf-fkin, frefh ftripped from the calf, and exactly equal in fize, were immerfed, one in an ounce and a half of the infufion of bark; the fecond in an ounce and a half of the fame infufion, with two drachms of white wine vinegar; the third in an ounce and a half of the infufion of Aleppo galls; the fourth in

(t) Macbride's Experimental Effays, p. 130

an

an ounce and a half of the infufion of galls, with two drachms of vinegar. At the end of feven days, they were taken out, and carefully examined. The pieces, which had been immerfed in the infufions of galls, and bark with vinegar, were much fofter and more fwoln, efpecially in the middle, than the other two pieces: And the cuticle very eafily feparated from the cutis, which was not the cafe with the others. So that the acid feemed greatly to diminifh the aftrictive powers of thefe two infufions. The pieces were all fo fhriveled, that I could not eafily meafure them, nor determine which was the moft con-tracted in fize.

VINEGAR, it is well known, hath the property of foftening animal fibres, in a very remarkable degree; and, diluted with warm water, it is fre-quently employed as a refolvent, in external topi-cal inflammations. But, when taken internally, or applied to any very fenfible membrane, it acts as an aftringent. Thus in the mouth, it corrugates the tongue and palate, and induces a palenefs in the lips, by contracting the fmall capillary arteries, which run upon their furface. And when injected into the *vagina*, it proves an excellent remedy in the *fluor albus*, but requires, in fome cafes, to be diluted with water, otherwife it would be too fuddenly aftrictive and corroborant. On what principles it produces fuch oppofite effects

F 3   on

on the dead and living fibre, would be difficult with certainty to determine. Perhaps its aftringent property may depend upon its ftimulus, which can only exert itſelf on the *ſolida viva*; as the ſimple ſolids are the proper ſubjects of its reſolvent power. But although the preceding experiments clearly prove, that vinegar, in combination with aftringents, diminiſhes their corrugating effects on the dead fibre; I would by no means infer that its action is the ſame, when applied to the living fibre, or that acids and the bark are improperly exhibited together, in the cure of hemorrhages. From the twenty-fourth experiment it appears, that the infuſion of galls is rendered much more auſtere to the taſte, by the addition of vinegar; and it is not improbable that its aftrictive power, as a medicine, is increaſed in the ſame proportion. For I apprehend that the taſte, with reſpect to the operation of this claſs of vegetables on the body, is the leaſt fallacious teſt of aftringency. I term it the leaſt fallacious teſt, becauſe it will be ſhewn afterwards, in the ſucceeding ſection, that neither the taſte, nor the property of ſtriking a black colour with chalybeates, nor yet the power of hardening animal fibres, whether ſeparately or collectively taken, are certain criteria of the aftrin-gent power of a medicine on the living body *(u)*.

I SHALL

(u) WHEN the twenty-eighth experiment was made, it did not occur to me to try the effects of the mineral acids,

I SHALL conclude this section with a few obvious practical inferences, from the foregoing
obfervations and experiments.

1. IT is the opinion of a very eminent phyfician, that the bark, when taken in fubftance,
difagrees with weak ftomachs, on account of its
fermenting quality (x). But I think the fixteenth,
feventeenth, and eighteenth experiments, which
prove its remarkably flow folubility, furnifh a
better explanation of the fact. When the ftomach is overloaded with a dofe of the *cortex*, in
powder, a fenfe of weight and oppreffion, not of
flatulency or diftenfion, is for the moft part
complained of. And it is a common, and I
believe ufeful practice, to join aromatics with the
bark, and that doubtlefs with a view to ftimulate
the digeftive powers, and quicken its paffage
through the *prima via*. For as it is evident, from
the experiments of Sir John Pringle himfelf, that
they are of a very fermentable nature, they cannot
correct, but muft rather promote that tendency in
the *cortex*, and add to the uneafinefs which it
occafions, by the frefh generation of air. But the

acids, in conjuction with the vegetable aftringents. But
I have fince found, by an experiment made with the
decoction of the bark and elixir of vitriol, that the
aftrictive power of the former is much increafed by the
addition of the latter.

(x) Pringle's Dif. Army. Append. p. 66.

F 4   beft

beft proof that the bark is not fo prone to run
into fermentation, and that it is in fome ftomachs
almoft indigeftible, is the cafe of a patient of the
late Dr. Alfton, who vomited up a dofe of it
almoft unchanged, eight days after taking it *(y)*.
A very ingenious friend of mine hath remarked, in
the courfe of his practice, that the bark, in fubftance, is lefs oppreffive, when given in draughts,
than either in the form of a bolus or electuary.
A confiderable quantity of unfixed air, he fays,
adheres to the particles of the powder, which
occafions difturbance, when carried into the ftomach. By combining the *cortex* with any liquid,
this air is in a great meafure, he thinks, feparated,
as appears by the bubbles which are formed, and
the frothynefs which is produced, during the act of
mixture.

THE fact is curious, and I doubt not, accurately ftated; but the explanation of it is more
plaufible than fatisfactory. The bark, when
adminiftered in draughts, is generally mixed
with fome agreeable aromatic water, which
renders it more palatable, dilutes it in the
ftomach, and by its grateful warmth, promotes
the more fpeedy digeftion of it. But when
given in a bolus or electuary, which are for
the moft part made up with fyrups, it is

(*y*) Cullen's Lect. on the Mat. Medica.

peculiarly

peculiarly naufeous, owing probably to the
unpleafant combination of fweet and bitter.
And it is a common obfervation, that what
is difgufting to the palate is generally offenfive to the ftomach. The more folid form
of thefe two preparations is likewife unfavourable to quick folution. Soap pills have been
known to pafs undiffolved through the whole
inteftinal canal. In a weak ftate therefore
of the ftomach and bowels, we need not
wonder that a large mafs of an electuary of
the bark fhould lie long unchanged, and
prove very oppreffive.

2. As it appears, from feveral experiments,
that bitters have the property of neutralizing
acids, their ufe, in acidities of the firft paffages,
is very obvious. In fuch cafes indeed, they
may be confidered as indicated on a double
account, to correct the difeafe when prefent,
and by their bracing and corroborant effects,
to remove the caufe, and prevent the return
of it. When given with fuch intentions,
they fhould be infufed in brandy, or in fome
of the ftronger wines. It has been long the
practice to exhibit bitters, in icterical complaints, as a fubftitute for the bile. But
though with this view they are improperly
employed, as being antifeptic, retarders,
and moderators of fermentation, and confequently

sequently very different from the bile, which
is posseffed of all the oppofite qualities ; yet I
cannot join with a very celebrated phyfician,
in opinion , that they do little or no fervice
in the jaundice *(z)*. This difeafe, when it
has been of fome ftanding, is almoft always
accompanied with lofs of appetite and indigeftion, and with acidities and flatulencies in
the *primæ viæ*. The ftomach and bowels,
from the defeét of bile, are deprived of
their ufual *ftimulus*, their periftaltic motion
is impaired, and the food, by long ftagnation,
runs with violence through its fucceffive ftages
of fermentation. In this ftate of the diftemper,
the *faliva* and *fuccus pancreaticus* probably acquire a morbid difpofition, and inftead of
affifting digeftion, and checking the generation of air, ferve rather to injure the one,
and promote the other, increafing the general
tendency to fournefs and crudity. Under
thefe circumftances, evacuants, antacids, and
antifermentatives are certainly indicated.
Vomits and purgatives anfwer the firft, and
bitters the two laft intentions. The former
are adapted to remove the caufe of the difeafe ; the latter only to palliate fome of its
moft troublefome fymptoms. In this view

(z) Pringle's Append. to Dif. Army, p. 72.

however

however they are of importance; and the ufe of them fhould by no means be difcouraged.

3. In a pofthumous work of the learned Dr. Boerhaave, publifhed by his pupil Van Eems, it is afferted, that the deleterious effects of fcammony, colocynth, and fpurge, are corrected by vinegar *(a)*. Thefe are all vegetable bitters, and probably the action of the acid confifts in neutralizing them. If this be the cafe, the ufe of vinegar, as an antidote, may perhaps be more extenfive than is commonly fuppofed. For many of thofe fubftances, which on account of their virulent and pernicious effects on the body, are termed poifons, have a confiderable degree of bitternefs; as may be inftanced in the *lauro-cerafus, nux vomica, helleborus, nicotiana, camphor, opium, euphorbium, afarum, bryonia, coloquintida, elaterium, chelidonium majus,* &c. And it is at leaft as probable that their noxious qualities refide in their bitter, as in any other part of their compofition *(b)*.

4. Dr.

(a) Boerhaave de Morb. Nor. Cap. de Paralyfi.

(b) On communicating this conjecture to my ingenious and learned friend Dr. Dobfon of Liverpool, he furnifhed me with the two following experiments in confirmation of it.

4. Dr. Hillary, in his treatife on the Yellow Fever of the Weft India iflands, dif-commends

Experiment I. "May 21, 1764. Twelve grains of opium, diffolved in half an ounce of water, were given to a pointer bitch, that weighed twenty-five pounds and two ounces. The natural ftate of her pulfe was from 110 to 115 pulfations in a minute; and it fhould be premifed, that in making the following experiments, I never examined the pulfe, but after fhe had been in my room 15 or 20 minutes, and was either afleep, or lay at reft.

Soon after giving her the opium, fhe looked heavy; flavered a great deal; and appeared to be much offended with the tafte of the opium.

When at liberty, fhe went out into the open air, but was dull and moved flowly.

One hour after; pulfe 75. Very uneafy and dif-treffed. An univerfal rigor and trembling every five or fix feconds.

Two hours after; pulfe 60. Had run out into the ftreet for half an hour; head rather giddy, with an un-fteadinefs in her gait; complains and groans frequently; heavy, but does not fleep much; flavers a great deal.

Three hours after; pulfe 59. In other refpects much the fame.

Five hours after; pulfe 60. Had been in the open air for more than an hour; rather ftaggered as fhe went down fome fteps; frequently kept her head very erect, but not fteady; flept very little; loft all her playfulnefs; flavers; refufes to eat bread; offended with the tafte of the opium; and has ftill the tremblings and twitchings.

Eight hours after; pulfe 80. More brifk, and feems to be coming to herfelf again.

Twelve

commends the ufe of the bark in that difeafe, chiefly on account of its difagreement with
the

TWELVE HOURS AFTER; pulfe 86. Had followed the fervant for more than a mile; ftill more herfelf.

SIXTEEN HOURS AFTER; pulfe 113. Not much different from her ufual appearance.

EXPERIMENT II. May 28, 1764. Twelve grains of opium, diffolved as in the former experiment, and with the addition of 30 drops of the acid elixir of vitriol, were given to the fame pointer. Much offended with the tafte; foams and flavers.

ONE HOUR AFTER; pulfe 90. Slavers very little; alert as ufual. As fhe lay afleep in my room, fhe had a little rigor and trembling.

TWO HOURS AFTER; pulfe 85. There were now given her 20 drops of the elixir of vitriol, in an ounce of water; flavered a little after this.

THREE HOURS AFTER; pulfe 80. The flavering foon ceafed; is not near fo much offended with the tafte of the opium, as in the former experiment. Rigor and trembling very obfervable, but only when afleep: 30 drops of elixir of vitriol were now given; and one hour after this, 20 drops more; fo that fhe has had, in all, 100 drops of the elixir of vitriol, within the four hours.

FIVE HOURS AFTER; pulfe 95. Brifk; fome of the twitchings, but only when afleep.

EIGHT HOURS AFTER; pulfe 126. Not much different from her ufual appearance; fome very flight twitchings, as fhe lay afleep.

THESE and fome other experiments were made, in order to afcertain the efficacy of acids in counteracting the deleterious qualities of opium. When an over dofe of opium has remained in the ftomach for fome time, the fenfibility
of

the ſtomachs of his patients. He acknowledges however, that it is ſtrongly indicated,
and ſeems to lament that, even under the
pleaſanteſt form, it cannot be retained. But
from the twenty-ſeventh experiment I ſhould
conclude, that it would ſit tolerably eaſy,
or at leaſt that it would not be rejected, if it
were combined with the vegetable acids. A
redundance and corruption of the bile are
the pathognomonic ſymptoms of this fever;
and notwithſtanding the incredible evacuation
of it, in the firſt ſtage of the diſtemper, there
ſtill continues, through the whole courſe of it,
both an inordinate ſecretion of that humour
in the liver, and a depravation of it in the
firſt paſſages. In ſuch circumſtances, the
bark, given by itſelf, cannot fail to diſagree;
for when mixed with putrid gall, it is obſerved greatly to increaſe the fetor of it *(c)*.

of that organ is almoſt entirely deſtroyed, ſo that the moſt
active emetics are ineffectual to evacuate the poiſon. It is
a matter of conſequence therefore, in this caſe, to know
what claſs of medicines we may next have recourſe to,
with the greateſt probability of ſucceſs. As the opium
cannot be rejected from the ſtomach, relief is only to be
expected from ſuch remedies, as will change the nature
of the opium itſelf: And how far this end is to be attain-
ed, by the liberal uſe of acids, the reader may judge by
comparing theſe two experiments.''

(c) Macbride's Eſſays, p. 140.

But

But when joined with acids, which have the power of neutralizing the corrupted bile, as will hereafter be proved, it can occasion no disturbance, and must be highly serviceable, not only as an antiseptic, but also as a corroborant. The truth of this remark is confirmed, even by the practice of Dr. Hillary himself, who exhibits an infusion of snake-root, as a substitute for the *cortex*, and accompanies it with the elixir of vitriol.

S E C T I O N   III.

HAVING frequently observed, during the course of my experiments, that the astringency and bitterness of vegetables are distinct and separate properties, I was desirous of tracing their differences, and of ascertaining the proportion, which they reciprocally bear to each other. To this end, I made a variety of trials, and though not with all the success that I wished or expected, yet as they throw some light on this intricate subject, I shall here faithfully relate such of them, as were most conclusive and satisfactory.

EXPERIMENT XXIX.   To equal quantities of strong infusions of Aleppo galls and gentian

root,

root, were added two drachms of a solution of green vitriol. The infusion of galls instantly struck a deep inky blackness: That of the gentian root was unaltered in colour. The former, it is well known, is very slightly, the latter very intensely bitter.

EXPERIMENT XXX. To equal quantities of strong infusions of rue, wormwood, gentian, green tea, bohea tea, bistort, and galls, was added a tea-spoonful of the solution of *sal martis*. The galls assumed the deepest black; the infusion of bistort was next in degree; then followed the green and bohea tea, between which I could perceive no difference; the tinge of the wormwood and rue was a little deepened, but the gentian was unaltered. Their degrees of bitterness were in the following order; 1. gentian. 2. wormwood. 3. rue. 4. green and bohea tea. 5. bistort. 6. galls. The two last were very slightly bitter. Twenty drops of white wine vinegar discharged the colour, induced by the green vitriol on the infusions of rue and wormwood: A hundred drops considerably diminished the blackness of the infusions of galls, bistort, and bohea tea. But the first, after standing twenty-four hours, recovered its inky colour, and a number of fine jet-black flakes floated about in it, without subsiding: The colouring particles of the two last, much diminished in their blackness, sunk to the bottom of

the

the glaffes. Twenty drops of oil of vitriol entirely difcharged the black colour of the green tea,
and it continued clear and pellucid.

EXPERIMENT XXXI. To determine the comparative antifeptic powers of bitters and aftringents, I put into ten phials marked 1, 2, 3, &c.
a drachm and a half of mutton, which had been
kept feveral days, but was perfectly fweet. To
the firft, which was intended for a ftandard, was
added an ounce of fpring water; to the fecond,
an ounce of a cold infufion of green tea; to the
third, an ounce of an infufion of common wormwood; to the fourth, an ounce of the decoction
of the bark; to the fifth, an ounce of the infufion
of galls; to the fixth, an ounce of a cold infufion
of the bark; to the feventh, an ounce of a cold
infufion of rue; to the eighth, an ounce of a cold
infufion of biftort; to the ninth, an ounce of a
cold infufion of bohea tea; to the tenth, an ounce
of a cold infufion of gentian. By miftake, only
the five firft phials were placed in the fand bath,
the other five were left in my ftudy window, which
has a northern afpect. I was called from home,
and was abfent three days and a half. On my return, I found No. 1, 2, 3, 4, the ftandard, the green
tea, the wormwood, and the decoction of bark, were
all putrid, but in different degrees, according to
the order in which they are marked down. No.
5. the infufion of galls was unchanged. The

mixtures, which had been left in my study window, were quite sweet; but they seemed to have some little fermentative motion in them. They were placed in the sand bath, and the next day, I examined them. No. 7. the infusion of rue was very offensive. No. 6. the infusion of bark was putrid, but in a less degree than the rue. No. 5. 8. 9. 10. were all sweet. The day following, No. 9. the infusion of bohea tea, was very putrid. No. 8. the infusion of bistort, was a little tainted. No. 5. the infusion of galls, and No. 10. the infusion of gentian, continued sweet; and as they remained unchanged several days longer, I removed them from the sand bath, fully satisfied with the proof of their strong antiseptic powers.

EXPERIMENT XXXII. Eight pieces of calf skin, just stripped from the calf, and exactly of equal sizes, viz. two inches long and an inch broad, were severally immersed in an ounce and a half of each of the following preparations. 1. *Decoct. cort. peruv.* 2. Cold infusion of the bark. 3. Cold infusion of galls. 4. Cold infusion of gentian. 5. Cold infusion of green tea. 6. Cold infusion of bohea tea. 7. Cold infusion of rue. 8. Simple water, as a standard. At the expiration of a week, they were taken out and examined. The piece in the water, was soft and putrid. That in the infusion of rue, was sweet, but soft. Those in the infusions of green and bohea tea, were

were hard and curled up; nor did there appear
to be any fenfible difference between them.   The
infufion of gentian feemed to poffefs no inconfiderable degree of aftringency; for the piece of fkin
immerfed in it, was nearly as hard, and as much
fhrivelled, as thofe in the infufions of green and
bohea tea.   The decoction and infufion of the
bark were, to all appearance, alike in their degree
of aftringency, which was rather greater than that
of tea, but much inferior to the galls.

THIS experiment affords a ftriking proof, of
the difference between the action of a medicine on
the dead, and on the living fibre.   Tea, when
applied to the former, is manifeftly aftringent;
and yet, when received into the ftomach, it is
highly dibilitating and relaxant, and the immoderate ufe of it, is attended with the moft pernicious
effects.   It is curious to obferve the revolution,
which hath taken place within this century, in
the conftitutions of the inhabitants of Europe.
Inflammatory difeafes more rarely occur, and, in
general, are much lefs rapid and violent in their
progrefs, than formerly (d).   Nor do they admit
of the fame antiphlogiftic method of cure, which
                                                        was

(d) THE decreafe in the violence of inflammatory
difeafes may, perhaps in part, be afcribed to the prefent
improved method of treating them.   Moderate evacuations, cool air, acefcent diet, and the liberal ufe of faline

was practifed, with fuccefs, a hundred years ago.
The experienced Sydenham makes forty ounces
of blood the mean quantity to be drawn, in the
acute rheumatifm; whereas this difeafe, as it now
appears in the London hofpitals, will not bear
above half that evacuation. Vernal intermittents
are frequently cured by a vomit and the bark,
without venæfection; which is a proof that, at
prefent, they are accompanied with fewer fymptoms of inflammation, than they were wont to be.
This advantageous change however is more than
counterbalanced, by the introduction of a numerous clafs of nervous ailments, in a great meafure
unknown to our anceftors, but which now prevail
univerfally, and are complicated with almoft every
other diftemper. The bodies of men are enfeebled and enervated, and it is not uncommon to
obferve very high degrees of irritability, under the
external appearance of great ftrength and robuft-
nefs. The hypochondria, palfies, cachexies, dropfies, and all thofe difeafes, which arife from laxity
and debility, are in our days endemic every where;
and hyfterical affections, which ufed to be peculiar
to the women, as the term indicates, now attack
both fexes almoft indifcriminately. It is evident, that

and antimonial medicines, are better adapted to check
the progrefs of fevers, than copious bleedings, ftimulating purgatives, and profufe fweats, excited by *theriaca*
or mithridate.

fo great a revolution could not be effected, without the concurrence of many caufes; but amongft thefe, I apprehend, the prefent general ufe of tea holds the firft and principal rank. The fecond place may perhaps be allotted to excefs in fpiritu-ous liquors. This pernicious cuftom, in many inftances at leaft, owes its rife to the former, which by the lownefs and depreffion of fpirits it occafions, renders it almoft neceffary to have re-courfe to what is cordial and exhilerating. And hence proceed thofe odious and difgraceful habits of intemperance, with which too many of the fofter fex, of every degree, are now, alas! chargeable.

FROM the twenty-feventh and twenty-ninth experiments, it appears, that green and bohea tea are equally bitter, ftrike precifely the fame black tinge with green vitriol, and are alike aftringent on the fimple fibre. From this exact fimilarity in fo many circumftances, one fhould be led to fuppofe, that there would be no fenfible diverfity in their operation on the living body. But the fact is otherwife. Green tea is much more fedative and relaxant than bohea; and the finer the fpecies of tea, the more debilitating and pernicious are its effects, as I have frequently obferved in others, and experienced in myfelf (e).

This

(e) I HAVE now under my care a lady, of a moft delicate conftitution, who has been long fubject to a

profluvium

This feems to be a proof that the mifchiefs, afcribed to this oriental vegetable, do not arife from the warm vehicle, by which it is conveyed into the ftomach, but chiefly from its own peculiar qualities *(f)*. And thefe qualities probably accompany the highly flavoured parts of the leaves, and depend upon the nicety and care obferved in the collection and preparation of them. When frefh gathered, they are faid to be narcotic, and to diforder the fenfes; and the Chinefe cautioufly abftain from the ufe of them, till they have been kept for twelve months *(g)*

It

profluvium menfium, to frequent diarrhæas, and to copious and fudden difcharges of urine. Bohea tea, of a moderate degree of ftrength, feldom fails to check the *catamenia*, and fhe has ufed it for this purpofe ten or twelve months. Green tea, whenever fhe drinks it, produces tremors, anxiety, and a large flux of urine, which fhe voids in the quantity of two or three pints at once. The bladder is not over diftended, previous to the difcharge; but fhe feels, (to ufe her own expreffion) as if the urine flowed from all parts of her body to the kidneys, during the time of micturition. - It fhould be remarked, that this lady never ufes bohea tea, but at a particular period, medicinally.

(f) THEÆ infufum, nervo mufculove ranæ admotum, vires motrices minuit, perdit. Smith, Tentamen Inaug. de actione mufculari, p. 46, exp. 36.

(g) Neumann's Chemiftry, p. 376.

A GENTLEMAN of veracity, who commanded an Eaft
India

It is remarkable that only one ſpecies of the tea plant is yet diſcovered, and that all the varieties of this dietetic article of commerce, are owing either to the difference of climate, or to the diverſity in the method of curing it. The fine green teas, which are the firſt crop of the ſhrub, are gathered with the utmoſt caution, and dried with the gentleſt heat, that their periſhable flavour may be preſerved. The bohea teas are more haſtily exſiccated, and even ſlightly parched over the fire, by which they acquire that brown colour which diſtinguiſhes them. And as their more volatile parts are diſſipated by this management, they become proportionably leſs injurious to the nervous ſyſtem.

An ingenious phyſician, who has done me the honour to adopt my ſentiments, and to quote my arguments againſt the uſe of tea, in his Inaugural Diſſertation, publiſhed at Leyden, 1769, has confirmed my teſtimony, by the following experiments *(b)*. " He injected into the cavity of the abdomen,

India ſhip ſeveral voyages to China, ſays that the Chineſe rarely drink the green tea; and that thoſe, who drink it to exceſs, are thrown thereby into a diabetes, or become tabid, and die emaciated.

Vid. Med. Muſeum, vol. II. p. 51.

(b) DISSERTATIO Medica Inaugularis, ſiſtens Obſervationes ad vires Theæ pertinentes, auctore J. C. Lettſom. As this Diſſertation is probably but in few hands,

abdomen, and into the cellular membrane of a
frog, about three drachms of a highly scented
and

the following extracts from it, which contain his experiments at large, may not be unacceptable to my learned
reader.

EXPERIMENTUM I. Sumpsi infusionis Theæ viridis,
& Boheæ, liquoris post distillationem superstitis; nec
non aquæ simplicis cujuslibet æqualem quantitatem, &
in quemlibet liquorem, in vase suo contentum, immisi
drachmas duas carnis bovis, ante duos dies mactati.

Caro bovina, immersa in aquam simplicem, post qua-
draginta octo horas corrupta, putridaque devenerat;
dum portiones carnis in reliquas tres Theæ infusiones
immissæ, post septuaginta demum horas putredinis indicia monstrabant.

EXPERIMENTUM II. Viridis atque Boheæ Theæ,
saturatis infusionibus addidi æquales portiones salis
martis, & protinus utrumque infusum colorem æqualem,
profunde nigrum, adquirebat.

Ex enarratis experimentis tuto concludere licet, Theam
& viridem & Boheam manifesta virtute antiseptica, ac
adstringente in fibris mortuis, & vi vitali carentibus,
gaudere; verumtamen propria, et etiam aliorum, experientia edoctus, certus scio, eam, in ventriculum in-
gestam, præsertim in subjectis tenerioris & delicatioris
compagis solidæ, insignem potestatem relaxantem ex-
serere.

1. Potum hunc usitatum forma aquæ calidæ, aut fer-
vidæ, sumendi mos invaluit, & inde nonnulli deducere
voluerunt effectum, atque vim debilitantem potius huic
vehiculo, quam herbæ ipsi tribuendam esse. Verum
enimvero omnia experimenta, curiosius capta, in eo
consentiunt, quod Thea viridis, & præcipue illa, quæ
subtilissimum,

and pellucid liquor, exhibiting no figns of aftringency, nor of oil floating on its furface, which had
been

fubtiliffimum, atque maxime penetrabilem, fpargit odorem, multo majori gradu virtutem relaxantem, quam
Thea Bohea dicta, præftet. Id quod animum mihi
addidit inveftigationes inceptas ulterius atque plenius
profequendi.

2. Hoc fine libram dimidiam herbæ Theæ viridis op-
timæ notæ, & admodum fragrantis, cum aqua fimplici
diftillavi, atque aquæ infigniter odoratæ, pellucidæ, un-
ciam unam, quæ nullum oleum in fuperficiem excu-
tiebat, neque ulla virtutis adftrictivæ exhibuit indicia,
elicui.

3. Eam partem liquoris, quæ finito ftillicidio in vafe
diftillatorio remanfit, ad extracti confiftentiam evaporavi,
quod levem odorem, attamen faporem valde amarum
adftringentemque habebat.   Extracti adquifiti copia
uncias quinque totidemque drachmas æquabat.

EXPERIMENTUM III.   In abdominis cavitatem, atque membranam cellulofam ranæ injeci circiter tres
drachmas aquæ ftillatitiæ odoratæ. (No. 2.) Poft viginti
minuta alterum ranæ crus, feu pes pofterior, multum
adficiebatur, dum parum mobilitatis, aut fenfibilitatis,
monftrabat, quæ adfectio per quatuor horas perfeverabat,
& rana in ftatu torpido infenfili univerfali ultra novem
horas manebat, donec gradatim ad priftinum vigorem
rediret.

Simili ratione liquorem a diftillatione Theæ viridis
(No. 2.) fuperftitem, atque ulteriori evaporatione magis
concentratum injeci, fed inde nullum effectum fenfibilem inductum vidi.

EXPERIMENTUM IV. Nervis Ifchiaticis ranæ denuda-
tis, atque cavitati abdominis, aquam ftillatitiam fragran-
tem (No. 2. & Exp. III.) adplicui, intra dimidiam horam
extremitates

been diftilled from half a pound of fine hyfon
tea. In twenty minutes the hinder extremities
of the frog were ftrongly affected, and continued
fo four hours, whilft the animal remained in a
torpid infenfible ftate upwards of nine hours,
and then recovered by degrees its former vigour.
He made the fame experiment with the *refiduum*,
left after diftillation, which produced no fenfible
effect.

" HE applied to the ifchiadic nerves of a frog,
when laid bare by diffection, and to the cavity of
the *abdomen*, the fame fcented, diftilled liquor

extremitates pofteriores, penitus paralyticæ infenfilefque
deveniebant, & poft horæ circiter fpatium rana vivere
defiit.

Liquorem a diftillatione refiduum No. 2. & Exper.
III.) eadem ratione alii ranæ admovi, fed nullos inde
natos obfervare potui effectus fedantes, immo virtutem
magis ftimulantem, quam fedativam, præftare videbatur.

Extractum (No. 3.) in aqua folutum, & fub iifdem
conditionibus, iifdem partibus admotum, nullum effectum fenfibilem produxit.

4. Experimenta hæc enumerata nullis commentariis
egent. Extra omnem dubitatiónis aleam ponere viden-
tur, quod effectus Theæ fedativus & relaxans a principio odorato, volatili, aromatico, potius, quam ab aqua
calida dependeat. (No. 1.) Non pauca utriufque fexus
fubjecta mihi innotuerunt, quæ maxima moleftia &
anxietate torquebantur, quotiefcumque unum tantum
poculum infufi Theæ potaverant; quæ tamen, confortio
gratificandi ergo, aquam calidam, loco & more infu-
fionis Theæ, fine ullo effectu incommodante hauferunt.

mentioned

mentioned above. In half an hour the hinder extremities became totally paralytic, and about an hour afterwards the frog died. The *refiduum*, after diftillation, was applied to another frog under the fame circumftances, but feemed to produce rather an aftrictive and ftimulating, than narcotic effect. He prepared an extract from this *refiduum*, which being diffolved in water, and ufed in a fimilar manner, had no vifible operation."

THESE experiments fhew, that the pernicious effects of tea depend on its more volatile parts, which are diffipated in a great degree by long keeping, by hafty drying, or by reducing it to the form of an extract. I have feen and tafted of fuch an extract, made in the Eaft Indies, which, though bitter and aftringent, was by no means unpalatable. A preparation of this kind, diffolved in hot water, would be a good fubftitute for the leaves of the tea plant.

BUT however cogent the objections may be, againft the general and too frequent ufe of tea, it muft be acknowledged, that it is capable of being applied to very important, medicinal purpofes. From its fedative power, and the weaknefs which it fuddenly induces, it might be adminiftered with advantage in ardent and inflammatory fevers, in order to abate the force, and leffen the inordinate action of the *vis vitæ*.

vitæ. In such cases it should be given, either in substance, or in strong infusion; and besides allaying the troublesome sensations of heat and thirst, which are the constant concomitants of those distempers, it would probably serve as a good substitute for some of the usual evacuations. And thus instead of producing watchfulness, which is a common effect ascribed to it in weak habits, it would in all likelihood prove the safest and most salutary opiate. After a full meal, when the stomach is oppressed, the head pained, and the pulse beats high, tea is a grateful diluent, and agreeable sedative. And as studious, sedentary men are particularly subject to indigestion and the head ach, it is on this account justly stiled " the poet's friend." Other uses, to which tea is applicable, might easily be pointed out; but I have already made too long a digression.

THE twenty-ninth experiment affords a further proof, that the astringent parts of the *cortex* are as well extracted by maceration as by decoction. But I am inclined to think from this, and many other trials, that the astrictive quality of this medicine is not so great as it is commonly reputed to be: and consequently the prejudice entertained against the use of it, in cases where powerful astringents are supposed to be contraindicated, is without sufficient foundation. Thus it hath been a commonly received rule, not to exhibit the bark

in

in intermittents, before the difeafe has in fome meafure fpontaneoufly abated; and then to adminifter
it only in the intervals of the fits *(h)*. But this
extreme caution, as it took its rife at firft from
falfe theory, is found, by later experience, to be in
moft inftances unneceffary; and the *cortex* is now
frequently given, with the utmoft fafety and fuccefs, after previous evacuations, not only at the
commencement of the diforder, but even juft
before the acceffion of the cold fit. This was
the common method of exhibiting the bark, when
it was firft introduced into Europe *(i)*. But
Sydenham informs us, that not long after, it came
into difufe, for two reafons; *Primò quia paucis*
horis ante adventum paroxyfmi, pro recepto id tem-
poris more, exhibitus ægrum nonnunquam è medio
tolleret. Funeſtior hic pulveris exitus, quamvis op-
pidò rarus, medicos tamen paulò cordatiores ab ejus
ufu meritò retraxit. Secundò quia æger ope pul-
veris, à paroxyfmo aliàs invafuro liberatus, quod ple-
rumque eveniebat, tamen intra dies 14. *recidivam*
ut plurimum pateretur, in morbo fcilicet recenti,

(h) CURANDUM eft ante omnia ne præmaturè nimis
hic cortex ingeratur, ante fcilicet quam morbus fuo fe
marte aliquantifper protriverit.

Sydenham. Opera. p. 57.

(i) THO. BARTHOLIN. Hift. Anatom. Medic. Cent. 5,
p. 108.

necdum

necdum temporis curſu ſuoque marte committigato (k).
The laſt objection would have been obviated by
a longer uſe of the bark; the firſt is totally without foundation. For the very few inſtances of
mortality (Sydenham only enumerates two) which
immediately ſucceeded the exhibition of the *cortex*,
were not to be aſcribed to the operation of the
powder, but to the violence of the cold fit, which, in
all likelihood, would have carried off the patients,
had no medicine been adminiſtered. For the
natural tendency of the bark is to moderate, and
not to increaſe, the force of the paroxyſms. And
ſo far is it from producing obſtructions, when
given with proper precautions, at the beginning
of intermittents, that it effectually prevents them,
by putting a ſpeedy ſtop to the diſeaſe, the continuance of which, in weak habits, is the true cauſe
of their formation. " I am convinced," ſays Mr.
Cleghorn, in his excellent treatiſe on the diſeaſes
of Minorca, " that the unhappy *metaſtaſes*,
" which ſome have obſerved to follow the uſe of
" the bark, are exceedingly rare, and ought
" rather to be aſcribed to other cauſes, than to
" this medicine. And I will venture to affirm,
" that more bad conſequences enſue from giving
" it too late than too ſoon; proſtration of ſtrength,
" ſudden death, or the moſt obſtinate chronic

(l) Sydenhami Opera, p. 265.

" diſeaſes,

" difeafes, being the ufual effects of delay.
" Whereas the worft that commonly happens,
" from the too early ufe of it, is that it does not
" at once reftrain the paroxyfms like a charm,
" without any fenfible evacuation, as it frequently
" does, when given after the fever has arrived
" naturally to its height, and begins to decline of
" its own accord *(n)*." In another part of his
work, the fame ingenious and accurate writer
obferves, " that the great advantages, which
" accrue from the early ufe of the bark in
" tertians, are that it invigorates the powers of
" the body, prevents or removes the dangerous
" fymptoms, and brings on a crifis foon, and
" with little difturbance. Inftead of fuppreffing
" any beneficial difcharge, as fome have afferted,
" we daily obferve a laudable feparation in the
" urine; warm, profufe, univerfal fweats; plentiful
" bilious ftools; and fometimes the hæmorrhoids
" and menfes coming on after it has been ufed;
" though it effectually reftrains the colliquative
" night fweats, to which perfons, weakened by
" tedious intermittents, are incident *(o)*." Morton, who had great experience of the innocence
and efficacy of the *cinchona*, frequently prefcribed
it, without premifing any evacuations; and he

(n) Dif. of Minorca, p. 206.

(o) Id. p. 189, 190.

afferts,

afferts that, after twenty-five years practice, he never knew the leaft bad confequence enfue from its exhibition, nor had ever occafion to repent the ufe of it. Dr. Lind informs us that, for three years paft, he has annually prefcribed upwards of one hundred and forty pounds weight of bark, and never obferved any bad fymptoms which could with propriety be afcribed to its ufe, except in two inftances; in one of which it was fuppofed, though perhaps without fufficient foundation, to have occafioned an obftruction of the *menfes*; in the other, it produced a fit of fuffocation in an afthmatic patient, probably owing to its being given in fubftance, and in too large a dofe *(p)*. A celebrated profeffor at Vienna has related a number of curious cafes, which fully evince the fafety and efficacy of the bark in femitertian, miliary, and malignant fevers. *Cortex peruvianus, vel declarante fe malignitate, aliquamdiu poft eruptionem exanthematum, vel cum ipfa exanthematum eruptione, vel etiam ante eruptionem eorum, vel ab ipfo morbi principio, illicò fummo cum effectu datus eft (q)*. In the inoculated fmall-pox, inftances have been known of fevere ague fits attacking perfons, between the in-

(p) *Vide* Lind on the hot Climates, p. 294.

(q) *Vide* De Haen. Rat. Medend. vol. I. p. 166, 264, 265. Paris.

fertion

fertion of the variolous matter, and the eruption of the pock, when the bark hath been given liberally and with fuccefs, the principal bufinefs in the mean time fuffering no injury or interruption (r). And in the confluent fmall-pox, a very free ufe of it has not appeared, in a variety of cafes, to have abated the fpitting (s). The retroceffion of the morbid acrimony, in the meafles, is prevented by nothing more powerfully than by the *cortex*, which obviates the fecondary fever, allays the cough, and continues the efflorefcence on the fkin, even to the twelfth day: Whilft the difeafe runs through its accuftomed ftages with the utmoft regularity, and creates much lefs difturbance and alarm than ufual (t).

I HAD lately under my care a patient, who was feized with an intermittent, whilft he laboured under a fevere *gonorrhœa*. The bark was given him in large quantity; and fo far was it from fuppreffing the difcharge, that it evidently increafed it, and at the fame time diminifhed its virulence. The late Dr. Whytt informs us that he fwallowed, in fixteen days, near four ounces of it in fubftance, when he laboured under a catarrh-

(r) *Vid.* Dimfdale on Inoculation, p. 12; *vid.* alfo the Monthly Review for Sep. 1766, p. 189.

(s) Medical Tranfactions, vol. I. p. 469.

(t) *Vid.* Dr. Cameron's Paper, Med. Mufeum, p. 281.

ous cough, without feeling any bad effects from its
aftringent quality. In a tertian, attended with a
cough and fpitting, after the ufe of vomits and
fome pectorals, he prefcribed the *cortex* in the
ufual quantity, without the breaft being any way
hurt by it. And he had repeated experience of
its virtues, in curing a hoarfenefs after the meafles,
when unattended with a fever, or difficult refpiration. In the hooping cough alfo, when given
early, he found it one of the beft remedies (*u*).
The bark has been fuccefsfully adminiftered, in
the quantity of a drachm every three hours, to a
woman two days after her delivery, without leffening the *lochia*; and it has been frequently given to
others, during their *catamenia*, without the leaft
interruption of them (*x*). Thefe facts fufficiently evince the common apprehenfions, concerning the aftringent quality of the *cinchona*, to be
groundlefs. And it may be hoped, that all fuch
prejudices againft the ufe of it will now vanifh;
as by its efficacy in the cure of fcrophulous,
glandular tumours, it is proved to be even a
powerful deobftruent.

THE property of ftriking a black colour with
green vitriol hath been afcribed to all vegetable
aftringents, without exception, and hath hitherto

(*u*) Whytt on Nervous Diforders, p. 241.

(*x*) Medical Tranfactions, vol. I. p. 469.

been

been regarded as an infallible teft of their aftringency (y). But from the twenty-ninth, thirtieth,
and thirty-firft experiments, it is evident, that
neither the one, nor the other are ftrictly and
univerfally true. For gentian appears to be endued with no inconfiderable aftrictive power, and
yet the infufion of it fuffers not the leaft change
from the addition of *fal martis*. On the contrary,
the infufion of rue has no degree of aftringency on
the dead fibre, and yet it ftrikes a faint black
with green vitriol.

THE action of acids in neutralizing vegetable
bitters, as defcribed in the laft fection, naturally
led me to try their effects on the animal bitters.
For this purpofe, I procured a quantity of frefh
ox-gall; but being prevented for feveral weeks,
by various avocations, from purfuing my experiments, I found the gall at the end of that term
extremely putrid. This accident pointed out to
me a train of inquiries, fomewhat different indeed
from what I had at firft propofed to myfelf, but
which afterwards appeared to be much more

(y) THE power by which they produce this blacknefs,
fays a celebrated chemift, and their aftringency, or that
by which they contract an animal fibre, and by which
they contribute to the tanning of leather, feem to depend
upon one and the fame principle, and to be proportional
to one another.

Lewis Com. Ph. Tech. p. 345.

interefting

interesting and important. I shall therefore make no apology for laying before the reader the result of them.

EXPERIMENT XXXIII. Putrid ox-gall, diluted with water, struck a green colour with syrup of violets, and sensibly effervesced with oil of vitriol, became turbid and of a light yellow colour. This experiment was repeated several times, and always with the same success; so that I am pretty confident there must have been some error in that trial of Dr. Macbride's, from which he concludes, " that putrid ox-gall shews no sign of alkali; it " neither effervesceth with acids, nor does it " change the colour of the blue juices; neither " does it throw down any precipitate from the " solution of corrosive sublimate (z)." At first it occurred to me, that the mistake, into which this very ingenious and accurate experimentalist hath fallen, might arise from his not diluting the gall before he added the acid; by which the latter would be so inviscated, as not to give sufficiently evident signs of effervescence. But afterwards the curious observations of M. Gaber of Turin, concerning putrefaction, suggested to me a still more probable source of fallacy, to which Dr. Macbride was exposed. That learned Italian hath clearly proved, " that the marks of alcalescence, in putrify-" ing animal substances, are greater or less, or

(z) Macbride's Essays, p. 101.

" none

" none at all, according to the time the experi-
" ment is made, after the putrefaction begins;
" that such substances, upon their first putrefaction,
" do not effervesce with acids; that afterwards
" they effervesce manifestly with them; but that
" at length they cease from doing it, though the
" putrefaction still continues *(a)*." Now it is not
unlikely that Dr. Macbride's trial on the ox-gall,
was made either before the volatile alkaline salt
was formed, or after it was evaporated; as Sir
John Pringle candidly acknowledges to have
happened, in his experiments on putrid substances.

EXPERIMENT XXXIV. To two drachms of
putrid ox-gall, diluted with half an ounce of
water, were added twenty drops of *ol. vitriol.*
A light yellow cloud instantly formed itself, and
the mixture slightly effervesced and became turbid: But though the peculiar fetor of the gall
was destroyed, yet it emitted a strong and dis-
agreeable smell, nor was its bitter taste entirely
corrected. Thirty drops rendered the mixture
rather sharp to the taste; but still the bitterness
was perceptible: Nor did forty drops entirely
destroy it, although that quantity made the
mixture very sour. After standing a while, it

(a) Vid. Miscellanea Phil. Mathem. Societat. Privat.
Taurinensis: *vid.* also, Pringle on the Diseases of the
Army, Append. p. 125.

H 3   assumed

aſſumed a deep green colour, a ſediment gradually formed itſelf, which in twenty-four hours ſubſided to the bottom of the glaſs, and left the liquor above almoſt clear.

EXPERIMENT XXXV. To the ſame quantity of putrid gall and water, as in the former experiment, were added forty drops of white wine vinegar. The putrid fetor was entirely deſtroyed, and no other diſagreeable ſmell was produced in its room. The mixture became turbid, but in a leſs degree than the former with the oil of vitriol; and the efferveſcence was likewiſe much more obſcure. Sixty drops of vinegar ſeemed nearly to neutralize the gall. For though ſome ſmall degree of bitterneſs remained, it was very trifling, and by no means unpalatable.

EXPERIMENT XXXVI. To a third glaſs of gall and water, mixed together in the above-mentioned proportions, were added forty drops of juice of lemons. The mixture became turbid, but the putrid ſmel! was not perceptibly covered. A hundred and twenty drops neutralized the mixture, entirely correcting both the odour and taſte.

I. FROM theſe experiments may be deduced, the great utility of acids, in all diſeaſes which either proceed from, or are accompanied by a redundance and depravation of the bile. And this ſeems to be the caſe with moſt autumnal

fevers,

fevers, and in general with the epidemics of all
hot countries, efpecially where heat and moifture
are conjoined. For the former promotes the
generation, and the latter the putrefaction of
the bile. I have been affured, fays Dr. Bryan
Robinfon, by a very knowing butcher, that
animals have leaft bile in January, and moft in
July*(b)*. And Hippocrates hath obferved,
Æftate fanguis adhuc viget, fed et bilis exaltatur;
per æftatem etiam ac antumnum bile corpus abundat;
autumno autem atra-bilis plurima eft et fortiffima(c).
Mr. Cleghorn, in his account of the difeafes of
Minorca, informs us, that he examined the
bodies of near a hundred perfons, who died of
tertian fevers, and that he conftantly found the
vefica fellea, and the ftomach and inteftines
overflowing with bilious matter *(d)*. The teftimony of Profper Alpinus likewife, ftrongly confirms the truth of this obfervation. He fays,
Alexandriæ autumno graffantur febres peftilentes
multæ lethales, quæ fere quamplurimos invadunt.
His vero notis pleræque dignofcuntur: In principio
enim vomitus multi, biliofi ac virulenti obfervantur,
à quibus cibum affumptum continere nequeunt,
affiduifque corporis agitationibus, inquietudinibufque
vexantur, ftomachique angore anguntur. In plerif-

(b) Robinfon on the Operation of Medicines, p. 48.
(c) Hippocrates lib. de. Nat. Hom. fect. 14.
(d) Dif. of Minorca, p. 165.

que etiam observantur multæ symptomaticæ dejec-
tiones liquidæ, biliosæ, variæ, admodum ægrè
olentes sive fœtentes (d). The yellow fever of the
West Indies is always at the beginning attended
with great sickness, violent reaching, and a
copious discharge of bile. The vomiting recurs
at short intervals, often becomes almost incessant,
and an incredible quantity of bile is sometimes
thrown up in a few hours *(e)*.

2. THE difference between the action of mineral and vegetable acids on putrid gall, as
evidenced in the preceding trials, is deserving of
particular notice. From the ignorance of this
distinction, or want of attention to it, I believe
the elixir of vitriol is often exhibited, when
vinegar, or the sour juices of vegetables, would
be much more serviceable. For though it is
the common property of all acids to *correct* the
putrid acrimony; yet the power of *sweetening*
it, seems to be peculiar to those of the vegetable
class. And as they are mildly aperient at the
same time, they will not only neutralize the
septic *colluvies*, which in some diseases lodges in
the stomach and flexure of the *duodenum*, but
will also gently tend to evacuate it; an advantage not to be expected from the mineral acids.

(d) Alpinus de Medicin. Ægypt. lib. I. cap. 14. p. 51.

(e) Vide Hillary's Observ. on the Dif. of Barbadoes:
Vide also Bisset's Medical Essays and Observations.

3. MR.

3. Mr. Browne Langrish, in his Modern Theory and Practice of Phyſic, relates the caſe of a poor man who, after eating heartily of ſtale mutton, which he bought on account of its cheapneſs, was affected with vomiting and purging to a ſtrange degree, and in all reſpects ſeemed as if he had been poiſoned.   Vinegar, diluted with water, contributed more than any other medicine towards his cure.

4. A table spoonful of the juice of lemons, unmixed with any thing, is ſaid, by an ingenious writer, (f) to have repeatedly proved a certain cure for a palpitation of the heart, after many of the medicines, called antihyſteric, had been tried in vain.   This effect he aſcribes to an uncommon diſpoſition in the nerves of the ſtomach. But I think it is not improbable, that the complaint proceeded from bilious acrimony, which the vegetable acid corrected and neutralized. This conjecture is confirmed by a ſimilar caſe, which Dr. Biſſet hath related, of a middle aged gentleman, who had a palpitation of the heart, accompanied with ſome ſymptoms of the jaundice, and who was completely cured by drinking, every evening, weak rum punch, acidulated with the juice of Seville Oranges. (g)

(f) Whytt on Nerv. Diſorders, p. 372.

(g) Biſſet's Medical Eſſays and Obſerv. p. 254.

5. I have

5. I HAVE been lately informed, by an ingenious practitioner, that he has seen four cases of
a suppression of urine, supposed to arise from
gravel in the kidneys, almost instantly removed
by the juice of lemons. Not long after taking
it, the patient voided a quantity of sabulous matter. In one case, a very painful chordee accompanied the complaint, which immediately yielded
to the same medicine. All the patients were
of bilious habits, and it is probable, the lemon
juice resolved the spasms of the urinary passages,
by correcting some putrid acrimony in the stomach, or by producing a grateful sensation in
that organ. Sydenham recommends the juice
of lemons, joined with manna, as a remedy for
the gravel, and found, in his own case, that it
rendered the purgative quicker in its action, and
more agreeable to his stomach.

6. FROM the effect of acids on the gall, we
may infer the reason why the immoderate use of
them so much impairs digestion. The bile, in
its natural state, is a saponaceous fluid, abso-
lutely necessary to chylification; and whatever
weakens its powers, must proportionably injure
the due concoction and assimilation of our food.
Hence the body is deprived of its proper nourishment and support, the blood becomes vapid and
watery, and a fatal cachexy unavoidably ensues.
This has been the melancholy lot of many unfortunate

fortunate perfons, who, in order to reduce their exceffive corpulency, have indulged themfelves in the too liberal ufe of vinegar.

7. It is not improbable that the acidities, to which infants are peculiarly fubject, arife as much from the weaknefs of their biliary fecretions, as from the acefcency of their food. The liver of a child is extremely lax, in its texture, and with refpect to his bulk, is much larger than the liver of an. adult: Hence the fecretions of the one will be proportionably greater than the fecretions of the other. But though the bile flows copioufly, yet the powers of nature, in the ftate of infancy, are too feeble for its due preparation; and it is a mere watery, inert fluid, unfit for neutralizing thofe acidities, which in the more advanced ftages of life, it is one part of its office to correct. And this, I apprehend, is a principal caufe of their redundancy in the *primæ viæ* of children.

The frequent opportunities, which the preceding courfe of experiments afforded me, of obferving the effects arifing from the combination of green vitriol and aftringents, naturally led me to examine into the principles of INK. And as the fubject is not only curious in itfelf, but alfo interefting and important, from its relation to the arts of dying and ftaining black, I was induced to inftitute a new fet of trials, in order to the more

clear

clear and accurate inveſtigation of it. That a ſolution of vitriol ſtrikes a deep black, with vege- table aſtringents, is a faɛt univerſally known; but Dr. Lewis is almoſt the only chemiſt who hath attempted to explain it. He is of opi- nion that the colouring matter of ink is iron, extricated from its acid in a highly attenuated or divided ſtate, and combined with a pecu- liar ſpecies of matter contained in aſtringent vegetables. Acids, he ſays, deſtroy its black- neſs, by rediſſolving the ferrugineous parti- cles; and alkalis, by uniting with the aſtrin- gent matter, and precipitating the iron, nearly in the ſame ochrey ſtate, as they do from the ſimple acid ſolutions of the me- tal *(b)*.

But from the following experiments, I think it will fully appear that this very inge- nious and uſeful chemiſt is miſtaken; and that the colouring matter of ink is iron, not extricated from, but in combination with an acid.

EXPERIMENT XXXVII. To half an ounce of the decoɛtion of galls, was added one grain of *ſal martis:* An inky blackneſs ſuc- ceeded. Sixty drops of *ſp. c. c. vol.* diſcharged the black, and rendered the liquor thick, and

(b) Lewis Comm. Ph. Tech. p. 340.

brown

brown coloured. A hundred and twenty drops of oil of vitriol reftored the blacknefs; two hundred again difcharged it, and gave the ink a yellow caft, incling to green. This experiment is illuftrated by the following one.

EXPERIMENT XXXVIII. One grain of green vitriol was diffolved in half an ounce of fpring water : Forty drops of *fp. c. c. vol.* were added; a greenifh yellow fediment formed itfelf, and prefently fubfided to the bottom of the glafs, with little white flakes, which I at firft judged to be calcareous earth, fepa-rated from the fpring water by means of the volatile alkali. But the *fp. c. c. vol.* mixed with the fame water, produced no precipitation. Oil of vitriol was then dropped in, to the point of faturation. When the effervefcence ceafed, the whole fediment was rediffolved, and the mixture became quite clear.

EXPERIMENT XXXIX. A piece of po-lifhed iron was immerfed in a cold infufion of the bark, made with diftilled water. In three hours, the liquor was juft perceptibly tinged with black. The piece of iron was then taken out, wiped clean, and again im-merfed in another infufion of the *cortex*, of equal ftrength with the former, made with common fpring water. In lefs than two

hours,

hours, the infusion assumed a deep purple colour, and the fluid in contact with the iron was of an inky blackness.

This experiment clearly proves, that an acid is necessary to the formation of ink. Spring water is generally impregnated with some of the mineral acids, in combination either with certain metallic substances, the fossil alkali, or calcareous earth. The water, employed in this trial, contained a considerable portion of selenitic salt, and hence it was capable of dissolving the iron, which was immersed in it, and of forming with it a perfect *sal martis*. This sufficiently accounts for the deep purple hue, which the infusion assumed. The distilled water was either not sufficiently pure (for I did not particularly examine it) or the *cortex*, which, like all other vegetable substances, is of an acescent nature, communicated to it a slight degree of acidity, by which the iron was corroded, and a faint and scarcely perceptible blackness produced.

Experiment XL. Three or four drachms of *sal martis* were dissolved in half a pint of boiling water. After standing a few days, that the ochre might precipitate, the solution was passed through brown paper. The filtered liquor was perfectly clear, discovered no marks of acidity to the taste, and struck a deep black with the
infusion

infufion of galls. In four or five days it let fall
a very fine, light, yellow fediment, was again
paffed through the filter, and ftruck as before
a deep black with the infufion of galls. I did
not profecute this experiment any further; being
fatisfied, from the trial I had made, that the acid
and the iron, the component parts of green vitriol, are not fo eafily feparated from each other,
as is commonly fuppofed. And it is probable
that the acid, after the precipitation of the ochre,
ftill retains as much ferrugineous matter, as is
fufficient to faturate it, when fo much diluted
with water.

Experiment XLI. From a large Copperas
Work, eftablifhed near Wigan, I procured a
quantity of the yellow ochre, precipitated from
green vitriol; and of a chocolate coloured pigment, made by expofing the ochre to fuch a
degree of heat, as is fufficient to feparate the
acid, and give it what the painters term a body.
Neither the ochre, nor the pigment were attracted by the magnet, a proof that they were
both in a ftate of calcination. Three grains of
the ochre, and the fame quantity of the chocolate coloured pigment were added to two glaffes,
each containing half an ounce of a decoction of
the bark. The pigment communicated to the
decoction its own peculiar colour; but the yellow ochre ftruck with it a deep purplifh black.

Twenty

Twenty drops of *sp. c. c. vol.* made no change in the decoction with the pigment; but the other instantly lost its black, and assumed a chocolate colour, exactly resembling that of the pigment.

EXPERIMENT XLII. THE result of the last experiment led me to imagine, that an alkali, dropped upon the ochre, would render it brown by abstracting its acid; and on the contrary, that oil of vitriol added to the chocolate pigment, would restore its yellow colour, and give it the property of striking a black with vegetable astringents. I therefore diffused four grains of the ochre, and the same quantity of the pigment, in two glasses of water. To one, I added twenty drops of *sp. c. c. vol.* to the other, the same quantity of *ol. vitriol.* The hartshorn immediately precipitated the ochre in fine, light flakes, but did not either effervesce with it, or alter its colour: The acid had no sensible effect on the pigment. Thus was I doubly disappointed in the issue of this experiment.

EXPERIMENT XLIII. A few drachms of the yellow ochre were well mixed with four ounces of spring water. As soon as the ochre subsided, the liquor above was carefully poured off, and passed through common filtering paper doubled. It had acquired a deep orange colour, was perfectly transparent, had an aluminous taste, and

was

was remarkably ſtyptic and aſtringent in the mouth. A drachm of it ſtruck a deep green, inclining to black, with half an ounce of the bark decoction. I inſtilled twenty drops of *ſp. c. c. vol.* into a table-ſpoonful of it: No effervefcence enſued, but a very copious, flaky, and yellow ſediment was inſtantly produced. I kept the remainder of the orange coloured liquor, in an open glaſs veſſel, for ſeveral weeks, without obſerving the leaſt ochrey precipitation, or any diminution of its tranſparency. And this I apprehend is a proof, that a firm and laſting combination takes place, between certain proportions of the component parts of green vitriol.

THE ſame ochre was macerated in freſh portions of water, till the filtered liquor had neither taſte, colour, nor the property of giving the leaſt black tinge to an infuſion of galls. The ochre was then dried by a very gentle heat, and two ſcruples of it were added to half an ounce of the ſame decoction of the bark, which was uſed in the former experiments; but no change of colour enſued, only the decoction aſſumed a lighter yellow, whilſt the particles of the ochre floated in it.

EXPERIMENT XLIV. Spirit of hartſhorn, dropped into a ſolution of green vitriol, occaſioned a copious precipitation, but no effervefcence. It cannot be alledged therefore, that the yellow ochre

contains no acid, becaufe it doth not raife a fenfible ebullition with the volatile alkali.

THUS it appears, that whatever deprives green
vitriol of its acid, whether it be heat, the addition
of an alkali, or repeated affufions of water, deftroys its power of ftriking a black colour with
vegetable aftringents. May we not then juftly
conclude, that an acid is effentially neceffary to
this property, which, it is more than probable,
depends upon the compofition of the copperas as
a mixt; and not upon either of its conftituent
parts feparately taken? Ink therefore is a combination of vitriolic acid, iron, and a certain proportion of vegetable aftringent matter *(i)*. But
as thefe principles bear but a weak relation to each
other, their bond of union is eafily diffolved, and
it has long been a defideratum in chemiftry, to

(i) AN ingenious friend (Dr. Falconer of Bath)
is of opinion, that a double elective attraction takes
place in the production of ink. The acid forfakes
the iron and combines with the vegetable aftringent,
feparating from it the phlogifton, which unites with the
iron. In fupport of this hypothefis he obferves, 1. that
mineral aftringents, fuch as earth of alum, &c. precipitate iron, as well as thofe of the vegetable clafs; but
affording no *phlogifton*, the precipitate is in an ochreous
ftate. 2. That the black fediment of ink is eafily foluble in acids, whereas the *calces* precipitated by alkalis
are of very difficult folution, owing to the almoft entire
lofs of their *phlogifton*. For a perfect calx is found to be
abfolutely infoluble.

render

render it more fixed and permanent. Acids by attracting the aftringent matter, with which it is evident, from many of the foregoing-experiments, they have a ftrong affinity, difcharge the black colour of ink. Alkalis, on the contrary, decompofe it, by abftracting the acid from the vitriol, and precipitating the iron. If the blacknefs hath been deftroyed by an acid, the addition of an alkali in due proportion will reftore it, and *vice verfa*. The reafon why they thus counteract each other's effects, is too obvious to require an explanation.

A RECAPITULATION OF THE

PRINCIPAL FACTS ASCERTAINED BY THE PRECEDING EXPERIMENTS.

1. THE PERUVIAN BARK, and many other vegetable bitters and aftringents, yield their virtues as perfectly to cold, as to boiling water.

2. As much of the refin of the bark is dif-folved by cold maceration, as by coction.

3. TRITURATION promotes and increafes the folution of the bark in water.

4. A STRONG

4. A STRONG infusion of the bark may, by means of triture, be prepared with great expedition.

5. QUICK LIME neither quickens, nor increases the solution of the bark in water.

6. THE BARK will not yield all its virtues either to cold water, boiling water, or rectified spirit of wine, nor probably to any other *menstruum* singly employed. After thirty cold macerations, and twenty-five coctions, in different portions of water, each *refiduum*, though perfectly infipid, yielded a bitter and aftringent tincture, when digested in rectified spirit of wine. On the contrary, after repeated digestions in rectified spirit of wine, when that *menstruum* acquired neither taste nor colour from the bark, cold water extracted from it a manifest degree of aftringency.

7. COLD WATER is a more powerful solvent of the bark, than rectified spirit of wine. But brandy is a stronger solvent than water, and rhenish wine than brandy.

8. THE DECOCTION, and INFUSION of the Peruvian bark are very perishable preparations.

9. ACIDS, BITTERS, and ASTRINGENTS neutralize each other, forming what the chemists term a *tertium quid*. When combined together in due proportion, their taste and smell is altered; the acids lose the property of striking a red colour with syrop of violets; and their antiseptic powers, in combination, are double the sum of them
when

when feparately employed. The bark likewife, with vinegar, hath the property of reftoring fweetnefs to putrid fubftances, which Dr. Macbride affirms it hath not alone.

10. THE VEGETABLE ACIDS, combined with aftringents, diminifh their aftrictive power on the dead fibre; the mineral acids increafe it.

11. ASTRINGENCY and BITTERNESS are diftinct properties, and are united together in very different proportions, in different vegetables.

12. NEITHER the tafte, nor the power of ftriking a black colour with chalybeates, nor yet the property of hardening animal fibres, whether fingly, or collectively taken, are certain criteria of the aftringent power of a medicine on the living body.

13. THE power of ftriking a black colour with green vitriol is not always a teft of aftringency on the dead fibre; nor is it common to all vegetable aftringents. Rue yields a faint black, on the addition of *fal martis* to an infufion of it, and yet is not aftringent: Gentian, on the contrary, ftrikes no black, although it is a pretty ftrong aftringent.

14. PUTRID GALL is neutralized by all acids. But thofe of the native vegetable clafs alone entirely fweeten it.

15. WHATEVER deprives green vitriol of its acid, whether it be heat, the addition of an

alkali,

alkali, or repeated affusions of water, destroys its power of striking a black colour with vegetable astringents.

16. An acid, contrary to the opinion of Dr. Lewis, appears to be essentially necessary to the above-mentioned property of green vitriol.

17. Ink seems to be a combination of vitriolic acid, iron, and a certain proportion of vegetable astringent matter.

ESSAY

E S S A Y IV.

ON THE

USES and OPERATION

OF

B L I S T E R S.

Certè hinc lucis aliquid erui poterit, qua id tandem, in quo
medicorum diligentiam defidero, effici queat, ut accurata de
veficantium in diuturnis affectibus præcepta tradantur,
quæ et perfpicuitatem habeant, et quafdam errare in me-
dendo non patientes vias.

FREIND.

THOUGH the action of cantharides, as veficatories, was not unknown to the ancients, their application did not prevail much in
practice, till the beginning of the laft century.
And as nothing hath tended more to enlarge the
boundaries of fcience, than the contentions of the
learned, we perhaps owe, in a good meafure,
our prefent more accurate acquaintance with the
virtues and operation of blifters, to a difpute
amongft the Italian phyficians, relative to their

I 4

ufe

ufe in a plague, which prevailed about the years 1575 and 1590. But though blifters are now almoft univerfally employed, and experience hath afcertained their utility in various diforders, the theory of their action, as well as the mode of their operation, is yet undetermined, and remains a fubject of litigation. Hence arifes that diverfity of opinion concerning the difeafes in which they are indicated, the time of their application, and the parts to which they ought to be applied. Nor can we ever hope for uniformity in this particular, amongft phyficians, either with refpect to their opinions or their practice, till a jufter idea be formed of their mode of action, deduced from experience, and an attentive obfervation of their effects on the human body. When this is accomplifhed, a fyftem of rules may be laid down for their right and advantageous application.

MEDICINES are generally divided into fuch as act, 1. on the folids, 2. on the fluids : And blifters may be confidered as belonging to each of thefe claffes; though their relation is chiefly to the former. But here a queftion occurs, whether veficatories produce their effects by their external action on the body, or by the abforption of their ftimulating particles into the fyftem? Baglivy furnifhes us with two curious, though cruel experiments, of the injection of two ounces of the
tincture

tincture of cantharides, into the jugular veins of a dog and a whelp. Great anxiety, violent pain, infatiable thirft, convulfions, and death, were the confequences in each inftance. But no certain or juft inferences can be drawn from thefe experiments; becaufe medicines are not adminiftered by injection into the blood veffels; and fubftances, much lefs acrid in their nature than cantharides, if conveyed directly and undiluted into the courfe of circulation, will be found to produce effects fimilar, or at leaft equally deleterious (k). When taken by the mouth, in an over-dofe, the moft dreadful fymptoms fucceed; an exulceration of the bladder and *urethra*, inflammation of the bowels, violent pains in the *hypogaftrium*, extreme thirft, a high fever attended with delirium; and at laft death clofes the melancholy fcene. The like effects, it is faid, though in a lefs degree, have been obferved to arife from the application of blifters. And it is upon thefe active powers of cantharides, when abforbed into the fyftem, properly modified and feafonably applied, that the effects of veficatories are fuppofed, by feveral learned writers, chiefly to depend (l). The quicker contractions of the heart and ar-

(k) New milk, injected into the veins of a dog, proves a mortal poifon. Young on Opium, p. 6.

(l) Baglivy, Freind, Glafs, Huxham, &c. &c.

teries,

teries, in confequence of their application in certain diforders, they afcribe, not to a fympathy
with the fkin, but to a ftimulus circulated with
the fluids, and acting immediately on the veffels
themfelves.　And as Baglivy hath afferted that
cantharides have the property of colliquating the
blood, when mixed with it out of the body, they
apprehend that the good effects of blifters, in
fevers attended with a glutinofity and lentor in
the fluids, arife principally, if not entirely, from
their attenuating and diffolving powers.　But
this theory of the operation of veficatories is
liable, I think, to many objections.

1. If their action depend upon the ftimulus of
the abforbed cantharides, they fhould in all cafes
quicken the contractions of the vafcular fyftem.
But this is contradicted by experience; for in
pleurifies, peripneumonies, and other inflammatory difeafes, when the heart and arteries are
already acting very ftrongly, they abate the
inflammation, and lower the pulfe *(m)*.

2. The fmall portion of cantharides, which
may be carried into the courfe of circulation by
the lymphatics of the fkin, cannot I apprehend be
adequate to the effects afcribed to it, whether we
confider the large mafs of fluids with which it is
mixed and diluted, or the coats of the veffels

(m) Whytt's Experiments, Ph. Tranfact. vol. L. p. 2.

lined

lined with a mucus, which muft defend them
from any flight degree of acrimony. It may indeed be faid, that the ufual effects of a blifter on
the urinary paffages fhew, that the particles of
cantharides are abforbed in fufficient quantity, to
irritate and vellicate the internal parts of the body.
But allowing this objection its full force, by
granting what is difputed by fome, that the
ftrangury arifes from the immediate action of the
flies on the urinary paffages, this by no means
proves their ftimulating power, when circulating
with the general mafs of fluids. All extraneous
bodies introduced into the blood, and not capable
of being animalized, pafs off by one or other of
the excretories. If they be of fuch a nature as
to be volatilized by the common heat of the body,
they are eliminated by the lungs and pores of the
fkin, along with the matter of infenfible perfpiration. Garlic, onions, afafœtida, fulphur, and
moft of the effential oils, afford examples of this
kind. But if the extraneous matter be lefs volatile, if it be incapable of chemical mixture with
the blood, or if it unite only with the ferum, it
will be carried to the kidneys, and pafs off by
urine. Of this nature are cantharides *(u)*; and

(*u*) Baglivy, on mixing cantharides with the ferum
of the blood, found the powder precipitated foon after
to the bottom of the veffel, without having produced
any change in the colour of that fluid.

when

when their acrid particles are, in continual fucceffion, applied to the highly fenfible and nervous membrane, which lines the urinary ducts,
can we wonder at the ftrangury, and other painful effects which they produce (o)?

3. THE fame objection may be made to the
attenuating power of cantharides, as introduced
into the blood by means of blifters. Is it at all
probable that a few grains of cantharides can act
fo powerfully, as to diffolve a general lentor and
vifcofity of the whole mafs of fluids? Mercury,
it is true, in a very fmall quantity, will excite a
falivation: But it does not produce this effect, by
breaking down the *crafis* of the blood, though
the continued ufe of it may have that tendency,
but merely, as I conceive, by its partial ftimulus
on the falivary glands. An eminent practitioner
informed me, that he had more than once ordered blood to be taken from patients under
falivation, which he found not in a diffolved, but

(o) IT is not improbable, that the nerves of the urinary paffages are difpofed to be more irritated by the
acrimony of the flies, than thofe which are diftributed
to the other organs of the body. For Dr. Whytt hath
ingenioufly proved, that the different operation of
medicines depends very much on the particular nature
and diverfified fenfibility of the nerves of different parts
of the body; by which they are differently affected by
the fame kind of ftimulating fubftances.
Vid. Effay on Nerv. Dif.

even

even in a buffy ftate. But it may be prefumed, I think, that cantharides are not poffeffed, in any confiderable degree, of a colliquative power; for they have no chemical relation to the animal fluids, and Sir John Pringle hath proved that they are by no means feptic *(p)*. As this, however, is a point of fome importance, the two following experiments were repeated, after Baglivy, in order to determine it.

EXPERIMENT I. Four ounces of blood, juft drawn from the arm, were divided into two equal portions; to one was added ten grains of *pulv. cantharid.* the other was kept as a ftandard. The portion with cantharides coagulated at the fame time with the ftandard, and neither affumed a fublivid, nor an afh colour. Its furface was covered with a thin pellicle, but without the veficles Baglivy defcribes. After ftanding a few hours, the craffamentum in part diffolved, as appeared from the colour of the ferum, which was tinged with red; owing perhaps to a flight degree of agitation, which was ufed to mix the cantharides with the blood when frefh drawn.

THE portion without the cantharides feparated into a clear, pale coloured ferum, and a tough, afh coloured craffamentum; the furface of which contracted into the compafs of a fhilling, and

(p) Append. to Dif. Army, Exp. 22.

retained

retained that form till the putrefaction began; which happened fooner in the ftandard, than in the other portion of blood.

EXPERIMENT II. Ten grains of *pulv. cantharid.* added to two ounces of ferum, tinged by the craffamentum of a light, florid, crimfon colour, rendered it more liquid, and changed it to a dull red. Contrary to the affertion of Baglivy, it coagulated with great eafe, and with lefs heat than an equal portion of the fame ferum, without cantharides.

5. THE chief fymptoms induced by blifters may be rationally accounted for, without having recourfe to the abforption of the acrid particles, of which they are compofed. Thefe fymptoms are a quick pulfe, drynefs of the tongue, thirft, ftrangury, &c. They quicken the pulfe in the low ftate of fevers, by their ftimulus on the fkin, with which the whole vafcular fyftem fympathizes. They occafion thirft, drynefs of the tongue, and an increafe of fever, in the fame way, viz. by their external irritation. But thefe effects ought to be afcribed to the improper and unfeafonable ufe of blifters. When the inflammatory *diathefis* prevails univerfally and ftrongly, without any partial obftruction, every ftimulus muft aggravate the fymptoms; and blifters raifed on the fkin, by a cataplafm of muftard, or by the actual or potential cautery, where the irritation is confeffedly

feffedly external, would operate in the fame manner as an epifpaftic of cantharides. But in cafes wherein veficatories are indicated, I have never found, on the ftricteft examination, the leaft increafe of thirft, or drynefs of the mouth, in confequence of their application *(q)*. The
ftrangury

(q) THE three hiftories, which Baglivy relates, of the effects of epifpaftics, carry very little authority with them; becaufe the blifters were either ill-timed, or laid on in too great numbers. The firft cafe is that of a young man, of a bilious temperament, who, after being heated, fuddenly expofed himfelf to the cold wind. He was feized with an *angina,* which terminated in a violent pleurify, attended with the ftrongeft fymptoms of inflammation. Six veficatories were applied at once, to different parts of his body; the confequences of which were, a fuppreffion of the *fputum,* tremors, convulfions, delirium, and death. The fecond hiftory is that of a cook, who was attacked with a convulfion of the lower jaw, which was foon after fucceeded by fpafmodic contractions of the abdominal mufcles. The *pulvis cornachini* was prefcribed, and the next day four blifters were applied. Vomiting, convulfive motions, and an oppreffed breathing enfued. On the fourth day he died. This cafe was probably a locked jaw; a difeafe too frequently fatal. The third hiftory is that of a young and flender woman, eight months advanced in pregnancy, who, after fuffering much pain, was at length delivered. The pain however ftill continued, accompanied with an uncommon tenfion of the belly. Four blifters were applied at one and the fame time, as in the former inftances.

ftrangury has by fome been fuppofed to arife,
not from an abforption of cantharides, but from
a fympathy between the fkin and the urinary
paffages. And it is urged, that a warm fomentation of milk and water, applied to a bliftered
part, very quickly relieves this complaint, by
removing or diminifhing the irritation on the
furface of the body. But I confefs the probability lies on the other fide of the queftion;
and feveral reafons incline me to think, that
the ftrangury is produced alone by the abforption and internal ftimulus of the flies.

1. Neither muftard, the actual or potential cautery, nor any other veficating ftimulus
but cantharides, excite this complaint. And
is it not ftrange, that the urinary paffages
fhould have fuch an univerfal fympathy with
all the different parts of the body, to which

ftances. The *lochia* were immediately fuppreffed, convulfions came on, and at laft the poor patient fell a vic-
tim to death. Baglivius de Veficant. p. 70.

From the application of fo many blifters, it is not to
be wondered, that the thirft, quicknefs of the pulfe,
and other fymptoms of acute difeafes were, according to
the experience of Baglivy, greatly aggravated. Befides,
it is more than probable, that veficatories are attended
with greater inconveniences in warm, than in cold climates, becaufe the inhabitants of the former are generally of more irritable conftitutions, and of more aduft
and bilious temperaments, than thofe of the latter.

cantharides

cantharides are applied, whilft no fuch confent takes place, when any other veficatory is
made ufe of ?

2. Drinking plentifully prevents the ftrangury; and furely it can produce this effect in
no other way, than by diluting, in the kidneys
and bladder, the acrimonious particles of the
flies.

3. A blister, laid upon the head immediately after fhaving, is almoft always fucceeded
by the ftrangury; whereas no fuch effect takes
place, if the application be delayed twenty-
four hours. How are we to account for this
fact, unlefs by fuppofing, that the fubtler
parts of the cantharides enter more readily,
and in greater quantity into the blood, after
the fcarf-fkin hath been removed by the razor?
The effect of a warm fomentation, in allevia-
ting the troublefome fymptoms of this
complaint, arifes partly, from its fedative operation on the whole fyftem, but
chiefly, I imagine, from its wafhing off all
thofe acrid particles adhering to the fkin,
which would otherwife enter into the blood,
and increafe, or at leaft continue the irritation
in the urinary paffages.

But though it be acknowledged, that the
ftrangury is occafioned by the ftimulus of the
cantharides, acting internally, yet the ex-

K planation

planation, given above, of this effect removes, I think, every objection to what has been advanced. I fhall proceed therefore to confider the operation of blifters, according to the divifion already laid down.

THE difeafes of the SOLIDA VIVA, in which they are indicated, are very numerous; but taking a more general view of them, they may perhaps be reduced to three kinds.

1. WHEN THE ACTION OF THE MOVING FIBRES IS, EITHER PARTIALLY OR UNIVERSALLY, TOO WEAK.

2. WHEN IT IS IRREGULAR.

3. WHEN IT IS PARTIALLY TOO STRONG.

IN the firft cafe veficatories are indicated, as a ftimulus to the languid folids, to roufe them to more vigorous contractions, to fupport the *vis vitæ*, and to promote the falutary fecretions. They tend to quicken the circulation, to raife the pulfe, and to animate the whole fyftem. Hence we may deduce their ufe and operation,

1. IN LOW NERVOUS FEVERS; when the fpirits fink, when the contractions of the heart grow languid, and the unhappy patient ftruggles under anxiety, reftleffnefs, delirium, difficulty of breathing, and a load and oppreffion about the *præcordia*. Thefe fymptoms arife from debility, and denote a kind of

nervous

nervous orgafm, or fpafm of the vitals, which requires cordial medicines, aided by the application of blifters (r). An eminent practitioner hath indeed obferved, that in thefe fevers, epifpaftics fometimes aggravate all the fymptoms, and by their irritation occafion a fmall and contracted pulfe. But this he afcribes to a miftake, either in the time, or place of their application. On the firft figns of a delirium, when the urine turns pale, when the patient fighs, is anxious, and becomes dull of hearing, or when his eyes fparkle and look ftaring, &c. he advifes to cover the whole head with a blifter. The epifpaftic will thus be applied as nearly as poffible to the part affected; and as the head is lefs fenfible to the ftimulus of cantharides, than any other part of the body, all the bad effects, arifing from too great irritation, will be prevented (s). Baglivy long ago remarked, that blifters fometimes excite a fmall and contracted pulfe; and I apprehend in the clafs of difeafes, now under confideration, their utility muft always be attended with a peculiar degree of uncertainty. This depends on the nature of thefe fevers, and the concomitant ftate of the nerves.

(r) *Vide* Huxham on Fevers, p. 82.
(s) *Vide* Med. Effays of Edinburgh, vol. IV. Art. 23.

Whenever

Whenever they are accompanied with little pain, but with a high degree of irritability, which is not unfrequently the cafe, blifters, I think, will be found to be prejudicial, by increafing the fpafm, and throwing the fyftem into confufion. But if the body, however languid and enfeebled, has been accuftomed through the courfe of the difeafe, to the ftimulus of pain, or if the nerves be not affected with an excefs of fympathetic fenfibility, epifpaftics may be applied with fafety and advantage.

2. In the advanced ftate of INFLAMMATORY FEVERS, when the patient becomes languid, or perhaps comatofe, blifters are highly ferviceable. And they are found to be very efficacious in removing thofe obftinate and oppreffive head-achs, which have refifted every previous evacuation, and which often continue to the laft period of the diftemper *(t)*. The fame obfervation holds true in every other fpecies of fever, where fuch a train of fymptoms occur as have been already defcribed.

Even in malignant PETECHIAL FEVERS, notwithftanding the great diffolution of the blood, and the fuppofed tendency of cantharides to increafe that diffolution, fome of the moft eminent

(t) Vide Pringle's Dif. of the Army, p. 134.

practitioners

practitioners have been bold enough to recommend blisters. Thus Riverius says, *Ubi maxima est malignitas, unicum veficatorium non fufficit, fed plura admovenda funt; foleo ego in magna morbi fævitiâ, quinque locis admovere, cervici nimirum, utrique brachio, parti interiori inter cubitum et humerum, et utrique femori, parti etiam inferiori inter inguina et genua, cum felici fucceffu (u).* Etmuller, treating of the fame fevers, afferts, *Si ulla eft febris in qua veficatoria conveniunt, eft imprimis petechialis (x).* And in the malignant, ulcerous fore throat, it muft be acknowledged that they are productive of the beft effects. But with deference to thefe great authorities, I think blifters fhould be applied with the utmoft caution, in all cafes, attended with an highly putrid, and diffolved ftate of the fluids: For under fuch circumftances, they often exhauft the ftrength of the patient, by exciting an immoderate difcharge of bloody ferum; and they fometimes occafion a fudden and fatal mortification.

3. In the SMALL-POX, when the patient is of a lax and weak habit, when the pulfe is low, feeble, and depreffed; and the fever infufficient for the expulfion and fuppuration

(u) Riverii Opera, p. 541.
(x) Etmuller. Op. p. 365.

of

of the puſtules, epiſpaſtics are certainly indicated (y). When the pocks are of the bloody
kind, and attended with delirium, Dr. Mead
aſſures us that bliſters may be uſed with equal
ſafety and advantage. And in this diſtemper,
whenever the maturation of the puſtules does
not regularly ſucceed their eruption, and
when anxiety, inquietude, difficulty of breathing, and delirium come on, the fever ſhould
be quickened by warm cordial medicines, and
eſpecially by the application of bliſters (z).
This is confirmed by the teſtimony of Dr.
Tiſſot, in a late publication, who, after point-
ing out the analogy between the action of opium
and cantharides in the ſmall-pox, ſays, *Unicum eſt ſymptoma in quo, dum hæc pulchra operantur,
à narcoticis caveo; ubi nimirum relicta cute, ad
pulmonem acre devolvit viru, cum frequentiſſimo,
celerrimo, debilique pulſu, cutis ſiccitate, orthopnæa,
anxietate, delirio. Gravis eſt ſanè caſus, et è
peſſimis in medicina variolosa, quem feliciter ali-
quoties, citò accerſitus, curavi, larga et accerima
veſicatoria ſuris applicando, largiſſimos et calidos.
hauſtus decocti hordei, et ſambuci melliti preſcribendo,
cum minimis doſibus ſulphuris aurati antimonii.
Quatuor vel quinque lapſis horis, remittit frequentia*

(y) Hillary on the Small-pox, p. 94, 95.
(z) Mead, Sydenham, Morton.

pulſus,

pulfus, recedit anxietas, madet cutis, increfcunt vires. Omnino liberato pectore, et demiffa febre, juvari poteft natura leni narcotico. Diu fluere crura juvat (a). It is always accounted a bad fymptom, when the fwelling of the hands does not follow the tumour of the face, and the fwelling of the feet that of the hands; and if the patient be threatened with this alarming circumftance, epifpaftics fhould be applied to the wrifts and ancles, a little before the inflammation of thofe parts may be expected to begin. For they will not only tend to draw the humours thither, but will give them alfo a falutary vent (b). When the fauces are covered with puftules, and both deglutition and refpiration are impeded by the fwelling of the throat, blifters applied to the neck are highly ferviceable, as I have frequently experienced. Dr. Tiffot relates the hiftory of a patient, under thefe circumftances, who was fuddenly relieved by the application of finapifms to the feet. *Vidi hoc anno collum horride turgidum, educta è lecto ægra, et finapifmis plantis pedum applicatis, intra viginti minuta, dimidiam diametri partem amififfe. Horrendos verum eft pedum patiebatur dolores, quos per bihorium tolerare fuafi; tunc tumentibus admodum cruribus, finapi removi;*

(a) Tiffot. de variolis, &c. *vid.* Sandifort. Thefaur. vol. II. p. 11.   (b) Huxham, p. 155.

omnia

omnia pacabantur (c). In this inftance, it is probable that blifters would have been no lefs
efficacious than the finapifm; and they would
have been more eligible, becaufe productive of
a lefs degree of pain and inflammation.

4. IN the APOPLEXY, whether arifing from over
diftended veffels, injuring the brain by preffure,
from the effufion of blood within the *cranium,*
or from a pituitous collection there; after attempting to relieve the head by bleeding, cupping the *occiput,* with deep fcarifications, and
ufing fuch other evacuations, as the ftate of the
patient may require, blifters may be applied,
both to the head and extremities, with great advantage. By increafing the circulation of the
blood externally, and by producing a confiderable difcharge of ferum, they will unload the
veffels of the brain; whilft by their ftimulus,
they roufe the torpid fyftem of nerves, excite the
heart and arteries to quicker and more vigorous
contractions, and thus powerfully contribute to
reftore the equilibrium between the *vis motrix,*
and *moles movenda.*

5. IN the PALSY. When this difeafe invades
the whole body, blifters are ufeful by their general
ftimulus. But they are moft efficacious when
the paralytic affection is not univerfal, but confined to fome particular member or organ. Thus

(c) Sandifort. Thefaurus, vol. II. p. 16.

in

in palſies of the upper extremities, veſicatories applied to the *vertebræ* of the neck, and going obliquely to the ſhoulders, are remarkably uſeful. And when the diſeaſe attacks the lower extremities, they are equally efficacious, when laid upon the extremities themſelves. As moſt of the nerves which go to the bladder, paſs through the *foramina* of the *os ſacrum*, veſicatories have been very ſuccefsfully applied to that region, for the cure of an incontinence of urine. And it is probable, that they would be much more certain and powerful in their operation, if a proper attention were paid, in their external application, to the origin and courſe of the nerves *(d)*.

6. In the GUTTA SERENA, when it proceeds from a paralytic affection of the retina, bliſters applied to the forepart of the head, ſo as to cover the nerves which iſſue through the *ſupra* orbital *foramina*, and ſpread themſelves on the forehead, are highly ſerviceable, as I have more than once experienced.

7. In the TYMPANITES, Celſus adviſes to make ulcers in ſeveral parts of the belly, and to keep them running. But we are furniſhed, by means of epiſpaſtics, with a much more effectual, as well as more humane remedy. Dr. Mead recommends their application in this diſorder: And it is probable they may do ſervice, both as ſtimulants

(d) Vide Lond. Medical Obſerv. p. 318.

and

and antifpafmodics, except when the cafe is complicated with a mortification of the bowels.

8. In the RICKETS, Boerhaave recommends blifters, to ftimulate the languid veffels, and refolve the mucous concretions.

9. In SCHIRROUS TUMOURS of the conglobate glands of the neck, blifters applied to the head, or behind the ears, have a good effect. The finer parts of the cantharides, being abforbed by the lymphatics, are carried immediately to the obftructed glands, and by their ftimulus tend to difcufs thofe indolent fwellings. A young lady, who had a hard, glandular tumour in her neck, which fucceeded the fmall-pox, and had refifted very powerful applications, was lately cured of it by a blifter behind the ear, which I directed on account of an inflammation in one of her eyes. If the tumour be feated in the inguinal glands, veficatories fhould be applied to the thighs. In fuch cafes I have laid blifters over the glands themfelves, but without any beneficial effect.

10. In thofe fchirrous, or œdematous tumours of the joints, ufually called WHITE SWELLINGS, which, after a tedious and ill conditioned fuppuration, corrupt the *fynovia*, fhorten the tendons, make the bones carious, and deftroy the articulation, blifters applied to the part affected, have

been

been fometimes highly ferviceable *(f)*. But
their operation fhould be affifted by the internal
ufe of the Peruvian bark, calomel, or other
alterative and deobftruent medicines *(g)*.

OTHER difeafes, arifing from the too weak
action of the folids, might be enumerated; but
what has been advanced will fuffice to prove the
efficacy and utility of blifters in fuch cafes.

2. WHEN THE ACTION OF THE MOVING FIBRES
IS IRREGULAR, veficatories are indicated, both
as ftimulants and antifpafmodics.

CONVULSIVE MOTIONS OR SPASMS feem generally to arife from fome peculiar irritation of the
nervous fyftem. And whether the brain be
originally, or only fympathetically affected, whatever roufes and engages the attention of the mind
will feldom fail to afford relief, by leffening, or
deftroying the fenfe of that irritation. Blifters
therefore are indicated in fuch difeafes, to ftimulate and excite pain, in a part of the body that
is found. For according to the aphorifm of
Hippocrates, " When two pains occur, but not

(f) *Vide* Medical Tranfactions, vol. I. p. 104.

(g) THE Abbe Chappe mentions an epidemic difeafe
in Ruffia, probably a fpecies of the bronchocele, which
the natives cure by the application of tobacco and fal
ammoniac well mafticated. The tumours are of the fize
of an apple, they rife fuddenly, and if neglected foon
become incurable. Travels into Siberia, p. 353.

in

in the fame place, the greater obfcures the lefs *(g)*."
Dr. Whytt relates the cafe of a patient, who had
an alternate motion of the mufcles of the *abdomen*,
which was cured by a circular blifter, of about
eight inches diameter, applied to the part affected *(h)*. The fame author acquaints us, that
where epilepfies take their rife from an uneafy
fenfation in fome part of the arm or leg, he has
found veficatories, applied to thofe parts, the
moft effectual remedies *(i)*.

In the convulfions which fometimes precede
the eruption of the fmall-pox, blifters act as
powerful antifpafmodics. But they fhould not,
upon flight occafions, be employed in this ftate of
the difeafe, as by their ftimulus they may aggravate the fever, and increafe the number of puftules. When fuch fymptoms occur in the in-
grafted fmall-pox, as indicate the ufe of veficatories, it is faid that they will fucceed the beft,
if applied to the arms, over the part where the
variolous matter was inferted. This I am informed is the prefent practice of an ingenious
phyfician, and celebrated inoculator, who merits
all the honours which have been conferred upon
him, by one of the wifeft potentates in Europe.

(g) Lib. II. Aph. 46.
(h) Whytt on Nerv. Dif. p. 460.
(i) Whitt on Nerv. Dif. p. 461.

In

In the idiopathic epilepfy, the application of veficatories to the head is recommended by Hoffman, Riverius, Pifo, and Mead; who fupport their recommendation by many authentic cafes and hiftories. Celfus mentions feveral remedies for the epilepfy, which are very fingular; fuch as drinking the warm blood of a gladiator juft flain, eating human or horfe's flefh, or the parts of generation of certain animals. If thefe things ever had any efficacy, it muft arife from the repugnancy of nature to them, and from the ftrong and painful fenfations of mind, which fuch fhocking and difgufting remedies could not fail to excite. Upon the fame principle, Boerhaave cured the epileptics, in the poor houfe at Haerlem (k).

Hoffman relates that he has found epifpaftics of excellent ufe, in the fpafmodic afthma (l); and Dr. Whytt confirms the teftimony of Hoffman by his own experience (m).

In fixed pains of the bowels, from fpafms, though there are no evident marks of inflammation, the application of blifters to the *abdomen*

(k) See the Account in Kaw Boerhaave.

(l) Hoffman de Veficant.

(m) Nerv. Dif. p. 495. Epifpaftics have alfo been found to be very ferviceable in the *tuffis convulfiva*.

Vide Ridley's Obferv. p. 91.

may

may be recommended. Sir John Pringle affures us, that he has oftener than once feen a patient relieved in his bowels, as foon as he felt the burning of his fkin; and at the fame time have ftools by a purge, or a clyfter, which had not operated before. In fevere, and continued vomitings, when the ftomach is affected with very painful, convulfive motions, I have obferved the moft falutary effects, from the application of a veficatory to the epigaftric region. Hence we may conclude, that blifters act not, in fuch cafes, as evacuants, but as antifpafmodics.

3. WHEN THE ACTION OF THE SOLIDA VIVA IS TOO STRONG.

IT is yet a fubject of difpute amongft phyficians, whether epifpaftics are ufeful, or detrimental, in inflammatory fevers. Hoffman bears the ftrongeft teftimony againft their application in fuch cafes (n); and Baglivy, from his own experience, afferts, *Quod delirantibus cum febre acuta, lingua arida, et indicijs magnæ vifcerum inflammationis, fi applicentur veficantia, omnia in pejus ruunt, et magna ex parte moriuntur convulfi (o).* Alpinus fays, *Nunquam probare potui, in acutis febribus, veficantium ufum, quod calorem febrilem augeant, vigilias doloremque conci-*

(n) De Veficant. ufu. § 17.

(o) Praxis, p. 102.

tent,

*tent, et deliria inducant, coctionem impediant, non
minus et motui humorum critico obfint, quum incer-
tus fit locus ad quem, vel per quem crifis, eft fu-
tura (q).* Sir John Pringle acquaints us, that
his firft practice, in every inflammatory fever was
to blifter; but afterwards, when he found that a
folution of the fever was not to be procured by
fuch means, he confined the ufe of epifpaftics to
thofe ftates of the difeafe, in which he could be
moft affured of their efficacy *(r)*. Huxham,
if I miftake not, obferves, that to blifter in the
beginning of inflammatory fevers is to add fuel to
the fire; and Dr Whytt exprefsly fays, that in
fevers, where there is no partial obftruction or
inflammation, veficatories are of little fervice,
and are fometimes hurtful; unlefs perhaps towards the end of the difeafe, when the pulfe
begins to fink *(s)*.

On the other hand Sydenham, whofe authority
muft have great weight, from his accurate atten-

(q) Medicin. Method. lib. V. p. 173.

(r) In the fecond ftage of the jail or hofpital fever,
when the pulfe is quick and full, Sir John Pringle hath
ufed blifters, but without fuccefs. Nay upon the firft
attack, the whole head has been bliftered, and the
oozing kept up for fome days, without relieving it, or
preventing any of the ufual fymptoms.

Dif. of the Army, p. 318.

(s) Philof. Tranf. vol. L. part II. p. 578.

tion

tion to the *juvantia* and *lædentia* in all difeafes, adopted the ufe of blifters in the continued acute fever, which prevailed in the years 1673, 1674, 1675. The fymptoms of this fever, as he defcribes them, indicate a very high degree of inflammation; and his practice was, firft to take away a fufficient quantity of blood from the arm, and then to apply a large epifpaftic to the neck: At the fame time he employed the cooling regimen. Dr. Freind fays, that in acute fevers, the fafeft and moft fpeedy relief is afforded by veficatories. Nor are we to be too fcrupulous about accommodating them to the conftitution, or ftate of the patient; for whatever his habit of body may be, if the fever rages beyond meafure, the flight inconvenience of a blifter is rather to be endured, than the life of the patient endangered; for in thefe cafes, the only hope is in blifters. They derive the febrile matter from the brain, and affift and promote the other difcharges, thofe efpecially by fweat and urine *(s)*. Dr. Glafs alfo, in his learned commentaries, recommends the application of blifters in inflammatory fevers. *In febribus inflammatoriis, poft debitam fanguinis miffionem, locum habet id remedij; atque licet motus arteriarum, etiamnum nimis veloces, ab eo intendantur, brevi tantum intervallo id fiet,*

(s) *Vide* Freind de Veficant.

poftea

postea quidem, eliquatis densis humoribus, pulsus sen-
tientur molliores, et febres erunt leniores (t). " I
" have more than once in an evening," says Dr.
Lind, in his valuable paper on fevers and infection,
" ordered eight or ten patients to be bliftered,
" and have left them with a quick pulfe, great
" heat, immoderate thirft, a pain, confufion, and
" heavinefs of the head, and what, to a phyfician
" converfant with fuch fevers, communicates a
" moft certain knowledge of the condition of
" the patient, fuch a lifelefs, funk ftate of the
" eyes, as denoted great danger. But the next
" morning I found thefe patients with a lively,
" brifk eye, a calm pulfe, and with a defire to get
" out of bed *(u)*." Other authorities to the fame
purpofe might be advanced.

How then are we to determine this difpute?
May not the truth in this, as in moft other liti-
gated points, lie in the middle way between the
oppofite opinions? If fo, the following conclufion
may perhaps be juftified: that whenever the inflammatory *diathefis* prevails ftrongly and uniformly throughout the fyftem, and no one part
is more affected than the reft, veficatories are
pernicious and detrimental. But when peculiar
fymptoms of inflammation attack the head, the

(t) Glafs, Comment. p. 235.
(u) Lind on Fevers and Infection, p. 9.

lungs, &c. and prevail more in thofe parts, than the reft of the body, blifters are indicated, and often prove remarkably ufeful. And in fuch cafes, they are found from experience to leffen the impetus of the blood upon the veffels of the inflamed part, to abate the fever and heat of the body, and to diminifh, very evidently the quicknefs of the pulfe (x). Whatever may have been the original caufe of a fever, it will be continued, and often greatly increafed, by any particular inflammation, which may happen to have taken rife from it. Under thefe circumftances, the application of a blifter to a neighbouring part will fometimes produce a refolution of the difeafe, by leffening the impetus of the fluids on the inflamed part, by making a confiderable derivation of ferous humours from it, and by rendering the mind

(x) To underftand more clearly the action of blifters in fuch cafes, it is neceffary to form a juft idea of the nature of inflammation, which feems to confift in an increafed alternate contraction of the veffels of the part affected. If the inflammation be large, or the part inflamed very fenfible, the whole nervous fyftem will be fo affected by the pain, as to render the heart and larger arteries more irritable; and the force of the circulation will, of courfe, be greatly increafed, through the whole body. This ftate is what is called the inflammatory *diathefis*. In the cure of inflammation therefore, two indications are to be attended to; 1. to diminifh the force of the circulation in general; 2. to abate the action

mind lefs fenfible of the painful irritation, which
excites and continues the inflammation. Upon
thefe principles, I apprehend, we may eafily explain the action, and deduce from them the ufes
of epifpaftics in the following difeafes.

I. IN the SYMPTOMATIC PHRENITIS or DELIRIUM,
which accedes indifferently to the bilious, malignant, or inflammatory fever. If the lownefs of
the pulfe admits not of venæfection, the cure
muft be attempted by leeches and blifters *(y)*.
On this fubject, Dr. Whytt furnifhes us with
a practical obfervation of importance: that in
fevers, where the fubftance of the brain is affected,
and not its membranes, he has never found any
benefit from the ufe of blifters. And he always
fufpects the brain to be affected, when a fever

action of the veffels in the part affected. The former is
to be attempted by venæfection, and the antiphlogiftic
regimen; the latter by emollient and fedative applications, and frequently by bliftering the neighbouring
parts. For the impetus of the fluids, in the veffels of
the part to which the veficatory is applied, is much
more augmented in proportion, than the force of the
circulation in general. And as theie feems to be only a
certain degree of nervous energy, exerted in the body
at one time, the increafe of its action in one part, will
neceffarily diminifh it in another. And thus the original inflammation is cured, by exciting another contiguous to it.

(y) Vid. Pringle on the Dif. of the Army, p. 138.

and delirium come on, without any preceding head-ach, or redness in the *tunica albuginea* of the eyes. This kind of fever he has met with several times, and has observed it to be generally fatal *(z)*. But I have lately had under my care a patient, whose case furnishes an exception to this valuable observation; and as there is something in it singular and curious, it may not perhaps be an useless digression, to give a detail of the most interesting circumstances which attended it.

M. B. a maid servant, aged twenty-four, being with child, was turned out of her place, and obliged to go into the poor house, where she remained several weeks after her delivery. But sunk with low diet, oppressed with uneasiness, and exhausted with nursing, she was taken back by her friends, who were assisted in their endeavours to recruit and restore her strength, by the charitable benefactions of a neighbouring gentlewoman, distinguished for her humanity. August 12th, 1766, a few days after her return home, she was seized with a fever, which began with a coldness and shivering, and was succeeded by heat. On the 18th I saw her, and found her in a delirium, with a low and feeble pulse. Her eyes were sunk, but without the least redness or in-

(z) Vid. Phil. Tranf. vol. L. part II. p. 578.

flammation,

flammation, nor had fhe complained of any preceding pain in the head. Her urine was fometimes pale, fometimes high coloured. Her fkin
had that kind of heat, which is not eafily defcribed, but which leaves a difagreeable fenfation
in the hand that feels it. Her tongue was dry
and blackifh; fhe had a flufhing every now and
then in her face, and her belly was immoderately
loofe; and to all thefe complaints an almoft total
deafnefs was added. In the afternoon, there was
generally a flight remiffion of the fymptoms.

A LARGE blifter was ordered to be laid betwixt
her fhoulders, and a cordial, diaphoretic, and
lightly aftringent mixture was prefcribed.

AUG. 20. The delirium ceafed. Her pulfe
and heat were natural, her loofenefs was abated,
but her deafnefs ftill continued. Two blifters
were directed to be applied behind her ears.

21. THERE feemed to be no appearance of
fever, and the deafnefs was going off, though the
blifters had not been applied. She complained
of a numbnefs in her right leg, which on examination I found to be cold and motionlefs. Directions were given to rub it well with the flefh
brufh, and a large cataplafm of muftard and oat
meal *ana p. æ.* was ordered to be applied to her foot.

24. THE palfy was almoft removed. In other
refpects fhe was well, except the pain occafioned
by the cataplafm.

L 3

30th.

30th. SHE had the perfect ufe of her leg.

SEPTEMB. 3d. Though the inflammation occafioned by the cataplafm was very inconfiderable,
yet fhe complained of great pain arifing from it.
Her foot was therefore fomented with a decoction
of camomile and poppy heads, to which a fufficient quantity of milk was added; and afterwards a white bread poultice was applied.

5th. THIS morning fhe was feized with convulfions of the epileptic kind, and had fix fits
fucceffively. She was cold, feeble, and languid,
and complained much of ficknefs and pain in
her head. The following medicines were prefcribed.

R. *Tinct. valerian. volat. tinct. fuliginis, ana*
ʒfs. laud. liquid. gutt. xl. *m. cap. cochl. parv.* ij.
omni hora, ex cyatho aquæ fpiritufque vini gallici.

R. *Rad. valerian. fylveft.* ʒfs. *aq. fontan.* ℥xij.
coque parum, et adde afafœtid. ʒifs. *m. f. enema*
ftatim injiciend.

6th. SHE was better, and had no return of the
fits; but complained ftill of violent pain in the
foot.

7th. SHE continued free from the fits. Her
head was eafier, but her foot was ftill painful.
Yefterday in the afternoon, fhe was fuddenly
deprived of her fight, without the leaft previous
pain or uneafinefs in her eyes. No inflammation,
                                    opacity,

opacity, or alteration of any kind appeared externally; except that the pupils were more than
ordinarily dilated. On holding a lighted candle
close to her eye, the pupil did not contract itself,
and she had not the least perception of the light.
As I apprehended her blindness to be a *gutta serena*,
arising from a paralytic affection of the retina,
I ordered her forehead to be frequently rubbed
with the *liniment. volatile*, made with equal quantities of *ol. oliv.* and *sp. salis ammon. cum calce
viva*; and afterwards a flannel, moistened with
the mixture, to be left upon the part. It was
hoped that by this stimulus, applied immediately
to the nerves which issue from the eyes, through
the *supra-orbital foramina*, the retina might be
restored to its proper sensibility. And the event
in some measure answered my expectations; for
before night, she was able to distinguish the light
of a candle. But the recovery of her sight was
both imperfect, and of short continuance.

8th. She was still blind, and more stupid and
heavy than usual. She was frequently sick, and
vomited her food, but refused all medicines. A
blister was ordered to be applied to her forehead.

9th. She had perfectly recovered her sight.
No sooner did the blister begin to operate, but
she had a glimmering of light, the pain occasioned
a flow of tears, and she was gradually, during

L. 4   the

the action of the veſicatory, reſtored to the uſe of her eyes.

10th. SHE ſtill retained the perfect uſe of her eyes; was more cheerful and lively, had no pain in her head, and complained leſs of her foot. As ſhe ſeemed to be in a fair way of recovering her former ſtate of health, I left her, after giving the proper directions with reſpect to her diet.

N. B. THE young woman continued to re-cover, and about ten days afterwards, I ſaw her perfectly well.

II. IN OPTHALMIAS. Inflammations of the eyes are frequently cured, by making a derivation from the part affected, either by means of leeches, or of bliſters. Perhaps both might be uſefully applied at the ſame time; the leeches near the external angle of the eye, and the bliſters behind the ears; or, according to the preſent more effi-cacious method of practice, upon the forepart of the head. To conſpire with their operation, if the flux of humours to the eyes be great, a briſk purge may be adminiſtered, to make a revulſion. And thus, I apprehend, a cure may be compleated, without draining the whole body by large and repeated venæſections. Hoffman diſſuades us from applying epiſpaſtics to the neck, in opthalmias. *In opthalmia egregij ſunt uſus; ſed obſervavi, quod in nucha non adeo conducant,*

ſed

fed potius dolor inde augeatur; quum contrà pedibus admota, fæpe fimulac humor ftillare incipit, dolorem levent (a).

III. IN NASAL HÆMORRHAGES, blifters applied to the back have been ferviceable *(b)*; and may we not from analogy conclude, that they would be equally ufeful in HÆMOPTOES?

IV. IN the INFLAMMATORY ANGINA, Sydenham recommends the application of a large and ftrong epifpaftic between the fhoulders, having premifed bleeding and purging. Sir John Pringle mentions another remedy, whofe mode of operation feems to be fimilar to that of blifters; viz. the application of a piece of flannel to the throat, moiftened with two parts of *ol. oliv.* and one of *fp. c. c. vol.* or in fuch a proportion as the fkin will bear. By this means the neck, and fometimes the whole body, is put into a fweat. But I imagine it is not by the *diaphorefis,* fo much as by the revulfion which it produces, that this application is fo efficacious: and upon this principle, perhaps a blifter would be ftill more ferviceable. Its operation indeed would not be fo quick; but the copious derivation of ferous humours, from veffels nearly connected with the

(a) De Veficant. ufu. § 12.

(b) Cullen's Clinical Lect.

inflamed

inflamed parts, would much more than balance the comparative flowness of its operation *(c)*.

V. In the firft ftage of the ANGINA MALIGNA, a blifter applied to the nape of the neck, or to each fide of the throat, produces very falutary effects. But as the fkin in this difeafe is particularly difpofed to inflammation, I have feen inconveniences arife from the two powerful ftimulus of the cantharides. Of late, therefore, I have directed the *emplaft. veficatorium*, of the London Difpenfatory, to be mixed with an equal or double proportion of the *emplaft. ftomachicum*, and to this compofition, have added a drachm or two of camphor, properly comminuted with rectified fpirit of wine. Such a plaifter I have repeatedly experienced to be fufficiently efficacious as a blifter; and the antifeptic ingredients it contains, coincide with the general indication of correcting putrefaction.

If a blifter plaifter, after being moderately warmed before the fire, be covered with a fine foft piece of muflin, it will occafion much lefs irritation; produce no ftrangury, or but in a flight

(c) On looking into the laft edition of Sir John Pringle's Difeafes of the Army, I find a note in which he informs us, that in later practice, befides a blifter to the back, in bad cafes he lays one acrofs the throat : at other times he has applied feven or eight leeches under the *fauces.* p. 173.

degree

degree; and, when it is to be removed, will feparate from the fkin, with great facility: nor will fuch a covering prevent its veficating effects. Hence blifters may, in this manner, be applied with advantage, whenever the fkin is difpofed to eryfipelatous inflammation, from its extreme fenfibility; or when their evacuating powers are wanted, with a diminution of their ftimulus. In puerperal cafes alfo, they may thus be ufed, without danger of inflaming the *uterus*, by their action on the urinary paffages.

VI. In a true PERIPNEUMONY, efpecially when the inflammation is great, repeated bleeding is the principal remedy; and Dr. Whytt diffuades us from the early application of blifters. But when the difeafe is of a mixed kind, when the lungs are not fo much inflamed, as loaded with a pituitous matter, when bleeding gives but little relief, when the pulfe though quick is fmall, when the patient is not able to bear evacuations, and the difeafe hath continued for fome time, in fuch circumftances epifpaftics will produce remarkably good effects *(d)*. Sir John Pringle fays that a pleurify, taken in the beginning, may often be cured by one large bleeding, and a blifter laid to the fide affected. If there be no particular ftitch, but only a general oppreffion, the veficatory

(d) Phil. Tranf. vol. L. part. II.

may

may be applied to the back, and afterwards, if the
difeafe be obftinate, firft to one fide, and then to
the other.   Whether applied to the cheft, or to
the extremities, it will relieve the breaft, promote
expectoration, and lower the pulfe.   In pulmonic
diforders, Huxham recommends bliftering the
legs; and he obferves that when they ulcerate the
extremities feverely, they commonly give great
relief *(e)*.

VII. IN the CHRONIC ASTHMA, when the patients
ftrength is very much reduced, blifters are highly
efficacious.   But they fhould never be applied to
the cheft, when the *dyfpnoea* is very fevere; becaufe they render the motion of the intercoftal
mufcles more difficult and painful, as well as
obftruct refpiration, by their preffure and tenacity.
In thefe cafes volatiles are peculiarly ufeful.

VIII. IN the SMALL-POX, when it is attended
with rawnefs, forenefs, and great heat in the mouth
and throat, and a fharp rheum or ftoppage in the
noftrils, blifters are found to be very fuccefsful.
And in this difeafe, whenever the *membrana
fchneideriana* is affected, a revulfion from it is
indicated; otherwife towards the clofe of it, the
patient will be in danger of fuffocation *(f)*.

(e) *Vid.* Effay on Fevers, p. 219, and Obf. de Acre.
et Morb. Epid. vol. II.

(f) *Vid.* Effay on Fevers, p. 219, and Obf. de Aere.
et Morb. Epid. vol. II. p. 140, 149.

9th.

IX. In coughs, attended with fever, pain in the fide, and a pituitous infarction of the lungs, blifters are highly efficacious, in abating the fever, lowering the pulfe, and removing the inflammatory obftruction. This Dr. Whytt hath fatisfactorily proved, by a detail of cafes, laid before the Royal Society, and publifhed in the Philof. Tranf. vol. L.

X. In the inflammation of the liver, one of the beft remedies is a large blifter laid over the part affected (g).

XI. In the inflammation of the stomach and intestines, in the ileus and inflammatory colic, epifpaftics are found to be ferviceable (h).

XII. In the dysentery, when the pains in the belly are too fixed to yield to fomentations, they are relieved by a blifter, applied to the abdomen (i).

XIII. Blisters are remarkably ferviceable in the diarrhoea, which fometimes attends the mèasles; probably becaufe they leffen the inflammation, which in this difeafe falls on the inteftines.

XIV. In the rheumatism, sciatica, and gout, Hoffman commends the ufe of veficatories, becaufe they fet in motion, and evacuate the

(g) Pringle's Dif. of the Army, p. 151.
(h) Ibid.
(i) Pringle's Dif. of the Army, p. 202.

fuppofed

supposed acrid matter, which is impacted in the nervous and tendinous parts. Pringle advises their application to the part affected, in the rheumatism and sciatica; and a celebrated Professor at Edinburgh asserts, that they seldom fail of success in the rheumatism, when applied before a swelling of the part comes on *(k)*. Huxham also bears testimony in favour of epispastics: *In crudelissimo rheumatismo, nihil magis prodest quam vesicatoria, inter scapulas superimposita (l).*

Thus much for the action of blisters on the MOVING FIBRES. Their operation on the FLUIDS depends upon their medicinal powers, as attenuants and evacuants; and these, perhaps, arise solely from their stimulus on the solids. By quickening the alternative contractions of the vessels, they prevent the stagnation of the juices; hence their attenuating effects: and by exciting an inflammation externally, they occasion a flux of humours to the skin, and a consequent evacuation of them. It seems therefore to be almost unnecessary, to consider vesicatories as belonging to this second class of medicines. But as some interesting particulars, relating to their operation as evacuants, have been omitted in the preceding part of this attempt to investigate their uses, I shall briefly consider them under this head.

(k) Cullen's Clinical Lectures.
(l) De Colico Damnoniorum.

I. In

I. In nervous fevers, blifters act not only as a ftimulus, but as a drain; and they fhould not be too foon dried up. Huxham fays, the more they difcharge, and the better it is for the patient: and when the firft blifters heal up, he recommends the application of others.

II. In dropsies, particularly in the *anafarca*, blifters applied to the legs produce a very copious difcharge of ferous humours; but they fhould be ufed with caution, becaufe they fometimes oc-cafion a fpreading, painful, and dangerous in-flammation. I was lately witnefs to a fatal cafe of this kind. The patient laboured under a dropfy of the *thorax*, and a general *anafarca*. His legs and thighs were fwoln to an amazing fize. Veficatories were applied to the extremities, a little above each ankle; and by unloading the cellular membrane, they at firft afforded great relief; but in a few days an eryfipelas enfued, which extended itfelf over the whole legs and part of the thighs, producing fuch excruciating pain, that the patient, whofe ftrength had been before nearly exhaufted, funk under the anguifh. — Whenever it is thought expedient to employ blifters, for the removal of anafarcous fwellings, they fhould be covered with fine, foft muflin, in the manner before defcribed.

III. In the lymphatic or crystalline small-pox, veficatories are recommended as evacuants, both

both by Huxham and Mead. For by the feafon-
able difcharge of the ferofities, the fever, which
increafes when there is no further derivation of
humours to the fkin, is happily moderated, if not
prevented.

IV. In the WARTY SMALL-POX, blifters are very
ufeful evacuants; becaufe the matter being too
thick, can neither fuppurate, nor pafs off by
urine (*m*).

V. In the CONVULSIONS to which children are
fubject, the beft practical writers advife the application of blifters, chiefly on account of the drain
which they produce. The plenty of nutrition,
which nature hath provided for the young animal,
from the time of its birth, neceffarily creates many
redundancies, which in a healthy ftate, are carried
off by the glands of the fkin, by urine, or by
ftool. Hence when the infant is arrived to a
certain growth, an eruption, called the red gum,
ufually appears on the furface of the body, and
frequently at the fame time, there is a difcharge
from the glands behind the ears, and in the groin.
During thefe excretions, the child, for the moft
part, is lively and well; but as the equilibrium
of health, in fuch delicate fubjects, is eafily difturbed, their continuance is very precarious. And
if fome new evacuation be not fubftituted in the
room of them, difeafe will unavoidably enfue.

(*m*) *Vide* Mead de Variolis.

For

For so exquisite is the sensibility of the nervous system in children, that a very slight degree of irritation will, in their tender bodies, excite convulsions. In such circumstances, the utility of blisters is obvious, and might be inferred even *à priori*, if experience had not given a sanction to their application. But their good effects are warranted by the most undoubted testimonies. And as a proof, how salutary it is to promote the discharge of the superabundant juices in children, Willis relates the case of a girl, who was subject to the epilepsy, and in one of her fits fell into the fire, and burnt her face and forehead in the most shocking manner. The accident however was attended with this good effect, that as long as the ulcers remained open, she was free from the disorder. Hollerius furnishes us with a similar example. A girl had, from her infancy, a running sore in her head: It was suddenly healed, and she became epileptic. Variety of remedies were tried to no purpose: Duretus was consulted, who recommended the application of beet leaves to her head, which brought on a large discharge, and removed her epilepsy *(n)*. Agreeable to this is the observation of Hippocrates, that running sores of the head, happening to children, prevent convulsions. *Quibus-*

(n) Boerhaave de Morb. Nerv. p. 820.

*cunque quidem pueris exiſtentibus, erumpunt ulcera
in caput, et in aures, ac in reliquum corpus ; et qui
ſalivoſi fiunt, ac mucoſi, hi ipſi in progreſſu ætatis
facillimè degunt : Qui vero mundi ſunt, et neque
ulcus ullum, neque mucus, neque ulla ſaliva prodit,
neque in uteris purgationem fecerunt, talibus peri-
culum imminet, ut ab hoc morbo (i. e. epilepſia)
corripiantur (o).* Dr. Mead, in his learned
treatiſe, *de imperio ſolis et lunæ,* furniſhes us with
a very remarkable hiſtory of the epilepſy, cured
by a diſcharge from the head, in conſequence
of the application of a bliſter. A child about five
years old, of a luſty and full habit of body, had
convulſions ſo ſtrong and frequent, that her life
was with difficulty ſaved by evacuants, and other
medicines. She continued well for a few days,
but was, at the full of the moon, again attacked
with a moſt violent fit ; after which the diſeaſe
regularly kept the ſame period with the tides.
She continued in this ſtate fourteen days, that is,
till the next great change of the moon, when a dry
ſcab, the effect of an epiſpaſtic with which the
whole *occiput* had been covered, broke out, and
from the ſore iſſued a conſiderable quantity of
limpid ſerum. This diſcharge was promoted by
proper applications ; and the patient grew up to
woman's eſtate, without ever ſuffering any return

(o) Hippoc. de Morb. Sacro.

of

of the dreadful difeafe, under which fhe had laboured. Celfus, in the epilepfy, recommends fcarification, and the application of cupping glaffes to the *occiput (p)*; and as this difeafe frequently arifes, efpecially in children, from plenitude, and a redundancy of humours in the head, a drain made from that part, may juftly be regarded as a probable means of cure.

(*p*) Lib. III. cap. 23.

M 2 *ESSAY*

ESSAY V.*

AN

INQUIRY

INTO THE RESEMBLANCE BETWEEN

CHYLE AND MILK.

—— *Probabilia conjeĉurâ ſequens.*
Cic. Tuſc. lib. I.

THE properties of milk have with great
ingenuity been inveſtigated, and with
equal preciſion aſcertained, by ſeveral medical writers; and if the nature of the chyle were
as well known, the ſubjeĉt of the preſent inquiry
would be obvious, and of eaſy ſolution. But
as this fluid cannot, without great difficulty, be
colleĉted in ſufficient quantity to undergo an
experimental examination, it is almoſt impoſſible
to determine its qualities, with any conſiderable
degree of certainty. Nor have I, in a great
variety of authors which I have conſulted, met
with one experiment, which has been made

* THIS Eſſay was read to the Royal Medical Society
of Edinburgh in the year 1763.

immediately

immediately on the chyle, taken from the lacteal veffels. We muft therefore content ourfelves with attempting to determine, *à priori*, its nature and properties; that by comparing thefe with the known qualities of milk, fome probable conclufions at leaft may be deduced. And thefe conclufions may be confirmed by other arguments, drawn from facts and obfervations.

I. THE chyle muft neceffarily be compofed of the food we eat; which, being mafticated in the mouth, and mixed with the fermentable faliva, is carried into the ftomach, where it receives the addition of the *fuccus gaftricus*, is further broken down, ferments, and paffes over the *pylorus* into the *duodenum*. Here it mixes with the bile, cyftic and hepatic, with the *fuccus pancreaticus*, and the lymph which is thrown out from the exhalant arteries, into the inteftines. At length, if the animal feed chiefly upon vegetables, it is changed into a white and faccharine fluid, which being imbibed by the lacteals, is carried into the courfe of circulation, to be further affimilated, animalized, and converted *in fuccum et fanguinem*.

THE fluid thus formed, in all probability, confifts of oil, mucilage, water, a coagulable part, and fixed air. That oil and mucilage enter into its compofition, may be prefumed from the whitenefs of its colour; for thefe two fubftances, when intimately combined with water, always

M 3   put

put on that appearance. The exiftence of a coagulable part in the chyle is rather more uncertain; but I think there is fome foundation for the hypothefis. Our food is mixed, in the *primæ viæ*, with a confiderable quantity of lymph, which, as it is compofed of the ferum of the blood, muft be of a coagulable nature. And the mucilage, contained in the aliment itfelf, poffeffes alfo in fome degree the fame property. So that we may with probability conclude, that the chyle is not deftitute of a coagulable part. This coagulable part of the chyle may poffibly owe its origin, as much to the peculiar procefs of fermentation, which takes place in the *primæ viæ*, as to the animal fluids which are mixed with our food, in its paffage through the ftomach and fmall inteftines. And this fermentation depends, in a great meafure, on the nature of the aliments ingefted. For it is obferved that a cow, which feeds upon rank and watery grafs, yields milk that contains very little *craffamentum*, and is therefore unfit for the purpofe of making cheefe. That fixed air enters into its compofition is acknowledged by every one, and has lately been very ingenioufly illuftrated, by the experiments of Dr. Macbride.

BOERHAAVE, and other chemical writers endeavour to explain the formation of chyle, by the inftance of an emulfion, which is made by triturating

turating any of the oleaginous vegetables with water. But the analogy between them is very imperfect, and perhaps only fubfifts in this fingle particular, that the white colour of each fluid arifes from the mixture of oil and water, by the intervention of mucilage.

II. MILK confifts of oil, mucilage, fugar, water, and air. The oil is obtained by a fpontaneous feparation, and is called cream. The mucilage is that coagulable part, of which cheefe is made. It has often been compared to the ferum of the blood; but differs from it in this effential particular, that it is not coagulated by heat. The water contains a quantity of fugar, which may be feparated from it, by evaporating with a gentle heat, and cryftallizing. That air is prefent in milk may be made evident to the fenfes, by placing a quantity of it, previoufly heated, under the receiver of an air pump.

THE bare enumeration of the above particulars is fufficient to fhew the fimilitude that fubfifts between the two animal fluids, which form the fubject of our prefent inquiry. And if it could be fatisfactorily afcertained, that the properties, and component parts of the chyle are juftly laid down, this exact refemblance would prove, beyond all doubt, that they are one and the fame. But, unfortunately, it cannot; and as my conclufion is founded upon hypothefis alone,

it

it is neceſſary to ſupport it by arguments, drawn
from fa&ts and obſervations.

I. Milk, as to its properties, depends upon
the aliment. *Pro vi et differentiâ aſſumptorum lac
diverſum eſſe ; ex illis enim chylus melior vel deterior,
dulcis vel amarus, ex hoc tale lac ; qualia enim ingeſta,
talis chylus, qualis chylus, tale lac, aſſertum quotidiana
confirmat experientia (a).* Dioſcorides relates,
that the milk of goats, which fed on the ſcammony
plant and ſpurges, proved cathartic ; and inſtances
have been known, of an animal yielding bitter
milk, from having eaten wormwood *(b)*. If a
nurſe take a purgative, the infant will be purged ;
if ſhe drink wine or ſpirituous liquors, it will be
intoxicated *(c)* ; and I have been informed, from
good authority, of one inſtance, where the eating
of cabbage, or other flatulent vegetables, always
gave the child the windy gripes. Milk, and the
butter made from it, are found to differ greatly
in colour, conſiſtence, taſte, and ſmell, according
to the food of the animal. Human milk is made
yellow by taking ſaffron, bitter by wormwood,
and impregnated with a garlic ſmell by eating
that root *(d)*. Boerhaave relates that thick ale,
taken by a faſting nurſe, hath in a ſhort ſpace of

(a) Crantz M. M. p. 80.
(b) Vid. Lewis's Mat. Med. p. 330.
(c) Vid. Boerhaav. Prælect. § 690.
(d) Vid. Neumann's Chemiſtry, p. 569. Notes.

time

time been difcharged through the breafts *(e)*. Thefe inftances fhew, that milk retains all the adventitious properties of the chyle; we may therefore conclude, by analogy, that the natural and peculiar qualities of that fluid remain alfo unchanged.

II. The milk is proportioned in quantity, to the quantity of chyle. If the animal faft for a long fpace of time, neither chyle, nor milk is generated. The milk, which is fecreted immediately after taking in food, is found to be crude and indigefted; becaufe it proceeds probably from the juices of the aliment, which are carried into the fyftem by the abforbent veffels, before the chylous fermentation, if that expreffion be allowable, is perfected. A nurfe yields the beft milk about four hours after a meal; for by that time, the procefs of digeftion is fully completed. In about eight hours, the chyle begins to be affimilated to the nature of the animal fluids, and then the milk affumes a yellowifh colour, and acquires an offenfive tafte and fmell. At length, when the chyle is converted into blood, the fecretion from the breaft no longer bears any refemblance to milk, but becomes acrid, fetid, and in every refpect the reverfe of that mild, fweet, and agreeable fluid.

(e) Prælect. § 688.

3. The

III. The faccharine fubftance, that may be obtained from milk by infpiffation and cryftallization, and the inflammable fpirit, procurable by fermentation and diftillation, together with its acefcent quality, in which it differs from all the other animal fluids, fhew that the vegetable nature of the chyle is unaltered in the veffels of the breaft *(f)*.

IV. That the chyle may pafs through the courfe of circulation, without immediately mixing with the animal fluids, appears from the example of water, which is fometimes fecreted by the kidneys of hyfterical perfons, perfectly pure and infipid. And that it really does is evident from venæfection: For the chyle hath been feen floating on blood, recently drawn from the arm. In the laft ftage of a diabetes, the urine manifeftly points out the prefence of chyle in it, by its white colour, faccharine tafte, and acefcency. If it be kept in a clofe veffel feven or eight days, it will become four, and ferment ftrongly with any of the mild alkaline falts. The learned Baron Van Swieten fays, that a milky difcharge hath been obferved in diarrhœas *(g)*.

(f) If an animal feed upon vegetable diet, the milk will be faccharine and acefcent; if upon animal, no fugar will appear in that fluid, but on the contrary it will be putrefcent. *Vide* Young, Differt. Inaug. Cap. viii. p. 55.

(g) Van Swieten Comment. § 1329.

And

And Mr. Patch, in the Edinburgh Medical Essays, relates the case of a boy, from whose groin issued, through a small and almost imperceptible orifice, four or five pints of a liquor like milk *(h)*.

V. The remarkable laxity of the vessels of the breasts, aided by the power of suction, in diminishing the resistance which the fluids might meet with in their passage through them, renders it probable, that the chyle may easily pass into the breasts, and be secreted there unchanged.

VI. But the following history, which fell under the inspection of a very celebrated physician *(i)*, and was communicated to me by his friend and correspondent *(k)*, puts the matter almost beyond dispute. I shall therefore conclude this inquiry with the detail of it. A girl, about eight years old, was tapped for an *ascites*. She had also an universal *anasarca*; and even her face was very much bloated, and exceedingly pale. Four quarts of liquor were drawn off, which was of a milky colour, full as white as milk mixed with an equal quantity of water. It would not coagulate by heat; but after standing a day or two, it was covered with a kind of thin cream, and in a few days more, it smelled, and tasted sour. The girl

(h) Edin. Med. Essays, vol. V.
(i) Dr. Huxham.
(k) Sir William Watson, M. D.

was greatly relieved by this evacuation; but the tumour of her belly soon increased again to such a degree, that it was necessary to renew the operation. A liquor the same as before, only somewhat more dilute, was drawn off, the swelling of her whole body subsided, and she recovered her appetite and strength. This girl, before she was attacked with these complaints, was very lively and active, and had a great appetite, in which she was too much indulged. Probably, by using violent exercise after a full meal, she had ruptured some of the lacteals.

THE

E S S A Y VI.

EXPERIMENTS AND OBSERVATIONS ON

W A T E R:

PARTICULARLY ON THE HARD PUMP WATER OF

M A N C H E S T E R.

Sapientis medici eſt, eorum locorum aquas ubi medicinam facit,
convenienti examine probè ſcrutari, quò poſtea cum fruſtu,
tam præſervandi quam ſanandi gratia, iis uti poſſet.
HOFFMAN.

I N T R O D U C T I O N.

THE extenſive influence of WATER on the
health of mankind will, it is hoped, appear ſufficiently evident, from the following Eſſay.
The author propoſed to have enlarged the ſubject
of it, by inquiring into the effects of hard and
ſoft water on a variety of the common arts of life,
ſuch as brewing, malting, dying, bleaching,
tanning, &c. &c. But he found the ſubject too
copious,

copious, to be reduced within the bounds which he had prescribed to himself; and that the prosecution of it, would too much abstract his attention from those favourite studies, which more immediately belong to his profession.

An analysis of the waters, which are the objects of this inquiry, by means of evaporation, crystallization, &c. might perhaps have ascertained their contents with more minute exactness. But even this method is attended with some disadvantages; because heat decomposes many saline bodies; and to determine the composition of the *residuum*, recourse must have been had to the same chemical tests, which the author employed in his experiments. And it would have been an almost endless trouble, thus to analyze thirty different pump waters.

This Essay was intended only for communication to the ROYAL SOCIETY; and many of the experiments contained in it, have been read before that learned body. But the importance of the subject, and a desire of rendering his little work more extensively useful, have induced the author to publish it. And he flatters himself, that he shall at least be justified by the motives, if not by the success of his undertaking.

MANCHESTER, NOV. 1, 1771.

S E C-

SECTION I.

IT is a maxim of the divine Hippocrates, that
whoever would apply with fuccefs to the ftudy
of phyfic, fhould acquaint himfelf with every
circumftance relating to the fituation of the place
wherein he practifes, the nature of the feafons,
the influence of the winds, and the particular
qualities of the water. The laft object is by far
the moft important; becaufe as a fixed and permanent caufe, its effects will be regular, uniform,
and conftant. For whether the fimple element
itfelf be ufed, or it be mixed with vinous liquors,
or brewed into beer, it will ftill retain in fome
meafure its peculiar properties, and if impure,
will gradually produce fome morbid changes in
the body. On the robuft indeed, its action may
perhaps be flow and imperceptible; but the tender and valetudinary will find themfelves fooner
and more fenfibly affected by it. Many of the
difeafes of children, it is more than probable,
owe their rife to this neceffary diluent and vehicle of their food. And if we confider that numberlefs chronic diforders have their foundation
laid

laid in the ftate of infancy and childhood, the influence of water on the health of mankind will appear to be very extenfive, and deferving of our ftricteft attention and regard. It would be no difficult matter to prove that a confiderable number of thofe diftempers, which, from their being peculiar to certain people and places, are termed endemic, are chiefly the effects of this powerful and active caufe. Thus the inhabitants of the Alps, the Pyrenees, and of many other mountainous countries, are fubject to a mon-ftrous, external fwelling of the glands of the neck, owing, as it is univerfally acknowledged, to the peculiar properties of the water they drink (a). " As you advance towards Mount Cenis," fays Mr. Sharp in his excellent Letters from Italy, " you find very few exempt from thefe tumours, which are fo enormous, and of fo loathfome an appearance, efpecially in ugly, ragged, half-ftarved old women, that the very fight of them turns the ftomach. I was curious in my exami-nation, whether any children are born with this malady upon them: I was informed that there is no fuch inftance; and even that the fwelling never begins to form till towards two years of age; fome examples of which I myfelf faw (b)".

(a) Quis tumidum guttur miratur in Alpibus?
Juvenal. Sat. 13.
(b) Sharp's Letters, p. 298.

Nor

Nor is this diftemper peculiar to the natives of thofe countries; for ftrangers become affected with it, after refiding there a few years *(c)*. And fuch is the influence of cuftom on the common people, that they regard this blemifh as a beauty, and even ridicule thofe who are without it. At Rheims, the capital of the province of Champagne in France, there is hardly an aged perfon free from the *bronchocele*, owing to the drinking, till of late, the common water of their wells, which runs through a kind of chalky quarry, with which it is ftrongly charged. The fame effect has been obferved to arife from the abufe of fea water *(d)*. The inhabitants of the village of Steinfeffein, in the diftrict of Schmiderberg, are faid to have freed themfelves from this malady, by abftaining from certain fountains, which were obferved to produce it *(e)*. In two cities of Hercynia, Wildeman and Andreafberg, which are built upon a large bed of minerals, fcarcely a woman is to be found, who does not labour under ftrumous fwellings of the throat, occafioned, it is juftly fuppofed, by the conftant ufe of hard, metallic, and calcareous water *(f)*. The men

(c) Hoffman. Op. tom. VI. p. 202.
(d) Vide Lucas on Waters, vol. I. p. 29.
(e) Hoffman. Op. tom. VI. p. 203.
(f) Id.

N too,

too, in all probability, are not exempt from them;
but as the female part of our species have more
delicate constitutions, and especially a much
greater degree of laxity in their glandular sys-
tems, the same causes, which but slightly affect
the one sex, may prove highly injurious to the
other. The people of Siberia, who live near the
river Kirenga, which is remarkable for its impurity, are almost universally affected with scrophulous diforders; and strumous swellings are
common, even amongst the cattle of that country (g). It is worthy of obfervation, that horfes,
by an instinctive sagacity, always prefer soft water,
to that which is hard. And when, by necessity or
inattention, they are confined to the latter, their
coats become rough, and they are subject to the
gripes.

HIPPOCRATES afferts, that hard waters, which
are unfit for boiling, dry and astringe the belly;
and that such as are stagnant and ill-fcented
injure both the belly and spleen (h). In confirmation of this it may be obferved, that in
Minorca, where the water, which the springs and
rivulets afford, is often brackish, and always
hard, obstructions, indurations, and swellings of
the abdominal vifcera, together with flatulency

(g) Comment. Lips. tom. II. p. 103.
(h) Hippoc. de Aere, Aquis, et Locis.

and

and indigeftion, are the moft common difeafes to which the inhabitants are fubject. And it is remarkable, that large fpleens and tumefied livers are not peculiar there to the human fpecies, but are incident alfo to brutes; efpecially to the fheep, which feed on the eaftern fide of the ifland, where the waters are particularly brackifh *(i)*. This fhews the wifdom of the ancients, in examining the livers of the cattle, which they offered in facrifice, wherever they propofed to build a town, or to pitch a camp. If they proved to be firm and found, there they planned fettlements, and erected fortifications. But on the contrary, if the livers appeared to be lax in their texture, or in any refpect difeafed, they fpeedily decamped; juftly concluding, that the fame food and water would produce a fimilar effect in human bodies *(k)*.

PLINY mentions a fountain in Æthiopia, about which a large quantity of native cinnabar was found, and which produced its deleterious effects chiefly on the brain *(l)*. And Athenæus fpeaks of a fpring in Paphlagonia, to which the inhabitants of the country frequently reforted, which had an inebriating quality. Ovid poetically defcribes fuch waters, in the following lines.

(i) Vide Cleghorn on the Dif. of Minorca.
(k) Vitruvius, lib. I. cap. 4.
(l) Plin. Hift. lib. XXXI. c. 2.

Cui

Cui non audita eft obfcenæ Salmacis undæ,
Æthiopefque lacus ? quos fi quis faucibus haufit,
Aut furit, aut patitur mirum gravitate foporem.

Metamorph. lib. XV.

THE *Plica Polonica,* a fingular difeafe to which
the inhabitants of Poland and Lithuania are fubject, and which confifts in a præternatural enlargement and convolution of the hair, is in part
afcribed by a very celebrated writer, to the ufe of
impure water. *Morbi hujus caufa valde perplexa*
& difficilis videtur, nihilominus eam, quantum fieri
poterit, indagare allaborabimus. Primo multum
fordidum vitæ genus confert, cui hi populi addicti
funt ; dum raro crines pectunt, in humidis et depreffis
locis dormiunt, et fpiritum vini liberaliffimè ingurgi-
tant. Suum quoque fymbolum AQUÆ *contribuunt;*
hinc non male Gehema in Epiftola ad Bontekoe,
de Plica Polonica pag. 10. *fentit, hærere vitium*
in nonnullis Poloniæ aquis, &c.

———— *Nos fupponimus quoddam vitium hære-*
ditarium, quod in nimia pororum et bulborum capil-
lorum fub cute in capite confiftit ; unde fuccus nutri-
tius, craffus, et glutinofus, pravâ diætâ ex CRUDIS
AQUIS *productus, calore, quem potus fpiritus vini*
conciliat, urgetur ad tubulos capillorum, ex quorum
poris exfudat, et monftrofam illam intricationem
efficit (m).—This fuppofition of the learned Hoff-

(m) *Vide* Hoffman. Op. tom. VI. p. 205.

man

man is confirmed by the following aphorifm of
Sanctorius. Heavy water and a foggy air con-
vert the matter of perfpiration into an ichor,
which, when retained in the body, induces a
cachexy (n).

DR. MEAD, in the firft edition of his Effay on
Poifons, relates the cafe of a lady, whofe life was
formerly imbittered by the frequent returns of
violent colic pains, till fhe was happily advifed by
her phyfician, not to drink, as fhe ufually did,
beer brewed with well water. And fo evidently
was the eftablifhment of her health owing to this
caution, that the neglect of it was always attended
with a return of her diforder. A fact fimilar to
this is recorded by Van Helmont, of the monks
belonging to a certain monaftery near Bruffels,
who were always affected with the gripes, by the
water which they ufed, unlefs they corrected its
effects, by boiling wild carrot feeds in their beer(o).

THE *Elephantiafis* is endemial amongft the
Egyptians (p), and is afcribed by Galen and
Avicena to the ufe of the impure waters of the
Nile. Lucretius alfo adopted the fame opinion,
as appears by the following lines:

(n) Sanctor. Med. Stat. fect. 2. Aph. 6.

(o) Helmont Lithiafis. — *Vide* alfo Hale's Stat.
Effays, vol. II. p. 248.

(p) Alpinus de Med. Ægypt. Lib. I. cap. 4.

Eſt

Eſt Elephas Morbus, qui propter
flumina Nili
Gignitur Ægypto in medio. ————

IT is an opinion which the father of phyſic
firſt advanced, and which has been almoſt univerſally adopted by his followers, and hath remained till lately uncontroverted, that the ſtone
and gravel are generated by the uſe of hard
water. *Damnantur imprimis fontes,* ſays Pliny,
quorum Aquæ decoɕæ, craſſis obducunt vaſa cruſ-
tis (q). And from this quality, which the waters
of certain ſprings poſſeſs, of depoſiting a large
earthy ſediment, either in the aquæducts through
which they are conveyed, or in the veſſels in
which they are boiled or preſerved, it was obvious
to infer, that in paſſing through the kidneys, and
eſpecially whilſt retained in the bladder, they
would let fall their groſſer particles, which by
the continued appoſition of freſh matter, connected by the animal gluten, and compacted by
the muſcular action of that organ, would in time
form a *Calculus,* ſufficiently large to produce
a train of the moſt excruciating ſymptoms. And
this reaſoning, *à priori,* has been ſuppoſed to be
confirmed by facts and experience; for not to
mention the authority of Hippocrates, Dr. Liſter
has obſerved, that the inhabitants of Paris, are

(q) Lib. XXXI. c. 3.

peculiarly

peculiarly fubject to the ftone in the bladder *(r)*. And it is well known, that the water of the river Seine, with which that city is fupplied, is fo impregnated with calcareous matter, as to in-cruftate, and in a fhort time to choak up the pipes through which it runs. But on the other hand, it is objected, that the human *Calculus* is of animal origin, and by chemical analyfis, appears to bear very little analogy to the ftony concre-tions of water. And though it is allowed, that more perfons are cut for the ftone in the hofpitals at Paris, than in moft other places, yet upon enquiry it is found, that many of thofe patients come from different provinces, and from towns and villages far diftant from the Seine.

I WILL not prefume to decide this difputed point: but if I may be allowed to indulge a conjecture, I fhould fuppofe, that though this difeafe may chiefly depend upon a peculiar dif-pofition to concrete in the animal fluids, which in many inftances is hereditary, and in no inftance can with certainty be imputed to any particular

(r) Vid. Lifter's Journey to Paris.

NICHOLAS DE BLEGNY has related the hiftory of one who was diffected at Paris, in whom the Pylorus, a great part of the Duodenum, and the ftomach itfelf, were found incruftated with a ftony matter, to the thicknefs of a finger's breadth. Zodiac. Med. Gallic. A. D. 1679. Mens. Feb. Obf. 3.

caufe;

caufe; yet hard water is at leaft negatively favourable to this *diathefis*, by having no tendency
to diminifh it. The urine of the moft healthy
perfon is generally loaded with terreous matter,
capable, in favourable circumftances, of forming
a *Calculus*; as is evident from the thick cruft
which it depofits on the fides of the veffels, in
which it is contained. And it feems as if nature
intended, by this excretion, to difcharge all the
fuperfluous falts of the blood, together with thofe
earthy particles, which are either derived from
our aliment, and fine enough to pafs through the
lacteals, though infuperable by the powers of
circulation, or which arife from the abrafion of
the folids, or from the diffolution of the red
globular part of our fluids. Now water, whether
ufed as nature prefents us with it, or mixed with
wine, or taken under the form of beer or ale,
is the great diluter, vehicle, and *menftruum* both of
our food, and of the faline, earthy, and recrementitious parts of the animal juices. And it is
more or lefs adapted to the performance of thefe
offices, in proportion to its degree of purity. For
it muft appear evident to the moft ordinary underftanding, that a *menftruum* already loaded, and
perhaps faturated, with different contents, cannot
act fo powerfully as one which is free from all
fenfible impregnation. Nor is this reafoning
founded

founded upon theory alone *(s)*: For it is obferved, that MALVERN WATER, which iffues from
a fpring, in Worcefterfhire, remarkable for its
uncommon purity, hath the property of diffolving
the little fabulous ftones, which are often voided
in nephritic complaints. And the folution too,
which is a proof of its being complete, is perfectly
colourlefs. Hence this, water is drunk with great
advantage, in diforders of the urinary paffages.
And during the ufe of it, the patient's urine
is generally limpid, and feldom depofits any fandy
fediment. Yet, notwithftanding this appearance
of tranfparency, it is certainly at fuch times
loaded with impurities, which are fo diluted and
diffolved as not to be vifible. For it is attended
with a ftrong and fœtid fmell, exactly refembling

(s) A GENTLEMAN of this place, who had been long
fubject to nephritic complaints, and often voided fmall
ftones, was advifed to refrain from his own pump water,
which is uncommonly hard, and to drink conftantly the
fofter water of a neighbouring fpring. And this change
alone, without the ufe of any medicine, hath rendered
the returns of his diforder much lefs frequent and painful. A lady alfo, much affected with the gravel, was
induced, by the perufal of the firft edition of this effay,
to try the effect of foft water ; and by the conftant ufe
of it, fhe has remained two years, entirely free from
her diforder.

that

that of afparagus *(t)*.   Hoffman mentions a pure,
light, fimple water, in the principality of Henne-
berg in Germany, which is remarkable for its
efficacy in the ftone and gravel ; and a water,
of fimilar virtues, was difcovered not many years
ago, in the black foreft near Ofterod, which upon
examination did not afford a fingle grain of
mineral matter.   Indeed it is worthy of obfervation, that moft of the fprings, which were formerly held in great efteem, and were called *holy*
wells, are very pure, and yield little or no fediment.

THESE remarks are fufficient to fhew the
utility and importance of the following chemical
inquiry into the nature and properties of the PUMP
WATER of MANCHESTER.   I therefore proceed to
lay before the reader the moft interefting of my

(t) Vid. Dr. Wall on Malvern Water.

IN nephritic cafes, diftilled water would be an excellent fubftitute for Malvern water, as the following ex·
periment evinces.

Two fragments of the fame Calculus, nearly of equal
weights, were immerfed, the one in three ounces of diftilled water, the other in three ounces of hard pump
water.   The phials were hung up clofe together, in
a kitchen chimney, at a convenient diftance from the
fire.   After fourteen days maceration, the calculi were
taken out, and carefully dried by a very gentle hea.
The former, viz. that which had been immerfed in
diftilled water, was diminifhed in its weight a grain
and half; the latter had loft only half a grain.

experiments

experiments on this fubject, with fuch inferences as are obvioufly deducible from them.

EXPERIMENT I. Near thirty different pump waters, moft of them collected from pumps common to a whole neighbourhood, were chemically examined. They all curdled foap; the volatile alkali occafioned a precipitation in many of them; the fixed alkali in all of them; and they became quite milky with a folution of *faccharum faturni*. The infufion of galls produced no change in their colour; but fyrup of violets turned moft of them green.

EXPERIMENT II. A three ounce phial, after being carefully counterpoifed in a very nice balance, was filled to the brim with diftilled pump water, which weighed twenty-one drachms and fifty grains. The fame phial, exactly balanced as before, was then filled to the brim with my own pump water, of the fame temperature with the diftilled water, which weighed twenty-one drachms and fifty-fix grains *(u)*. Several other pump waters were examined in the fame way, and very little difference was found in their fpecific gravities. The water of a pump, belonging to a public brewery in this place, weighed indeed, in the quantity above-mentioned, only twenty-

(u) THIS experiment was afterwards tried by the hydroftatical balance, with no other difference in the refult, but a fmall fraction of a grain.

one

one drachms and fifty-three grains. But on inquiry, I learned that this water is contained in a refervoir, fupplied by means of pipes, either from the rain which falls in the neighbouring grounds, or from the fuperficial fprings which run through them.

From the foregoing experiments it is obvious, that the pump water of Manchefter is, in general, very impure. It is impregnated with a large quantity of felenite; an earthy aftringent falt, compofed of the vitriolic, nitrous, or marine acid, and calcareous earth; and at the fame time contains no inconfiderable portion of alum, as may be reafonably inferred, from the green colour which it ftrikes with fyrup of violets. For though it be acknowledged that Buxton, Briftol, Pyrmont, Spa, and other fprings, which are not aluminous, produce a fimilar effect, yet thefe are all impregnated with mineral alkali, or with other fubftances, of which the Manchefter pump water appears to be deftitute, by the chemical tefts employed in its examination (x). But what puts this conclufion beyond difpute is, that the earth of alum is frequently

(x) Dr. Lewis afferts in his *Materia Medica*, p. 71, " that the blue juices of vegetables are changed red by " alum;" and again, in his excellent notes on Neumann's Chemiftry, p. 252, " that fyrup of violets is changed red by waters impregnated with alum."
The

frequently found in the wells of this town. I have now in my poſſeſſion ſome of this earth, which

The faƈt was otherwiſe in my trials; for two grains of alum, diſſolved in an ounce of diſtilled water, ſtruck a pea green with twenty drops of the ſame ſyrup of violets, which was uſed in the above recited experiments. A tea-ſpoonful of lime water, added to a part of the ſolution, conſiderably deepened the green colour; whereas two drops of elixir of vitriol produced, in the other part, a ſenſible though faint redneſs. A ſolution of alum alſo, in lime water, was turned at once into a deep green, by the addition of a ſmall portion of ſyrup of violets. The lime water was added, in the firſt experiment, to render the water employed more analogous to the hard, calcareous pump water of Manchelter.

In a later trial I have found that the blue or purple juice of radiſhes is changed to a red, ſo ſlight however as barely to be perceptible, by a ſolution of alum in water. But this does not invalidate my concluſion, that many of the pump waters of Manchester are aluminous, becauſe they are turned green by an admixture of ſyrup of violets. For it appears that a ſolution of alum produced a green colour in the ſame ſyrup of violets, which was employed in the before-mentioned experiment. And to ſecure againſt all fallacy, I repeated· that experiment ſeveral times: Nor had I reaſon to ſuſpeƈt the genuineneſs of the ſyrup, as it was prepared at the Apothecary's Hall, and never failed to become red on the addition of an acid. The reſult of it is alſo corroborated by the teſtimony of Neumann, who aſſerts that the common ſorts of alum change the ſyrup of violets green. Dr. Rutty ſays that ſyrup of violets, when new, is turned red, but when kept ſome time green, by alum.
by

by the addition of oil of vitriol, has been converted into true alum.—From the fecond experiment it is evident, that a quart of water contains upwards of fixty grains of adventitious
matter; and fuppofing this quantity to be daily
confumed, in one way or other, by every individual, which is a moderate computation, about
forty-fix ounces, troy weight, of crude, earthy,
indigeftible, and by no means inactive falts will,
in the courfe of twelve months, be received into
the body. And how pernicious this may be to
health thofe can beft conceive, who know the
powerful influence of flight, but continued caufes
on the human frame. It would be foreign
to my prefent purpofe, to enter into a detail of
the endemic difeafes of Manchefter. But one
obfervation I cannot omit, that the inhabitants
of this place are peculiarly fubject to glandular
obftructions, and fcrophulous fwellings. And
that water, loaded with aftringent, earthy falts,
hath a direct tendency to produce fuch complaints, has been already, I hope, fully evinced.

BUT hard and impure water may be confidered,
in a further view, as injurious to the human body.
It was before obferved, that this univerfal *menftruum* is defigned by nature to be the diluter, vehicle, and folvent both of our food, and of the
recrementitious parts of the animal fluids. And

in

in the performance of thefe falutary offices, it
immediately promotes the general health of the
body, and at the fame time counteracts the influence of various caufes of difeafe.   The Spa-
niards, it is faid, are for the moft part exempt
from the itch and the fcurvy, notwithftanding
they indulge themfelves in the daily ufe of pork,
the leaft perfpirable of all foods.   And the reafon
affigned for this remarkable fact is, that the air of
Spain is clear, thin, and ferene, and the water
light, pure, and wholefome *(z)*.   Hence the
minuteft feries of veffels are continued permeable
and unobftructed, perfpiration is free and copious,
all the excretions are duly and regularly performed, and every thing putrid and acrimonious
is carried out of the fyftem, before it has time
to create difturbance or diforder.   But water, impregnated with auftere, earthy, and indigeftible
falts, is ill qualified to anfwer thefe important

(z) Vid. Hoffmani Opera, Tom. VI. p. 204.

HERODOTUS, whofe teftimony is not always to be depended upon, relates that in Æthiopia the inhabitants
live to be an hundred and twenty years old, that they
eat flefh, and drink milk ; that the water of the country
is fo light, that nothing will float upon it, not even
wood, and that the ufe of this water makes them long
lived.   Lib. III. c. 125.

ends,

ends. Already nearly faturated with its heterogeneous contents, it is rendered lefs capable of
diffolving our food, of mingling uniformly with
our fluids, or penetrating the fineft ramifications
of the vafcular fyftem, and of paffing off copioufly
and eafily by the feveral emunctories. And thus
it becomes negatively the caufe of difeafes.

It is therefore of the utmoft confequence,
where nature hath denied the benefit of pure
water, to difcover fome means of correcting its
pernicious qualities. And with this view, the
following experiments were made.

Experiment III. A ftrong folution of *fal
tartari* was inftilled into hard pump water, 'till
no lactefcency enfued. The fame experiment was
repeated with a fmaller quantity of falt of tartar,
fo as not to deftroy the infipidity of the water;
but the foftening effect of the vegetable alkali
was then fcarcely perceptible. Hence it appears,
that the Manchefter pump waters are too hard
to be much improved in this way, without rendering them offenfive to the palate.

Experiment IV. To half an ounce of hard
pump water, juft boiled, were added five drops
of a folution of *faccharum faturni*. To an equal
quantity of the fame water unboiled, were alfo
added five drops. The boiled became much lefs
milky than the cold water. But fuppofing this
effect to arife from the heat of the water, I poured

half

half an ounce of it into a glafs, and when cold, inftilled five drops of the folution of fugar of lead into it, as before, without any increafe of its lac-tefcency. I then took equal quantities, viz. half an ounce, of unboiled water, and of water which had been boiled over a brifk fire during the fpace of twenty minutes, and poured into each a few drops of the folution of *faccharum faturni*. The raw water became twice as milky as the boiled water, and depofited a much larger fediment. And I thought the water, which had been boiled twenty minutes, was lefs changed by the addition of fugar of lead, than that which had undergone only a flight coction. Ten drops of *fp. fal. ammon. vol.* added to half an ounce of raw fpring water, turned it milky; but when added to an equal quantity of the fame water, which had been boiled twenty minutes, no change was produced. Three grains of fixed alkali (*fal tartari*) diffolved in half an ounce of the fame boiled water, occafioned no fenfible cloudinefs; but when mixed with an equal quantity of raw water, a great lactefcency and copious precipitation immediately enfued. The boiled water ftill continued to break and curdle with foap, though in a lefs degree than the fame water unboiled. The former, alfo, felt to the touch much fofter than the latter.

THIS experiment clearly shews, that hard water is freed from some of its earthy salts, and rendered considerably softer by boiling. And it appears likewise, that the coction should be continued some time, in order to produce its full effect. Dr. Heberden is, indeed, of a contrary opinion ; for notwithstanding he acknowledges that the unneutralized lime stone and selenite are separated by boiling from pump water, yet he thinks it becomes more strongly impregnated with the saline matter, and consequently less salutary. But in this instance the Doctor appears not to reason with his usual judgment and accuracy ; and I apprehend, his observation is neither confirmed by analogy, nor supported by experiment. For though heat generally increases the dissolving power of any *menstruum*, at the same time it tends, in many instances, to destroy the texture, and disunite the component parts of the solvend. Thus hot water suspends a much larger quantity of nitre than cold water ; but if the solution be boiled over the fire, a considerable portion of the salt-petre will be dissipated. If then the nitrous acid be volatilized and separated from its alkali by coction, may we not justly infer, that it will be disengaged, by the same cause, from an earthy basis, to which it bears comparatively but a weak affinity ? And this reasoning may be applied with equal force to the volatile

vitriolic

vitriolic or muriatic acids, which in all probability fly off by means of the boiling heat, leaving behind them an indiffoluble, petrifying earth, that fubfides to the bottom, and incrufts the veffel.

EXPERIMENT V. A quantity of hard pump water, which had paffed through a filtering ftone, when compared with the fame water unfiltered, was found to be confiderably foftened. Each curdled with foap, but the former in a lefs degree than the latter. The volatile alkali occafioned no cloudinefs in the filtered water, but a vifible one in the other : the fixed alkali produced a precipitation in both, lefs however in the former, than in the latter; and the folution of *faccharum faturni* rendered the unfiltered water much more lactefcent, than that which had foaked through the filtering ftone.

THESE two experiments point out an eafy and obvious method of purifying hard water, by freeing it, in fome meafure, from the unneutralized felenite, and groffer falts which it contains. The water fhould firft be boiled for the fpace of fifteen or twenty minutes, then paffed through the filtering ftone, and afterwards fuffered to ftand a few hours, till it has attracted from the atmofphere a due proportion of air. Thus it will be rendered tolerably pure, falutary, and potable, and at the fame time much better adapted to a va-

O 2

riety

riety of culinary ufes. If a filtering ftone cannot eafily be provided, the following fimple contrivance may be fubftituted. Let a large funnel be made of wood; fill the narrow neck of it with fponge, and above the fponge fpread a layer of fand and gravel; cover this with a piece of thick flannel, and place over the whole another layer of fand, leaving fufficient room for the water, which is to be filtered. Care muft be taken to change the fponge, fand, &c. as often as they become loaded with the impurities of the water (a).

EXPERIMENT VI. Mr. Boyle afferts that fome pump waters, barely by ftanding a few days, will become foft enough to mix uniformly with foap (b). A quantity of hard pump water was therefore expofed to the fun and air, but fo as to be fheltered from the rain, for the fpace of a week. It curdled with foap, and became as milky with a few drops of a folution of fugar of lead, as water juft drawn from the well. The volatile alkali, indeed, produced no cloudinefs in it, and this was the only mark which it afforded of being in the leaft degree foftened.

EXPERIMENT VII. A ftrong infufion of malt was not more mifcible with foap, than the boiled water with which it was prepared; nor did it

(a) *Vid:* Lind on the health of feamen, p. 92.
(b) Boyle's Works, Shaw's edit. vol. I. p. 141.

suffer

fuffer a lefs precipitation, on the addition of a few grains of *facharum faturni*.

EXPERIMENT VIII. Strong table beer, drawn from the barrel about ten days after it had been brewed, curdled with foap as much as the hard water boiled, which was employed in its preparation.

HENCE it appears, that fermentation hath not the power of foftening hard water; and that the wholefomenefs of malt liquors muft greatly depend upon the purity of the water, which is ufed in brewing them. This coincides with the following obfervation of Hoffman: *Bonitas cerevifiarum primò à falubri aqua dependet. Quo falubrior aqua fontana eft, eo præftantiorem exhibet cerevifiam; & quo fubtilior aqua, eo plus ingredientia extrahit, eoque melius fermentefcit (c)*. As a feafon for brewing, the month of March is preferable to October, becaufe the fprings are then increafed by the winter rains, and are proportionably fofter and more falutary.

EXPERIMENT IX. Strong infufions of green and bohea tea, in boiled hard water, curdled with foap, and were as much changed by the addition of fugar of lead, as the boiled water itfelf. So that thefe fafhionable and favourite articles of diet, notwithftanding the foft tafte which they communicate to the hardeft water, do not really alter

(c) Hoffman. Op. vol. I. p. 113.

or

or improve its nature. It were well however, if tea could be confidered, in this refpect, merely as innocent or ufelefs; but it imparts many pernicious qualities to its aqueous vehicle; and the daily ufe of it, by infenfible degrees, enfeebles the conftitution, and brings on a train of nervous diforders.

EXPERIMENT X. Two or three pieces of common brick were fteeped four days, in a bafon full of diftilled water. The water was then decanted off, and examined by various chemical tefts. It was immifcible with foap, ftruck a lively green with fyrup of violets, was rendered flightly lactefcent by the volatile alkali, and quite milky by the fixed alkali, and by a folution of *faccharum faturni.* The infufion of tormentil root produced no change in it.

EXPERIMENT XI. An experiment, fimilar to the former, was tried with a rough piece of freeftone, *(faxum arenarium)* which did not appear to have communicated any impregnation to a bafon full of diftilled water, in which it had been feveral days immerfed.

THE tenth experiment affords a ftriking proof of the impropriety of lining wells with brick, a practice very common in many places, and which cannot fail of rendering the water hard and unwholefome. Clay generally contains a variety of heterogeneous matters. The coloured loams

often

often participate of bitumen, and the ochre of iron: Sand and calcareous earth are ftill more common ingredients in their compofition; and the experiments of Mr. Geoffroy, and Mr. Pott prove, that the earth of alum alfo may in large quantity be extracted from them. Now as clay is expofed to the open air for a long fpace of time, is then moulded into bricks, and burnt, this procefs refembles, in many refpects, that by which the alum-ftone is prepared. And it is probable that the white efflorefcence, which is frequently obfervable on the furface of new bricks, is of an aluminous nature *(d)*.

It hath long been a prevailing opinion, that water, flowing through leaden pipes, acquires certain noxious qualities. Hippocrates, and his commentator Galen, exprefsly condemn the ufe of fuch water; and Vitruvius, in his treatife on Architecture, remonftrates ftrongly againft that means of its conveyance. *Multo falubrior ex tubulis aqua quam per fiftulas: quod per plumbum videtur effe ideo vitiofa, quod ex eo ceruffa nafcitur: hæc autem dicitur nocens effe corporibus humanis. Itaque mini-*

_____

(d) The long expofure of clay to the air, before it is moulded into bricks, the fulphureous exhalations of the pit coal ufed in burning it, together with the fuffocating and bituminous vapour which arifes from the ignited clay itfelf, fufficiently account for the combination of a vitriolic acid with the earth of alum.

mè

mè fiſtulis plumbeis aqua duci videtur, ſi volumus eam habere ſalubrem (e). Neumann, whoſe authority as a chemiſt is of great weight, gives it as his opinion, that the waters conveyed by pipes may corrode ſome of the matter of the pipe or of its cement, and thus contract diſagreeable qualities. And he aſſures us, that having examined the aquæducts at Rome, thoſe between Marly and Verſailles in France, and thoſe by which London is ſupplied with the New-river water, he found them in ſome places liable to this inconvenience *(f).* Doctor Falconer, in his ingenious and uſeful Treatiſe on the Waters of Bath, informs us that the leaden ciſtern, which ſerves as a reſervoir for the ſpring at its firſt riſe, is very much corroded on the inſide, as appears by the long furrows which are very viſible in every part of it. And he, with great propriety, imputes the failure of cure of many bowel diſorders, and the obſtinate coſtiveneſs ſo much complained of on drinking the Bath waters, in ſome meaſure to this cauſe *(g).* Baron Van Swieten alſo relates, *Vidi integram familiam hoc morbo (ſcilicet Colica Pictonum) laboraſſe, dum ad culinares uſus*

(e) Vitruvius, lib. VIII. c. 7.

(f) Neumann's Chem. by Lewis, p. 248.

(g) The waters of the hot bath are obſerved rather to open, than bind the body. The reſervoir there is made of ſtone. Falconer on Bath Waters, p. 184.

adhibebatur

adhibebatur aqua, in magno receptaculo plumbeo col-
lecta, & diu hærens. But a celebrated writer,
who has lately favoured the public with an excellent Treatife on the Poifon of Lead, thinks the
caution of Vitruvius and of Galen unneceffary,
except in fuch cafes where a quantity of vegetable
acid might be fuppofed to render the metal dif-
foluble in water *(b)*. I cannot however agree
with him in this opinion, notwithftanding his experiments, at firft fight, appear to be fo conclufive.
For I apprehend the water he employed in his
trials either contained no acid, or that the acid
was combined with other fubftances, by which
it was more powerfully attracted than by lead.
This metal diffolves very readily in weak *aqua
fortis*, in the volatile vitriolic acid, or in oil of
vitriol well diluted with water *(i)*. And from
Dr. Cullen's table of Elective Attractions it appears, that the laft of thefe acids has a much
ftronger affinity with lead, than with the earthy
bafis of alum. As fpring waters are, therefore,
fo frequently found to be aluminous, may
we not with reafon fufpect, that in their paffage
through leaden pipes, the vitriolic acid will depofit the earth with which it was combined, and
diffolve fome portion of the metal. And thus

(b) *Vid.* Medical Tranfactions, No. 13.
(i) Shaw's Notes to Boerhaave's Chem. vol. I. p. 85.

the fountain will become impregnated with a
metallic falt, of the moſt poiſonous and deleterious quality. It is a common obſervation, that
hard water renders pewter black; and this, moſt
probably, ariſes from a ſolution of the lead and
tin, of which this mixed metal is compoſed.
But as a point, of ſo much importance to the
health of mankind, ought to reſt on better evidence than theoretical reaſoning, the following
experiment was made to determine, whether
water, impregnated with alum, be capable of diſ-
ſolving lead.

EXPERIMENT XII. Two clean and bright
bits of lead, weighing 327 grains, were immerſed
ſixteen days in a phial of water, in which a drachm
of alum had been previouſly diſſolved. The
volatile tinɛ̍ture of ſulphur produced no blackneſs
in this water, until a few drops of the ſolution of
ſaccharum ſaturni were added to it, and then a
duſky colour immediately ſucceeded. The bits
of lead, carefully wiped and dried, were not found
to have ſuffered any ſenſible loſs of weight.

THE ſame experiment was repeated with hard,
aluminous pump water. I conceived that the
lead had communicated ſomewhat of a ſweetiſh
taſte to the water; but when a few drops of the
volatile tinɛ̍ture of ſulphur were inſtilled into it,
it did not exhibit any appearance of a ſaturnine
impregnation; nor had the bits of lead loſt any
part of their weight.   THOUGH

THOUGH the refult of this experiment feems to overturn the theory before advanced, yet it does not afford me full conviction, that lead is totally infoluble in aluminous waters. For the volatile tincture of fulphur may not perhaps, in every inftance, be a certain criterion of the prefence of this poifonous mineral, as I have proved that green vitriol is not of the aftringency of vegetables (k). Befides a proportion of lead, too inconfiderable to be detected by any chemical examination, may poffibly, in irritable habits, and under certain delicate circumftances, prove highly injurious to health (l). This is confirmed by the account which doctor Tronchin has given of the colic of Amfterdam, the caufe of which long eluded the refearches of the learned : At laft however it was difcovered to arife from the ufe ot water, flightly impregnated with lead. But confcious of the influence of a preconceived hypothefis, I have fairly ftated both the reafons and facts, relating to this point, and fhall leave the decifion concerning them to the more unbiaffed judgment of the reader. The ufe of leaden pumps however may be pernicious, though the conveyance of water through pipes of this metal fhould not be efteemed fo : For by the friction of

(k) Experiments on Aftringents, fecond edit. p. 150.
(l) *Vide* Dr. Falconer on Bath Waters, p. 187.

the

the bucket againſt the ſides of the pump, ſome portion of lead will be rubbed off, and ſuſpended in the water.

SECTION II.

FROM the ſubject of this Experimental Inquiry into the different properties of hard and ſoft water, we are naturally led to conſider their influence on many of the operations of PHARMACY. And we ſhall find, that the moſt innocent vehicle is, alſo the moſt powerful *menſtruum* for extracting the virtues of medicines.

EXPERIMENT XIII. Two drachms of green tea were ſeparately macerated, without heat, an equal length of time, the one in three ounces of hard pump water, and the other in the ſame quantity of diſtilled water. The latter infuſion had a more bitter taſte, and ſtruck a much deeper black than the former, with three grains of *ſal martis.*

EXPERIMENT XIV. A drachm of bark, finely powdered, was macerated two days, without heat, in three ounces of diſtilled water; and the ſame quantity, during the ſame ſpace of time, in three ounces of hard pump water. The infuſion made

with

with diftilled water, was of a paler colour than
the other, but yet tafted more intenfely bitter,
though fomewhat lefs rough and ftyptic.   Two
grains of *fal martis* were added to half an ounce
of each infufion, carefully filtered.   The latter
ftruck a much deeper black than the former.

DISAPPOINTED in the refult of this experiment,
I repeated it again, but with nearly the fame
fuccefs as before.   Twenty drops of a ftrong
folution of *fal martis* produced at firft no fenfible
change in half an ounce of the infufion, made with
diftilled water, whilft the fame number of drops
almoft inftantly ftruck an inky blacknefs with the
other infufion, prepared with hard pump water.
By degrees, indeed, the former affumed a dufky
hue, but after ftanding many hours, did not half
equal the blacknefs of the latter.

EXPERIMENT XV.   Thirty drops of a folution of alum, in lime water, were inftilled into
half an ounce of the infufion of bark, made with
diftilled water.   By this addition the fame quantity of *fal martis*, employed in the laft experiment,
immediately produced a very dufky colour; and
in lefs than an hour, the mixture affumed an inky
blacknefs.

EXPERIMENT XVI.   Two drachms of tormentil root bruifed were macerated in equal
quantities, viz. three ounces of hard pump water,
and of diftilled water, during the fpace of twenty-
four

four hours: The latter infufion was of a deeper orange colour than the former, and had a rougher and more ftyptic tafte. But when twenty drops of a folution of *fal martis* were added to equal portions of each infufion, an inky blacknefs, to all appearance precifely the fame, enfued in both.

EXPERIMENT XVII. An experiment, fimilar to the former, was tried with Aleppo galls, by macerating two drachms of the powder in equal quantities of hard pump water, and of diftilled water; but the refult was fomewhat different. I could not, by comparing their taftes, determine which infufion was moft aftringent or ftyptic. The one made with diftilled water was of a paler colour than the other, yet it ftruck a much deeper black with green vitriol.

EXPERIMENT XVIII. Equal quantities of Peruvian bark powdered were macerated, without heat, forty-eight hours, in three ounces of hard pump water, and of the fame pump water boiled. The latter infufion had a ftronger tafte of the *cortex*, but did not ftrike fo deep a black with the folution of *fal martis*.

FROM thefe experiments it may be inferred, that foft water, and efpecially diftilled water, acts far more powerfully as a *menftruum* on vegetable bitters and aftringents, than hard pump water. And the conclufion may, in all probability, be extended

extended to many other claffes of vegetables. The fourteenth experiment, indeed feems at firft view to prove, that the Peruvian bark yields its aftringency more perfectly to hard, than to foft water; but the fucceeding experiment fhews the fallacy of this inference: For the addition of thirty drops of a folution of alum in lime water could not give any real increafe to the ftrength of an infufion of the *cortex*, previoufly prepared, although it enabled it to ftrike a deeper black with green vitriol. But from this curious fact we may conclude, that hard, aluminous waters are likely to anfwer beft in the dying of black; and this is confirmed by the obfervation of Dr. Lewis, that alum heightens the colour of the watery tinctures of madder and brazil*(n)*. Mr. Chambers, in his ufeful Dictionary, informs us, that well-water is preferred for dying red, and other colours which require aftringency, and alfo for dying ftuffs of a loofe contexture, fuch as callico, fuftian, and cotton. Dr. Rutty alfo afcertained, by experiment, that hard water extracts a tincture of a deeper hue than foft water, from logwood, brazil, fena, rhubarb, and cale.

It is found that hard, calcareous waters render the mixture of refinous bodies, by the intervention of mucilage of gum arabic, difficult, and

(n) *Vid.* Neumann's Chem. by Lewis, p. 187.

fometimes

fometimes impracticable *(o)*. This naturally led
me to conceive, that foft or diftilled water might
poffibly diffolve thofe fubftances, without the
affiftance of any medium, or at leaft with a much
fmaller proportion of gum, than is commonly employed.   On fuggefting this hint to a fenfible and
ingenious apothecary of this place, he very ob-
ligingly undertook to make the experiments for
me; and has fent me the following account of
the refult of them, which I fhall deliver in his
own words.   The letter contains fome further
trials, which do not relate to the prefent fubject;
but as they lead to feveral ufeful and important
conclufions, I fhall, without any apology, infert
them.

(o) Vid. Lond Med. Obferv. vol. I. p. 435.

JUNE 29, 1768.

DEAR SIR,

I HAVE made the experiments you defire, of diffolving refinous fubftances in diftilled and common pump water, the refult of which feems to be much in favour of the former.

ONE fcruple of balfam of tolu, rubbed with half an ounce of diftilled rain water, added gradually to it, for fifteen minutes, formed a mixture which, on ftanding about a minute, fubfided, but reunited by fhaking: Being fet by a few days, the balfam became a concrete mafs, not again mifcible by fhaking up the bottle.

THE fame quantity required more trituration to mix it with common pump water. The mixture was not kept.

ONE fcruple of the fame, rubbed with fifteen grains of gum arabic, was nearly as long in perfectly uniting with half an ounce of diftilled water, as that without the gum. This was perhaps owing to the latter piece being more refinous; however, though on long ftanding there was a fmall fediment, it immediately reunited, a week after, by agitation.

FIFTEEN grains of balfam *capivi* united very fmoothly with half an ounce of diftilled water, by the medium of three grains of gum

VOL. I. P arabic.

arabic. Five grains of the gum were not fo effectual with pump water.

BALSAM of Peru ten drops, with gum arabic three grains, diftilled water half an ounce, formed a neat, white emulfion, but with common water a very unequal mixture.

GUM myrrh powdered, that there might be no difference in the feveral quantities ufed, half a fcruple, diffolved readily with gum arabic three grains, in both kinds of water, and even mixed with them, by longer trituration, without any me-dium, but more eafily with diftilled than common fpring water. Olibanum, maftich, gum guaia-cum, and galbanum may likewife be mixed with water by rubbing, without any gum arabic or egg.

THE fpring water, which was made ufe of, was from my own pump, and is very aluminous.

IN the making of all the faline preparations, when any confiderable quantities of water are ufed, diftilled or pure rain, or river water is greatly to be preferred: For the calcareous, alu-minous, and felenitical matter, which fo much abounds in moft fpring water, will render any falts diffolved in it very impure. For feveral years before I came to refide in this town, I had prepared *Magnefia Alba*, even fuperior to that fold by Mr. Glafs; but on attempting to make it here, I was furprized and difappointed to find it of greater fpecific gravity, and more coarfe

than

than 'ufual. I was for fome time unable to account for the difference, as I had conducted the
procefs in every refpect fimilar to my former
practice; but at laft difcovered it to depend
wholly on the variation of the water: And I
always obferve the magnefia to be light and pure,
cæteris paribus, in proportion to the purity and
foftnefs of the water I make ufe of. Nor will
this be wondered at by any one who obferves the
quantity of calcareous earth and felenites, which
is generally depofited by the pump water of this
town, when it has been boiled and has ftood fome
time to cool.

THE folution of crude mercury with mucilage
of gum arabic being fo eafily accomplifhed, and
it being very difagreeable to many patients, and to
fome almoft impoffible, to fwallow pills, boluffes,
or electuaries; I was induced to try whether
calomel, cinnabar, and the other heavy and metalline bodies, commonly adminiftered only under
thefe forms, might not by the fame means
be rendered mifcible with water, fo as to be
given more agreeably in a liquid form.—I had
indeed fometimes feen injections made with calomel and gum arabic, but had not obferved
whether it fufpended the calomel fo uniformly
as to be given by the mouth.

I ACCORDINGLY rubbed ten grains of cinnabar
of antimony, and a fcruple of gum arabic, with

P 2   a fuffi-

a fufficient quantity of diftilled water to form a mucilage, and added a drachm of fimple fyrup, and three drachms more of water.

THIS makes an agreeable little draught, and having ftood about half an hour without depofiting any fediment, I added three drachms more of water to it, and notwithftanding the mucilage was rendered fo much more dilute, very little of the cinnabar fubfided, even after it had ftood fome days.

STEEL, fimply prepared, and prepared tin were both mixed with water by their own weight of gum arabic, and remained fufpended, except a very fmall portion of each, which was not reduced to a fufficiently fine powder.

FIVE grains of calomel were mixed with two drachms of diftiiled water, and half a drachm of fimple fyrup, by means of five grains of gum arabic, which kept it fufficiently fufpended: A double quantity of the gum preferved the mixture uniform ftill longer. In this form it will be much more eafily given to children, than in fyrups, conferves, &c. as a great part of it is generally wafted, in forcing thofe vifcid vehicles into them, and it may be joined with fcammony, and other refinous purgatives by the fame method, and of thefe perhaps the gum arabic would be the beft corrector.

GUM

GUM ARABIC likewife greatly abates the difagreeable tafte of the corrofive fublimate, mixed
with water inftead of brandy; and (from the few
trials I have made) fits eafier on the ftomach,
and will not be fo apt to betray the patient, by
the fmell of the brandy.

MR. PLENCK, who firft inftructed us in the
method of mixing quick-filver with mucilage,
obferves (and experience confirms the truth of
it) that this preparation is not fo apt to bring
on a fpitting as the *argent. viv.* mixed by any
other medium, or as the faline and other mercurial preparations.—How far the theory, by which
he accounts for it, may be juft, is not of much
importance; but it may perhaps be worth while
to inquire, whether it would not be equally effectual in preventing calomel, and the other preparations of mercury, from affecting the mouth.
—If fo, is it not improper, where a falivation is
intended, to give emulfions with gum arabic and
other mucilaginous liquors, for the patient's common drink, as by that means the fpitting may
be retarded? And on the contrary, may it not
be an ufeful medicine to diminifh the difcharge
when too copious *(p)*?

BUT

(p) THE following cafe may in fome meafure ferve
to confirm the above obfervation.

A GENTLE-

BUT—*Ne futor ultra crepidam.* And though
I am sure your friendly candour will excuse these

A GENTLEMAN, always easily affected by mercurials,
having taken about twenty-six grains of calomel, in
doses from one to three grains, notwithstanding he was
purged every third day, was suddenly seized with a
salivation. He spat plentifully, his breath was very
fœtid, teeth loose, and his gums, fauces, and the margin of his tongue greatly ulcerated and inflamed. He
was directed to use the following gargle :

R. *Gum. arab. semiunc. solve in aquæ font. bullient-selib.
& adde mel. rosac. unc. unam. M. ft. gargar.*

AND to drink freely of a ptisan prepared with *aq.
hord. lib. ij. gum. arabic. unc. ij. nitr. pur. drachm. ij.
sacchar. alb. unc. j.*

His purgative was repeated the succeeding morning.

THE next day his gums were less inflamed ; but the
sloughs on his tongue, &c. were still as foul ; his spit-
ting was much the same : he had drunk about a pint of
the ptisan.—Some *sp. vitrioli* was added to the gargle.

FROM this day to the fourth, he was purged every
day without effect—his salivation still continued, his
mouth was no better—he had neglected the mucilaginous drink—this evening he was persuaded to drink
about a pint of it which remained, and he had it repeated, and drank very freely of it that night.

On the fifth morning, the purgative was again repeated. Though it operated very little, yet the change
was very surprizing, his mouth was nearly well, and
his ptyalism greatly decreased — the ptisan was repeated,
and on the sixth day being quite well, he was permitted to go abroad.

SEE also Dr. Saunders's Appendix to the second
edition of Mr. Plenck's Treatise, since published.

trifling

trifling obfervations, which have occurred as I was writing, yet I fear I trefpafs upon time which you would fpend much more ufefully, than in perufing thefe indigefted thoughts of, dear Sir,

Your very obliged and humble fervant,

THOMAS HENRY.

EXPERIMENT XIX. It has been remarked by Profeffor Whytt, and many others, that different kinds of quick lime impregnate water with different degrees of ftrength. This fuggefted to me, that a diverfity in the *menftruum* may alfo confiderably vary the qualities of the lime water. And my conjecture has been confirmed by the enfuing experiments.

EQUAL quantities, viz. a quart, of diftilled water, of boiled pump water grown cold, and of the fame hard pump water unboiled, were feverally added to half a pound of quick lime. After an infufion of twenty-four hours, the waters were decanted off, and filtered through paper. Ten drops of fyrup of violets ftruck a deep green with the lime water made with diftilled water, a lighter one with that prepared with boiled water, and the lighteft with the raw pump water. Sixty drops of a folution of falt of tartar in diftilled

water,

water, added to each lime water in the foregoing order, occasioned the largeft precipitation from the firft, the next in degree from the fecond, and the leaft from the third. The taftes of the different lime waters correfponded alfo with the above-mentioned tefts. For that made with diftilled water was by far the moft pungent, and yet the leaft difagreeable; whereas that prepared with raw pump water, was extremely harfh and naufeous, without being proportionably impregnated with the acrimony of the quick lime.

EXPERIMENT XX. Three fragments of human *calculi*, numbered, for the fake of diftinction, 1, 2, 3, were immerfed in equal quantities of different lime waters; the firft in lime water made with diftilled water, the fecond in lime water prepared with hard pump water, and the third in lime water made with the fame hard pump water poured boiling hot upon the quick lime. (No. 1.) was of a brown colour and hard texture, was fmooth on one fide and rough on the other, and weighed twenty-fix grains and a half. (No. 2.) was a fragment of the fame *calculus*, and weighed twenty-five grains and a half. (No. 3.) a fragment of a different *calculus*, was of a loofer and more fpongy texture than the former, and weighed twenty-feven grains. The phials, which contained the *calculi* and four ounces by meafure of lime water, were all nearly full, and clofely

clofely corked. After continuing the maceration eight days without heat, the *calculi* were taken out, carefully dried, on filtering paper, before a gentle fire, and then weighed. (No. 1.) had loft a grain and a half, and was covered over in many parts with a foft, white, cretaceous matter. (No. 2.) had loft only half a grain: Many little cryftals fhot from its furface. (No. 3.) had loft a grain. But it fhould be remembered, that this fragment was much fofter than the other two. The lime, employed in this experiment, was common ftone quick lime; that, ufed in the former experiment, was brought out of Derbyfhire, and made of a fpecies of marble containing a great many fhells in its fubftance. I was not aware of the difference of the lime, till after my trials were completed.

THESE two experiments, I think, fatisfactorily prove, that foft water is a much more powerful diffolvent of quick-lime, than hard water *(q)*, at the fame time that it covers and meliorates

(q) To afcertain more fully this important point, I have fince repeated the experiment above recited, by immerfing again the fragments of the fame calculus, (No. 1. and 2.) in equal quantities of frefh lime water, prepared with diftilled water, and with hard pump water. In twelve days, (No. 1.)was entirely reduced to a chalky powder, whilft (No. 2.) preferved its texture, to all appearance unchanged.

the

the harfh tafte of that acrid fubftance. Where diftilled water cannot conveniently be provided, rain water, freed by filtration from its impurities, may with equal efficacy be fubftituted in its room. Had a different kind of lime been employed in the laft experiment, or had the digeftion been made in a fand bath, it is probable the folvent power of cach *menftruum* would have been increafed. The little pointed cryftallizations, which were obferved to fhoot from the fragment of the *calculus*, (No. 2.) remind me of a fimilar appearance which occurred in one of the trials of the late Dr. Whytt, and which he informs us furprized him greatly. He afcribes them to the fea falt adhering, even after calcination, to the oyfter-fhells which he employed *(r)*. But the Doctor muft have been miftaken in his explanation, as in the experiment juft recited, common ftone quick lime alone was ufed, which cannot be fuppofed to contain any fea falt. And the cryftallizations were perceived only in that phial of lime water, which had been prepared with hard pump water.

(r) Whytt's Effay on Lime Water, third edit. p. 74

SECTION III.

A COMPARATIVE VIEW OF THE DIFFERENT PRO-
PERTIES OF SNOW WATER, RAIN WATER,
SPRING WATER, &c.

SNOW WATER is faid by Mr. Boyle to be
the lighteft of all waters; and if received
upon the tops of high mountains muft, one fhould
conceive, be free from all foreign impregnation.
And yet the fame accurate chemift found, on
examination, that it is not entirely deftitute of
faltnefs. But notwithftanding the fuperior purity
of fnow water, I fhould apprehend, that it is not
the moft wholefome liquor for common drink,
both from its extreme coldnefs, and becaufe its
properties as a *menftruum* are changed by the
congelation it hath undergone. For freezing
decompofes water, by feparating from it a confiderable portion of air. And that this alters
its qualities is evident from the following facts.
1. Water when frefh, diffolves a larger quantity
of falt, than when exhaufted of its air. 2. Water
faturated with any falt, when placed *in vacuo*
under the receiver of an air pump, will depofit
part of its folvend. 3. Snow water is obferved
not to boil greens or peafe fo well as common
water.

water.   4. The nitrous acid generates a much lefs degree of heat with fnow water, than with common water.   5. Snow, mixed in a certain proportion with flour will, like eggs, render it when baked or boiled, perfectly light and ad-hefive.   Hippocrates condemns the ufe of fnow or ice water, becaufe, after congelation, it never re-affumes its former nature; the clear, light, and fweet part of it being diffipated, whilft the moft turbid and heavy is left behind.   And he adduces an experiment in fupport of this reafoning.   Expofe, fays he, a veffel containing a certain quantity of water to the cold air in winter time, fo as that it may be frozen hard; then bring it into a warm place, where it may thaw; and when the ice is diffolved, meafure the water again and you will find it evidently dimi-nifhed.   But this lofs of bulk is not, as Hippo-crates fuppofes, to be afcribed to the diffipation of the thinner and finer parts of the water by congelation, but chiefly to the feparation of the air which it contained; and therefore his reafon for condemning the ufe of fnow water is founded on a falfe hypothefis.   This however does not invalidate his objection to it, which at firft, in all probability, he deduced from experience, and afterwards attempted to explain and confirm, by what now appears to be miftaken theory.

THE

THE fertilizing effect of snow on the ground is universally known, and may in part arise from the covering which it affords to the earth, by which the ascent of vapours is repressed, and a fermentation promoted in the soil. But I apprehend it depends not less upon the snow being destitute of air, so that like lime, when dissolved and sunk into the earth,. it abstracts air from the soil, occasions an intestine motion in its particles, and thus pulverizes them.

ICE WATER : What has been said of snow water is equally applicable to ice water, except that its specific gravity is greater, and that it is less free from saline impregnation, and consequently still less salubrious.

RAIN WATER, When collected in clean vessels, at a distance from large towns, is light, soft, and wholesome. But as it passes through the atmosphere, which is a chaos of different exhalations from the animal, vegetable, and mineral kingdoms, it must wash down some of those floating, volatile particles, and be impregnated with them. Hence rain will differ in some slight degree, according to the season of the year, as well as the country in which it falls. That it contains a quantity of adventitious matter is evident from the curious experiments of M. Mar graaf, from its tendency to putrefy, from the green weed which springs up on its surface, and

from

from the mucilaginous or ropy fubftance which grows copioufly on it, and which Boerhaave compares, on viewing it through a microfcope, to a grove of little mufh rooms. It is obferved alfo, after ftanding a while, to be full of the *ovula* of different animalcules; fome of which may have been carried down with it, in its paffage through the air, but the greater number are probably depofited in it, during its ftagnation. But although thefe circumftances prove, that rain water is by no means an homogeneous fluid, or free from impurity, yet it is univerfally acknowledged to be the moft falutary of all kinds of water. And by percolation through fand or ftone, or by boiling and decanting, its foulnefs would in a great meafure be feparated, and it would be rendered a grateful, potable, and very wholefome liquor. Its levity is fo great, that diftilled rain water is not lighter than the natural, as Boerhaave affirms, after weighing them in the hydroftatical balance. Nor need we wonder at this, as the exhalation of aqueous vapours from the earth and fea is exactly analogous to diftillation; if it be not an impropriety to compare the vaft and ftupendous operations of nature, with the trifling efforts of art. Hippocrates gives his teftimony in favour of rain water, but directs that it fhould be boiled or ftrained; otherwife it has an ill fmell, finell, and occafions a hoarfenefs, and deep voice in thofe who drink it *(s)*.

SPRING WATER: This muft vary in its properties according to the nature of the foil, and different ftrata of earth, through which it paffes. The pureft is that which flows, at no great depth, through a light gravel, or fand. Dr. Hales mentions feveral fprings remarkable for their levity, and freedom from calcareous impregnation. The water, conveyed by pipes to Hodfon in Hertfordfhire, which rifes from a gravel, and gufhes out of a fine white fand, he informs us, left no incruftation in a boiler, which had been ufed fifteen years. And that of Comb in Surrey, a hill, the foil of which is gravel almoft to the furface, is alfo uncommonly light, foft, and free from all adventitious ingredients. As the fprings iffue from the brow of the hill, out of the gravel; the Doctor juftly obferves, that the water muft partake greatly of the nature of rain water; fince the dew and rain, which fall on that hill, receive probably no other alteration from percolating through the gravel, than that of being rendered more pure and free from foulnefs *(t)*. Hippocrates lays a great ftrefs upon the choice of fprings, which have an eaftern afpect. Such waters, he fays, are chiefly to be commended,

(s) Hippoc. *de Aere, Aquis et Locis.*
(t) *Vid.* Statical Effays, vol. II. p. 242.

that

that gush out towards the rising of the sun; because they are clearer, lighter, and of a better smell than others. But I apprehend there is no foundation for this opinion: For water, which flows through clay, marl, black mould, or beds of minerals, will be equally hard and unwholesome, in whatever exposure it first bursts out. The purity and salubrity of it may however, with sufficient accuracy be ascertained, by its levity, transparency, and perfect insipidity; by its mingling uniformly with soap, and boiling pulse tender. And these are common tests, which it is in the power of every one to apply.

RIVER WATER: This is generally much softer, and better adapted to œconomical uses than most spring water. For though rivers proceed originally from springs, yet by their rapid motion *(u)*, and by being exposed, during a long course, to the influence of the sun and air, the earthy and metallic salts which they contain are in part decomposed, the volatile acid flies off, and the terrestrial or ochrey particles, with which it was

(u) THE Rhine and the Rhone, which flow from the Alps, whilst they preserve the rapidity of their course, are observed to be light and pure. The difference betwixt the Rhine and the Maine is obvious to those who navigate these rivers: For the barges, which sail from the latter into the former, sink considerably deeper in the one, than in the other. Lucas, vol. I. p. 35.

combined,

combined, become infoluble, and are precipitated. To this it may be added, that rivers are alfo rendered fofter by the vaft quantity of rain water, which, paffing along the furface of the earth, is immediately conveyed into their channels. But all rivers carry with them a great deal of mud, filth, and other impurities. And when they flow near large, populous, and manufacturing towns, they become the receptacles of all the common fewers, and are impregnated with an heterogeneous mixture of copperas, alum, foap lyes, logwood, and the refufe of numberlefs other fubftances, employed in different arts. In this ftate, river water is certainly unfit for the common purpofes of life : And yet if it be fuffered to remain a while at reft, all the feculencies will fubfide, and the water will become fufficiently pure, grateful, and potable.

STAGNANT WATERS: Thefe of all others are the moft impure and infalubrious. Hippocrates afferts that they enlarge and obftruct the fpleen; and his obfervation is almoft daily confirmed, by the diffection of thofe who die of the fcurvy; a difeafe, which putrid, ftagnant water hath a powerful tendency to produce. Dr. Hoffman, by means of a glafs water-poife, divided by lines, examined hydroftatically feveral different kinds of water. Rain water he found to be the lighteft; river water was one line heavier; the water com-

monly

monly ufed at Hall, in Saxony, was heavier by two lines; the fpring water of the fame place was four lines heavier; that of a particular fpring was fix lines heavier; and water, which had been long kept in an open veffel, in a cellar, was fix lines and a half; but ftagnant water, drawn out of the town ditch at Hall, was feven lines heavier than rain water *(x)*.

I SHALL conclude this Effay with the following obfervations of Celfus, which, in many refpects, coincide with what has been advanced. *Aqua leviffima pluviatilis eft; deinde fontana, tum ex flumine, tum ex puteo; poft hæc ex nive, aut glacie; gravior his, ex lacu; graviffima, ex palude. Facilis etiam, et neceffaria cognitio eft naturam ejus requirentibus. Nam levis, pondere apparet, & ex his, quæ pondere pares funt, eo melior quæque eft, quo celerius et calefit & frigefcit, quòque celerius ex eâ legumina percoquuntur (y).*

A REVIEW OF THE PRINCIPAL FACTS ASCERTAINED
BY THE PRECEDING EXPERIMENTS.

I. THE Manchefter pump water is in general very hard and impure. It is impregnated with a large quantity of felenite, and contains alfo no inconfiderable proportion of alum.

(x) Vide Hoffman Obf. Chem. p. 140.
(y) Celfus lib. II. cap. 18.

2. THE

II. THE hardeft water will become foft and mifcible with foap, by the addition of falt of tartar. But fuch a quantity of the vegetable alkali is required, to produce this effect on the Manchefter pump water, as renders it offenfive to the palate, and unfit for common ufe.

III. HARD WATER is confiderably foftened by boiling. For though heat generally increafes the diffolving power of any *menftruum*, at the fame time it tends, in many inftances, to deftroy the texture, and difunite the component parts of the folvend. Thus the groffer falts contained in hard water are decompofed by the boiling heat; the volatile vitriolic or muriatic acids fly off, leaving behind them an indiffoluble, petrifying earth, which fubfides to the bottom, and incrufts the veffel. But the coction fhould be continued fifteen or twenty minutes, to produce its full effect. The water fhould then be fuffered to remain a few hours expofed to the atmofphere, to recover its due proportion of air, before it be ufed. For the lofs of this air, by boiling, alters the properties of water, and probably may render it lefs falutary.

IV. HARD WATER is foftened by being filtered through ftone. And if it were firft boiled a fufficient length of time, and then filtered, it would be rendered tolerably pure, potable, and

falutary.

salutary, and at the same time much better adapted to a variety of culinary uses.

V. Mr. Boyle asserts, that some pump waters, by exposure to the sun and air for a few days, will become soft enough to be miscible with soap. But this is not the case with the hard water of Manchester.

VI. Neither malt nor tea produce any softening effect on the hard water, in which they are infused. Nor does fermentation improve or alter its nature. So that the wholesomeness of malt liquors must greatly depend upon the purity of the water, which is employed in their preparation.

VII. Bricks harden the softest water, and give it an aluminous impregnation. The practice of lining wells with them, which is common in many places, is therefore very improper. Free-stone communicates no pernicious qualities to water.

VIII. Though by the tables of elective attractions it is shewn, that the acid of vitriol hath a stronger affinity to lead, than to the earth of alum, yet this metal does not appear, by experiment, to be soluble in aluminous waters. But perhaps the volatile tincture of sulphur may not, in every instance, be a certain criterion of the presence of lead, as green vitriol is not of the astringency of vegetables. And a proportion of this poisonous mineral, too minute to be discovered by any chemical examination, may, in irritable habits,

and

and under certain delicate circumſtances, prove highly injurious to health.

IX. Soft water, and eſpecially diſtilled water, acts far more powerfully, as a *menſtruum*, on vegetable bitters and aſtringents, than hard pump water. And it diſſolves reſinous bodies without any medium, or at leaſt with a much ſmaller proportion of mucilage of gum arabic, than is commonly employed.

X. Hard, aluminous waters are likely to ſucceed beſt in the dying of black, red, and other colours, which require aſtringency; and alſo in the preparation of ink.

XI. Soft water is a much more powerful diſſolvent of quick lime, than hard water; and it covers and improves the harſh taſte of that acrid ſubſtance. The fragment of a human *calculus* was entirely reduced to a chalky powder, by being immerſed twelve days in lime-water, prepared with diſtilled water; whereas another fragment of the ſame *calculus* ſuffered no viſible change in its texture, by being macerated an equal length of time in lime-water, made with common pump water.

XII. In nephritic caſes, diſtilled water would be a good ſubſtitute for Malvern water; for it is a powerful ſolvent of the human *calculus*.

ESSAY

E S S A Y VII.

ON THE DISADVANTAGES OF

INOCULATING CHILDREN

IN EARLY INFANCY.

Non quæ mihi suggessit phantasiæ imaginatricis temeritas, sed
quæ phænomena practica edocuere.
SYDENHAM.

THE advantages arising from inoculation are
now so universally acknowledged, that arguments in support of it seem to be entirely
unnecessary. The rapid progress it hath made
affords the strongest presumption, in favour of
its safety and utility; and the well-attested accounts, we every day read, of the success with
which it is practised, justly remove every prejudice against it, whether political or religious.
The patrons of inoculation, therefore, have nothing
to fear from its avowed enemies, if any such there
be; but they have the utmost reason to guard
against the mistaken zeal of its friends, which may
prove

prove perhaps more dangerous to its real intereſt, than oppoſition itſelf. Credulity, faſhion, the love of novelty, and a propenſity to ruſh from one extreme to another are principles, which have too much influence on the generality of mankind. And how unfavourable theſe have been to the advancement and perpetuity of improvements, might be demonſtrated by numerous examples. That the artificial method of communicating the ſmall-pox, ſo happily introduced amongſt us, may not hereafter be added to this diſgraceful liſt, every ſincere advocate for it ſhould exert his warmeſt endeavours to diſcourage the wanton levity, with which it is at preſent, in many places, adopted. For the indiſcriminate uſe of remedies, exceſs in the cooling regimen, and a total diſregard to age, temperament, and habit of body cannot fail, in the iſſue, to injure the reputation, and check the progreſs of one of the moſt important diſcoveries in the whole circle of phyſic.

In the third volume of the MEDICAL OBSERVATIONS and INQUIRIES, Dr. MATY, a learned and ingenious phyſician in London, hath inſerted an Eſſay on the advantages of very early Inoculation. He propoſes that people ſhould be induced by perſuaſion, and by other encouragements, if neceſſary, to inoculate their children as ſoon as poſſible after their birth. And this he conſiders as the *maximum*, to which the art of

Q 4   inoculation

inoculation can be brought, both with respect
to individuals, and to the public. But the doctor's reasoning in support of his hypothesis, appears to me to be more ingenious and plausible,
than solid and satisfactory. And I apprehend the
practice which he recommends, would considerably diminish the benefits arising from inoculation,
and would be of dangerous and fatal consequence
to mankind. I shall endeavour, therefore, to point
out the disadvantages which would attend the
ingraftment of the small-pox on new-born children; and shall also make some strictures on Dr.
MATY's arguments in favour of it.

I. THE number of diseases to which infants
are incident, render them unfit subjects for inoculation. HIPPOCRATES, two thousand years ago
remarked, *Ætatibus morbosissimi sunt juniores.*
And when we consider the great and sudden
changes, both external and internal, which they
undergo at birth; the laxity and wonderful delicacy of their frame, and their extreme irritability perhaps depending upon it; the copiousness
of glandular secretions, with the difficulty of preserving that equilibrium, the least deviation from
which affects them; it is matter of real astonish-
ment that life itself can be supported, under a
series of such apparently unfavourable circumstances. Scarcely hath the little stranger been
ushered into the world, but he discovers signs of
                                                indisposition,

indifpofition, by his reftlefsnefs, anxiety, crying, and vomiting; by the fwelling of his belly; and fometimes by convulfions. Thefe fymptoms arife from the load of *meconium* with which the ftomach and bowels are oppreffed, and generally ceafe when thofe organs have been gently evacuated. The jaundice next fucceeds, and is fometimes complicated with a very acrimonious ftate of the fluids, as appears by the eruption of little red puftules, with which the fkin is every where loaded. The thrufh, watery gripes, and convulfions, obferve no regular order of time, but attack moft infants, either fingly or collectively, according as they are more or lefs obnoxious to the caufes which produce them. The quick growth of children in the firft period after birth, is likewife a fource of numerous ailments; notwithftanding the provifion which nature hath made, to guard againft the inconveniences refulting from it, by the laxity of the glandular fyftem. The fudden enlargement of the fœtus, in the womb of the mother is truly furprizing. Dr. HARVEY relates, that in the deer kind, he obferved the *punctum faliens*, on the 19th or 20th of November. On the 21ft he faw the *vermiculus* or embryo of the animal; and on the 27th the fœtus was fo perfect, that the male might be diftinguifhed from the female; the feet were formed, and the hoofs were cloven. This rapid

growth

growth muft be afcribed to the foft and yielding ftructure of the fœtus; to the plenty of nutrition it receives; to its exemption from all difcharges; and to the proportionably ftrong action of its little heart. And as moft of thefe caufes continue to exert their influence after birth, though in a lefs degree, the increment of the young animal proceeds apace, and redundances are formed, which in a healthy ftate are carried off by one or other of the glandular excretions. But a deficiency or excefs in any of thefe, neceffarily produces difeafes. And in fuch feeble, delicate, and irritable fubjects, the equilibrium cannot long be preferved. If they are defective, all the complaints which arife from plenitude enfue; the child grows feverifh, dull, and comatofe; his ftomach is difordered; his bowels are oppreffed with wind; and if his belly be conftipated, he falls into convulfions. On the other hand, if they are exceffive, a *diarrhœa* is produced; *aphthœ* and fevere gripes fucceed; and the violent irritation feldom fails to occcafion epileptic fits. From this fhort view of the firft period of infancy, I think it muft appear evident, that inoculation is ill adapted to that tender feafon of life. Nature, feeble and irritable as fhe then is, can fcarcely ftruggle with the difeafes to which fhe is ordinarily expofed. It is therefore equally cruel and unjuft to add to the number with which fhe is already oppreffed.

oppreffed. For it is demonftrable from the bills of mortality, that two thirds of all who are born, live not to be two years old; and I think it is more than probable, that a confiderable proportion of thefe, die under the age of fix weeks.

II. THE fears and anxiety of the mother, excited at a time when her ftrength hath been exhaufted by the pains of labour, and when every uneafy impreffion fhould be cautioufly avoided, cannot fail to injure her milk. And this is a powerful objection to the early ingraftment of infants. If a hired nurfe be employed, her milk may difagree with the child, fhe may fall into fome difeafe during the time of inoculation, may be guilty of excefs in eating or drinking, or may be under the influence of violent paffions; each of which will aggravate the fymptoms, and increafe the danger of the artificial diftemper, under which the infant labours (a).

3. IT

(a) INFANTES ex affumpto lacte nutricis, quæ brevi ante ira vel terrore perculfa fuit, in graviffima pathemata, convulfiva, epileptica, & fæviffima alvi tormina incidant.
Hoffman. Op. vol. I. p. 196.

A CHILD, whofe mother was its nurfe, became feverifh on the third day of eruption, which caufed violent anxiety in the mother; a rafh with coftive belly, was then obferved, and the child died on the fecond day after it. Monro's Acct. of Inoc. in Scot. p. 25.

.A NURSE

III. It hath been obferved, by a very able and experienced practitioner *(b)*, that young children have ufually a larger fhare of puftules from inoculation, than thofe who are a little farther advanced in life: And that, from this circumftance, fo many have died, as to difcourage the practice of ingrafting the fmall-pox on fuch delicate fubjects. This fact is not eafy to be explained. Whether the greater irritability of infants fubjects them to be more affected with the variolous *miafma* than children of two or three years old; or whether the larger eruption, to which they are liable, be owing to the proportionably greater quantity of their fluids, I will not prefume to determine. Both caufes may poffibly confpire to produce this effect; the former by exciting a quicker, and increafed contraction of the heart and vafcular fyftem; the latter by affording a more copious *pabulum* for the variolous ferment.

A NURSE of an inoculated child who died, was difcovered to have drunk immoderately of malt liquor, during the procefs of inoculation.

Monro's Acc. of Inoc. in Scot. p. 33.

THE nurfe of an inoculated child who died, was fufpected to have been tainted with the Lues Venerea, by her hufband, who was afterwards difcovered to have had the difeafe, and at the time fhe was nurfing the child.

Monro's Acc. of Inoc. in Scot. p. 33.

(b) BARON DIMSDALE.

By

By the fame principles we may perhaps account for the greater virulence of the *lues Venerea*, in infancy, than in the more advanced ftages of life.

IV. A CONSIDERABLE number of thofe who die of the natural difeafe, before the expulfion of the variolous eruption, are infants, or very young children *(c)*. This does not arife, as Dr. KIRK-PATRICK fuppofes, from the extreme weaknefs of the *vis vitæ* of infants; for the contraction of their hearts is proportionably ftronger than in adults, as the quicknefs of their growth evinces; but from the high degree of irritability with which their nervous fyftem is endued. Hence the con-vulfive paroxyfms, which often precede the ap-pearance of the poftules, and which, though re-garded by SYDENHAM as no unfavourable figns, are always alarming, and when they happen to very young infants, are frequently fatal.

V. IF the number of puftules be fo great in the mouth or throat as to obftruct fuction, the difeafe, in all probability, will prove fatal. Even a few pocks, in thofe parts, are highly trou-blefome and dangerous to infants; for befides the pain and reftleffnefs which they produce, they often terminate in ill conditioned ulcers *(d)*. Under fuch circumftances the mute wailings, or fhrieks, of an infant occafion equal embarraffment and diftrefs.

(c) KIRKPATRICK's Analyfis.

(d) *Vide* SCHULTS on Inoculation.

VI. THOSE

VI. THOSE who are affected with cutaneous difeafes, have been generally regarded as unfavourable fubjects of inoculation *(e)*. Infancy, therefore, which is feldom unattended with eruptions on the fkin, muft be an improper period for receiving the fmall-pox by ingraftment.

VII. THE thicknefs of the teguments of infants, which arifes from the quantity of fluids interpofed between their fibres, by which the fkin is rendered foft and œdematous to the touch, and their perfpiring lefs than children who are capable of ufing exercife, are further objections to very early inoculation.

VIII. BUT the moft forcible argument againft this practice, is deduced from the ill-fuccefs which hath attended infant inoculation in general. For it appears by Dr. JURIN's account of the progrefs of inoculation in Great Britain from 1721 to 1726, and by Dr. SCHEUCHZER's continuation of it to 1728, that of fifty-eight children under two years old, who received the fmall-pox by ingraftment, fix died; whereas of two hundred and twenty-one, inoculated between the ages of two and five, only three died.

HAVING thus pointed out fome of the principal objections to the early inoculation of infants, I fhall make a few remarks on Dr. MATY's inge-

(e) DR. JURIN's Account of Inoculation.

nious

nious Effay in favour of it. After enumerating
the advantages which infancy has with regard to
the fmall-pox, the Doctor fums up the whole by
faying: " If there is a period in which the
" machine is in a perfect ftate, it certainly is im-
" mediately before it begins to be fpoiled, or at
" the firft period after nativity *(f)*." This affertion, I apprehend, is repugnant to reafon, ana-
tomy, and experience. It feems to be a general
law of nature, that all organized bodies fhould
advance by progreffive ftages to their acme or
ftate of perfection; and fhould-then decline by
the fame regular gradation. A plant, when it firft
fprings out of the ground, is frail and tender ; by
degrees the ftem thickens, the leaves expand
themfelves, the juices are concocted, the flower
opens, the feed is formed, ripened, and fhed; and
when the office affigned it by the fovereign Crea-
tor is thus accomplifhed, it droops, withers, and
falls into decay. The animal world furnifhes ftill
more ftriking proofs of the truth of this obfervation. And I know nothing which contributes
more to the beauty and harmony of the univerfe,
or affords a more admirable difplay of the wifdom
of its great Author, than the order and uniformity
with which thefe fucceffive changes are carried on,
amongft the different claffes of beings.

(f) Medical Obfervations, vol. III. p. 290.

FROM

From the researches of anatomists into the structure of the human body, it is evident that our machine, in infancy, is comparatively imperfect; that its parts are disproportionate; and its organs incapable of those functions, which they are destined in future life to perform. The head of a new-born child, bears a much larger proportion to the bulk of his body, than that of an adult; the former being as one to three, the latter only as one to eight. And this, joined to the remarkable laxity of the fibres in infancy, is the reason perhaps of the excessive irritability with which the body is then endued, and which lays a foundation for numerous diseases. The liver and pancreas are so immensely distended, as to fill up almost the whole cavity of the abdomen; and the copiousness of their secretions is equal to their bulk. The bile, cystic and hepatic, is almost insipid, and so inert that it is incapable either of promoting digestion, or of neutralizing those acidities, which the weakness of the stomachs, and the acescency of the food of infants, generate in the *primæ viæ*. Hence, probably, arise the crudities, flatulency, gripes, aphthæ, and convulsions, to which children, at that tender age, are peculiarly exposed. The heart, with respect to the vascular system, is both stronger and more bulky

in

in infancy, than in after life. *(g)* By this means the blood is propelled with greater force; and as the arteries, at that period, have lefs firmnefs and denfity than the veins, as appears by Sir CLIFTON WINTRINGHAM's experiments, they are then moft yielding and diftenfile. And both thefe caufes equally confpire to promote and quicken the growth of the young animal. But wife and neceffary as this provifion of nature is, it unavoidably expofes the infant to all the dangers which arife from a *plethora,* and muft be confidered as a prefent imperfection, however well adapted it may be to thofe progreffive changes, which advance him from childhood to maturity. For, by degrees, the heart abates of its proportional force, and the arteries acquire their greateft amplitude. At this period, the moving powers of the machine are equally balanced, and the body feems to enjoy, for a while, a ftate of reft.

(g) BY the curious tables of Dr. BRYAN ROBINSON, it appears, that the weight of the heart, with refpect to the weight of the body, is greater in a child than in a man, in the proportion of three to two : that the quantity of blood, which flows though the heart in a given time, is greater in a child than in grown bodies, in the proportion of twenty to feven, which is the proportion of their pulfes in a minute : and that the velocity of the blood is greater in a child than a man, in the proportion of eighty to feven.

VOL. I.   R   But

But the delicate equilibrium cannot long be maintained : The heart grows feeble and languid ; the arteries gradually contract themfelves ; a venous plenitude enfues ; and old age clofes the fcene.

But analogy may deceive us, and the obfervations of anatomifts may be doubtful ; experience however carries conviction along with it, and inconteftibly demonftrates, that the human body, contrary to the affertion of Dr. Maty, is moft imperfect in the firft period after nativity. For it is univerfally acknowledged, that infancy is liable to a much greater variety of maladies, than any other ftage of life. This can arife only from the extreme delicacy of the ftructure, and difproportion of the parts of new-born children ; and both the caufe and effect, in this inftance, are marks of frailty and imperfection.

" Convulsions in young babes, fays Dr.
" Maty, feem to be not fo much a difeafe,
" as an indication of fome diforder in the
" bowels, or the effort of nature to expel fome
" enemy (h)." The obfervation is, in general, juft ; for I believe the true idiopathic convulfions happen very rarely. But though fomewhat lefs alarming on this account, thefe fits are always attended, in fuch feeble and delicate fubjects,

(h) Medical Obfervations, vol. III. p. 292.

with

with imminent danger. Many, it is well known, have expired under them; whilft others, who have ftruggled through with great difficulty, have been fo debilitated, and their faculties fo impaired, that the effects have been perceptible during the remaining part of their lives *(i)*. The convulfions about the time of the eruption, and fubfiding of the inoculated fmall-pox, fays Dr. Monro, are the moft frequent bad fymptom in this difeafe; and by them more of thofe, in the column of dead, loft their lives, than by any other caufe *(k)*.

" THAT difpofition in the inteftinal tube to " excoriate, which arifes from the too great " acefcency of milk or vegetable aliments, is " eafily corrected by magnefia, lime water, oil, " and by fmall quantities of broth or other ani- " mal food *(l)*." The remedies, which Dr. MATY hath here pointed out, are very judicious and proper; but their effects are much more uncertain than he feems to apprehend. The ailments of children are generally very compli- cated; and the indications of cure are often ob- fcure and doubtful. In their irritable bodies, one fymptom frequently brings on a variety of

(i) DIMSDALE on Inoculation.
(k) Monro's Account of Inoculation in Scotland, p. 25.
(l) Medical Obfervations, vol. III. p. 293.

R 2   others

others, fometimes connected with the original
one; at other times, to all appearance, totally
diffimilar. And thefe fymptoms of fymptoms,
as they are termed, do not always ceafe, when
the caufe, which firft produced them, is removed.
This every phyfician experiences, who is converfant with the difeafes of infants; and it neceffarily occafions, in his treatment of them, fome
degree of difficulty and confufion.

FROM the lifts of Dr. JURIN, and DR SCHEUCH-
ZER, Dr. MATY finds that nine out of two hundred and feventy-three, i. e. one out of thirty,
inoculated under five years of age, died between
the years 1721, and 1728. But if the doctor
had confined himfelf, as he ought to have done,
to the lift of thofe who died by inoculation under
one year old, he would have found the proportion to be vaftly greater, viz. no lefs than one in
twelve. But as even one in thirty is a great mortality, and as the operation in grown people,
during that period, appears to have carried off
only one in fifty; Dr. M. endeavours to obviate this objection, in the following manner:
" As fo many more children, under five years,
" die of different diforders, than at any other
" age, it is more than probable that feveral, per-
" haps moft of thefe nine would have died,
" though they had not been inoculated (m)."

(m) Medical Obfervations, vol. III. p. 295.

But

But though the Doctor has given fome good reafons for prefuming upon this probability, I would afk him, wherein confifts the juftice or propriety of ingrafting the fmall-pox, at a period when, from the inftances he himfelf adduces, the rifque appears to be fo great of other dangerous, and fatal diftempers acceding to it? For flightly as this artificial difeafe is now regarded, it is of itfelf fufficient for the powers of nature to ftruggle with, in early infancy.

THE fecond part of Dr. MATY's Effay difplays the political advantages, which would accrue from the early inoculation of infants. But if it be evident, from what has been advanced, that the practice he recommends, is prejudicial to individuals, it will require no arguments to prove that it muft be equally fo to the public. The abfurd cuftom of feparating, in the bills of mortality, the ages of thofe who die, from the difeafes by which they are carried off, renders it impoffible to afcertain, with precifion, the rifk of the natural fmall-pox, which is incurred by delaying inoculation. But from my own experience, as well as from the obfervations of the moft intelligent of my medical friends, I fhould conclude this rifk to be very trifling; and that the fmall-pox is a diftemper to which children, in the firft period of life, are rarely liable. For, at that tender age, they are neither in the way of infection, nor

R 3 are

are they much difpofed to receive it. Dr. Monro informs us, that of twelve infants, inoculated within a fortnight after their birth, not one had the variolous eruption *(n)*.

To conclude: Though infants are lefs proper fubjects for receiving the fmall-pox by ingraft-ment, than children a little further advanced in life, yet it muft be confeffed, that fuch circum-ftances may occur, as to render the inoculation of them highly expedient and advifable. In fuch cafes however, I think the age of two or three months is preferable to the period which Dr. MATY recommends. For it will then be too early to apprehend any difturbance from den-tition; and yet the child will have furmounted fome of the difeafes, peculiar to the firft ftage of its exiftence. The chylopoietic organs will alfo, by that time, have been fo ftrengthened by exercife and habit, as to difcharge their functions with fome degree of regularity. But the fitteft feafon for inoculation feems to be, between the age of two and four years, in healthy children, and of three and fix in thofe who are extremely tender and delicate. The powers of nature are then fufficiently vigorous; perfpiration is free and copious; the irritability of the body is greatly diminifhed; the vifcera are found and unob-

(n) Monro on Inoculation, p. 25.

ftructed;

ftructed; the mind, though active and lively, is
not difturbed by violent emotions; the teguments
are properly extenuated; and the fibres are neither
too tenfe, nor too lax, for the variolous eruption.
To thefe important advantages may be added,
that, at this age, the child is both a proper fubject
for preparatory medicines, and for fuch as may
be deemed neceffary during the courfe of the
diftemper. It is no wonder therefore, that the
practice of inoculation is attended with moft fuccefs at this period. And it is ferioufly to be
lamented, that the precious opportunity fhould
ever be neglected.

E S S A Y VIII.

ON THE

EFFICACY OF EXTERNAL APPLICATIONS

IN THE

ANGINA MALIGNA,

ULCEROUS SORE THROAT.

THE Angina Maligna is, for the moſt part, ſo rapid in its progreſs, that it requires all the aſſiſtance of art to counteract its malignity, and to prevent its fatal termination: And when children are attacked with it, we are often reduced to the moſt diſtreſſing perplexity, from the difficulty of perſuading, or the danger and impoſſibility of forcing them to uſe thoſe means which are neceſſary for their relief It has been my misfortune lately to attend ſeveral ſuch froward patients, whoſe caſes, independent of their perverſeneſs, afforded the moſt unfavourable prog-
noſtics,

noftics, and obliged me to depend entirely on external applications.   The following method of cure I have hitherto fuccefsfully purfued.

A PLASTER, compofed of *Emplaft. Stomach.* or *Emplaft. è Cymino p. ij. Emp. Vefic. p. j. Camph. S. V. R. trit. ʒifs,* is directed to be applied to the nape of the neck, and a cataplafm of *Cort. Peruv. & Flor Chamæm.* boiled in vinegar, with the addition of two drachms of camphor, to be laid acrofs the throat, and renewed every four hours.   Sometimes, inftead of this cataplafm, a flannel, moiftened with equal parts of camphorated fpirit of wine and vinegar, is recommended, which is highly refrefhing and grateful to the patient.

A PEDILUVIUM, confifting of the above-mentioned ingredients, viz. bark and chamomile flowers, boiled in vinegar and water, is prefcribed to be ufed three or four times in a day.   When the weaknefs of the patient renders him unable to fit with his feet in the bath, cloths, lightly wrung out of the decoction, are ordered to be wrapped round his legs and thighs.

To medicate the air, both for the benefit of the patient and of his attendants, fuch a compofition as Dr. Huxham recommends, viz. chamomile flowers, rofemary, and myrrh, with vinegar, is advifed to be kept boiling over the lamp of a tea-kettle, fo that the vapour, which

is

is by no means difagreeable, may be diffufed through the room; and the lamp is fometimes placed near the bedfide of the fick perfon, that he may infpire the antifeptic fteams more copioufly.

My reafon for prefcribing a bliftering plafter, under the form above directed, is becaufe I have found by experience, that the fkin, in this dif-order, is very eafily inflamed and veficated; and that a fufficiently copious difcharge of ferum is procured by this compofition, which at the fame time coincides with the general indication of cor-recting putridity. And I muft here take leave to remark, that early bliftering, in the *angina maligna*, has a peculiarly good effect; though I am no advocate in general for the application of veficatories, in the beginning of fevers.

The cataplafm feems to me to anfwer feveral ufeful purpofes: It tends to foften and relax the glands of the neck, which are often tumefied in this diforder; it continually exhales an antifeptic vapour, which is drawn into the mouth and fauces, at every infpiration; and no inconfiderable portion of it is carried into the fyftem, by abforp-tion. And it appears not improbable, from the common methods of preventing putrefaction in animal flefh, that fome part of it may pafs to the feat of the difeafe, by penetrating through the interftices of the mufcular fibres, when the cellular membrane is not loaded with fat.

THE

THE ufe of the *pediluvium,* in every fpecies of fever, is acknowledged to be highly ferviceable, and is peculiarly fo in this diforder, in which the fkin is hot and dry, and the efflorefcence on the furface of the body apt to difappear, from the flighteft caufes, producing an aggravation of all the fymptoms. Befides its relaxing and antif-pafmodic effects, it tends to bring on a fwelling of the feet, which I have fometimes obferved to be fo beneficial to the patient, as almoft in-clined me to think it a critical derivation. By the addition of bark, chamomile flowers, and vinegar, the *pediluvium* is rendered powerfully antifeptic, without any diminution of its other effects. An ingenious writer has propofed a method of conveying a very large portion of nitre into the body, as a corrector of putrefaction ; but in the fore throat, and every putrid difeafe, could fuch a quantity be introduced into the courfe of the circulation, it would probably difappoint our expectations, and by weakening the *vis vitæ* increafe the feptic ferment.

THESE means, affiduoufly purfued, have hitherto fucceeded to my wifhes, though I fhould not chufe to truft to them alone, when other remedies could be employed. However fuch is my con-fidence in their efficacy, that I would never fail to recommend them, along with frequent gargling, and the internal ufe of the *cortex,* wine, &c.

AN

AN eminent practitioner has very judiciously recommended, in the first stage of the disorder, the washing of the stomach with a gentle emetic. This advice I have generally pursued, and have always observed, that it mitigated the violence of the symptoms, and, in some instances, has entirely removed the disease. The efficacy of emetics, in this distemper, is not to be ascribed solely to the evacuation, which they produce, of the contents of the stomach, but to their unloading the glands of the throat, promoting an equal circulation, and increasing perspiration.

I DO not recollect that any authors have taken notice of a symptom, which has not unfrequently attended the sore throat, as it has appeared in this neighbourhood; I mean a very fœtid, ichorous discharge from the ears. In the beginning of the present summer, (1770) this symptom occurred only in the worst cases, and such as generally proved fatal: I have lately observed it several times when the patient has recovered; but indurated parotids, and deafness have ensued.

I HAVE met with cases, in which all the symptoms of the *angina maligna* have appeared, excepting the ulcers of the throat: Nor could there be any doubt concerning the nature of the disease, as the patients had been exposed to the infection of it. These instances, I apprehend, incontestibly prove the ulcerous sore throat to be a

distemper

diftemper of the whole habit, and not almoft entirely a local affection, as may be inferred to be the opinion of a very learned and eminent phyfician, (whofe writings contain a treafure of medical knowledge,) from his laying *the chief ftrefs of the cure on gargling.*

THOUGH we fhould be cautious in the ufe of the vegetable acids, on account of their tendency to renew or increafe the *diarrhœa,* yet the mineral acids are not liable to this objection, and I think may be adminiftered with great advantage. I frequently direct the dulcified fpirit of nitre to be given freely, in an infufion of red rofe leaves, mixed with port wine. It is cordial, antifeptic, and gently diaphoretic, and thus anfwers feveral very important indications.

E S S A Y S

MEDICAL, PHILOSOPHICAL,

A N D

EXPERIMENTAL:

P A R T II.

------------ Sicut formica,

Ore trahit quodcunque potest, atque addit acervo.

Hor. Lib. I. Sat. I.

THE

P R E F A C E.

THE great Lord Verulam recommends the collection and collation of facts, obfervations, and experiments, as the beft method of promoting the improvement of phyfic; and experience hath fully evinced the utility of fuch a plan. In this way, I am ambitious of contributing my mite to the general ftock of medical knowledge; and fhall think myfelf happy, if I can thus render the purfuit of my own inftruction and amufement, fubfervient to the interefts of my profeffion, and to the general good of mankind.

THE Obfervations on the COLUMBO-ROOT have been read at the College of Phyficians, and before the Royal Society; and have been communicated to a confiderable number of my friends and correfpondents,

VOL. I.   S   to

to some of whom this remedy was unknown, and by others applied only to the cure of the *cholera morbus*. During the course of the last year (1772) I have had the satisfaction of receiving from them the strongest testimonies of its efficacy, in a variety of disorders. What I have advanced, therefore, in its favour, may be regarded, not as the conclusions of an individual, partial to a favourite remedy, but as facts supported by the experience of many learned and ingenious physicians.

THE dissertation on the ORCHIS ROOT has been honoured, by Dr. Hunter of York, with a place in the Georgical Essays, a useful and entertaining work on the subject of agriculture. But as it contains some experiments and observations on the medicinal qualities, as well as on the culture and preparation of this root, it is here reprinted, with a few corrections and additions.

THE papers on FACTITIOUS AIR form a part of an experimental inquiry into this interesting and curious branch of physics,

in

in which the friendſhip, and too favourable opinion of Dr. Prieſtley firſt engaged
me, in concert with himſelf. But this
learned philoſopher, who poſſeſſes a hap-
pier genius, more leiſure, and better
health than I am bleſt with, has carried
his reſearches far beyond the limits of
mine; and his pleaſing and wonderful
diſcoveries, in theſe almoſt trackleſs regi-
ons of ſcience, will reflect the higheſt
honour on his induſtry and abilities.

To theſe Experimental Eſſays, I have
annexed a few ſelect HISTORIES of
DISEASES, agreeably to the plan of
Lord Bacon, who adviſes phyſicians
" to revive the Hippocratic method
" of compoſing narratives of particu-
" lar caſes, in which the nature of the
" diſeaſe, the manner of treating it, and
" the conſequences are to be ſpecified;
" to attempt the cure of thoſe diſeaſes,
" which have been too boldly pronounced
" incurable; and to extend their inquiries
" into the powers of particular medicines,
" in the cure of particular diſorders (a)."

(a) De Augment. ſcient. L. IV. cap. 2.

THE

THE PROPOSALS, for eſtabliſhing more accurate and comprehenſive BILLS of MORTALITY, were ſuggeſted by the peruſal of a Treatiſe on Reverſionary Payments, lately publiſhed by my friend Dr. Price; who employs his great mathematical knowledge, not in idle ſpeculation, or in the ſolution of amuſing problems, but in diſquiſitions at once curious, inſtructive, and of the higheſt importance to the intereſts of mankind. The Plan has been honoured with his approbation, and is likely to be carried into execution at Mancheſter.

I CANNOT take my leave of the candid reader, without intimating that, though the experiments contained in theſe ſheets were made with great care, and are related with the ſtricteſt fidelity, I am ſenſible many inaccuracies may have eſcaped me; which thoſe will moſt readily excuſe, who have experienced the difficulties incident to ſuch reſearches. The philoſopher has frequent occaſion to lament both the fallacy of his ſenſes, and the limited

powers

powers of his underftanding.   " You will
" wonder," fays Mr. Boyle, in the preface
to his Philofophical Effays, " that I
" fhould ufe fo often *perhaps, it feems,*
" *'tis not improbable,* words which argue
" a diffidence of the truth of the opinions
" I incline to.   But I have hitherto not
" unfrequently found that what pleafed
" me for a while, was foon after difgraced
" by fome further, or new experiment."
Such is the imperfection of human knowledge, even when derived from evidence,
which is ufually regarded as the moft
clear, and inconteftible.   And fo true is
the fentiment of the comic poet,

Nunquam quifquam ita bene fubducta ratione ad vitam fuit,
Quin res, ætas, ufus, femper aliquid apportet novi,
Aliquid admoneat, ut illa, quæ te fcire credas, nefcias;
Et, quæ tibi putaris prima, in experiundo repudies.

TERENT.

MANCHESTER,
Jan, 1, 1773.

S 3   *E S S A Y*

E S S A Y I.

OBSERVATIONS AND EXPERIMENTS

ON THE

C O L U M B O - R O O T.

- - - - - *Symbolum aliquid, utcunque exiguum, in commune medicinæ ærarium contribuerem.*

SYDENHAM.

THE Columbo-root, though a medicine of confiderable efficacy, is not yet generally known in practice. Books, fo far as my reading extends, are filent about it; and I have not hitherto been able to obtain any fatisfactory information concerning its Natural Hiftory. The celebrated Linnæus is unacquainted with it. Dr. Watfon made particular inquiry concerning it of an Eaft-India Governor, and alfo of Mr. Loten, who was feveral years Governor of Ceylon. Thefe Gentlemen informed him only that the root was brought to Ceylon, and to our fettlements, where it is called, in the Portuguefe language, *Rajis de Mofambique.* Dr. Hope, Profeffor of Botany at Edinburgh, has

S 4   tranfmitted

tranfmitted to me the following account, which he received from Dr. Rainey, a Phyfician who refided a long time in the Eaft-Indies. The Columbo-root grew originally on the continent of Afia, and was thence tranfplanted to Columbo, a town in Ceylon, which now gives name to it, and fupplies all India with it. The inhabitants of thefe countries have for a long time ufed it, in diforders of the ftomach and bowels. They carry it about with them, and take it fliced or fcraped, in Madeira wine.

THE Columbo-root comes to us in circular pieces, from half an inch to three inches in diameter; and divided into *frufta*, which meafure, in length, from two inches to one quarter of an inch. The fides are covered with a thick, corrugated bark, of a dark brown hue on its external coat, but internally of a light yellow colour. The furfaces of the tranfverfe fections appear very unequal, higheft at the edges, and forming a concavity towards the centre. On feparating this furface, the root is evidently feen to confift of three *lamina*, viz. the cortical, which in the larger roots is a quarter of an inch thick; the ligneous, about half an inch; and the medullary, which forms the center, and is near an inch in diameter. The laft is much fofter than the other parts, and when chewed feems very mucilaginous: A number of fmall fibres

run

run longitudinally through it, and appear on the furface. The cortical and ligneous parts are divided by a circular black line. All the thicker pieces have fmall holes drilled through them, for the convenience of drying.

THIS root has an aromatic fmell; but is difagreeably bitter, and flightly pungent to the tafte, fomewhat refembling muftard-feed, when it has loft, by long keeping, part of its effential oil. Yet though ungrateful to the tafte, when received into the ftomach it appears to be corroborant, antifeptic, fedative, and powerfully antiemetic.

IN the CHOLERA MORBUS it alleviates the violent *tormina,* checks the purging and vomiting, corrects the putrid tendency of the bile, quiets the inordinate motions of the bowels, and fpeedily recruits the exhaufted ftrength of the patient. Mr. Johnfon of Chefter, a furgeon of eminence, who ferved ten years on board one of his Majefty's fhips in the Eaft-Indies, and in 1756 had the care of an hofpital-fhip, gave the Columbo-root in that climate to a great number of patients, often twenty in a day, attacked with this difeafe. He feldom employed any means to promote the difcharge of bile, or to cleanfe the ftomach and bowels, previous to its exhibition: And he generally found that it foon ftopped the vomiting, which was the moft fatal fymptom, and that the purging, and remaining complaints, quickly

yielded

yielded to the fame remedy. The mortality on board his fhip, after he ufed this medicine, was remarkably lefs than in the other fhips of the fame fleet; and this difference he attributes entirely to the good effeéts of the Columbo-root, in this fatal diforder. The dofe he gave was from half a drachm to two drachms of the powder, every three or four hours, more or lefs according to the urgency of the fymptoms.

THOUGH Columbo-root does not feem to poffefs much, if any degree of aftringency, yet I have often obferved very falutary effeéts from its ufe, in DIARRHOEAS, and even in the DYSENTERY. In the firft ftage of thefe diforders, when aftringents would be hurtful, this root may be prefcribed with fafety and advantage, for by its antifpafmodic powers, it correéts the irregular aétion of the *primæ viæ.* But as a cordial, tonic, and antifeptic remedy, it anfwers better when given towards their decline.

I HAVE more than once experienced its efficacy in the vomitings which attend the BILIOUS COLIC; and in fuch cafes where an emetic is thought neceffary, after adminiftering a fmall dofe of ipe-cacuan, the ftomach may be wafhed with an infufion of Columbo-root. This will anfwer the purpofes of an evacuant, as well as chamomile tea, and will tend to prevent thofe violent and convulfive reachings which, in irritable habits,

abounding

abounding with bile, are fometimes excited by the mildeft emetic. The efficacy of ipecacuan in the colic, given in fmall dofes, is well known; and perhaps its operation as an antifpafmodic may, in fome meafure, depend on the naufea which it produces. But unfortunately it often occafions very fevere ficknefs and vomiting, and thus aggravates the diforder, by inducing a new and moft diftreffing fymptom. Perhaps (for I fpeak not from experience) if it were combined with fome grateful aromatic, and adminiftered in an infufion of Columbo, prepared with mint water, this troublefome effect might be obviated.

In bilious fevers, fifteen or twenty grains of this root, with an equal or double quantity of vitriolated tartar, given every four, five, or fix hours, produce very beneficial effects. The neutral falt abates the febrile heat, allays thirft, and brings on a gentle falutary *diarrhæa*; whilft the Columbo-root fupports the ftrength of the patient, obviates the naufea and ficknefs to which he is fo much difpofed, and powerfully checks the feptic ferment in the *primæ viæ*. When the belly is fufficiently foluble, an infufion of it may be directed, in conjunction with the dulcified Elixir of Vitriol (*a*). Is it not probable, that the Columbo

(*a*) Dr. Haygarth, a very ingenious phyfician at Chefter, has lately, by my recommendation, made trial of the

Columbo-root may be highly ferviceable in the malignant, YELLOW FEVER of the Weft-Indies? This fever is always attended with great ficknefs, violent reachings, and a copious difcharge of bile.

the Columbo-root, in a fever of the bilious kind, which has been epidemic at Namptwich, and in other parts of Chefhire; and he has favoured me with the following account of his fuccefs. "After the *primæ viæ* have " been fufficiently unloaded of their bilious, and other " putrefcent contents, I find the Columbo-root a moft " ufeful remedy, in allaying the naufea and reachings, " to which the patients are liable. In this fever, " though the remiffions are very evident, and the ac- " ceffions generally marked with chills, and other fymp- " toms of an intermittent yet the bark appears to do " more harm than good, as it occafions an increafe of " feverifh heat, and a parched tongue. The Columbo, " in thefe cafes, feems to fupply its place moft admi- " rably, by correcting the bile, reftoring the proper " tone of the ftomach, and of the whole habit. It alfo " prevents relapfes, to which, in this fever, the patients " are particularly difpofed.

" Such have been the good effects of the Columbo- " root in the cafes which have fallen under my own " obfervation; but a judicious Apothecary informs me, " that he has often feen it fail of fuccefs in this fever, " which in no refpect feems wonderful. It is not fup- " pofed that Columbo has any febrifuge quality, fimilar " to antimony, or Peruvian bark. By correcting the " putrid bile it deftroys the *fomes* which aggravates the " fever, and produces many of its moft dangerous fymp- " toms. When bilious fevers are epidemical, does it " not feem a probable remedy to prevent the difeafe?"

The

The vomiting recurs at ſhort intervals, often becomes almoſt inceſſant, and an incredible quantity of bile is ſometimes evacuated, in a few hours.

CHILDREN, during DENTITION, are frequently ſubjeƈt to ſevere vomitings and diarrhœas. In theſe caſes the Columbo-root is an uſeful remedy; and I have ſeen almoſt inſtant relief procured by it, when other efficacious medicines had been tried in vain. The more effeƈtually to correƈt the acidities, which at ſuch times uſually prevail, a little chalk or magneſia may be combined with it.

THE Columbo-root is extremely beneficial in a LANGUID STATE of the STOMACH, attended with want of appetite, indigeſtion, nauſea, and flatulence. It may be given either in ſubſtance, with ſome grateful aromatic, or infuſed in Madeira wine, and during the uſe of it, gentle doſes of the tinƈture of rhubarb, or of any other ſtrengthening and cordial purgative, ſhould occaſionally be preſcribed. If the bile appear to be defeƈtive, a ſufficient quantity of ox gall, carefully evaporated to the conſiſtence of an extraƈt, may be mixed with the powder of Columbo, and the maſs reduced into pills. In this manner I have frequently taken the Columbo-root myſelf, and have generally found my appetite increaſed, and my digeſtion improved by it.

HABITUAL

HABITUAL VOMITING, when it proceeds from a weaknefs, or irritability of the ftomach, from an irregular gout, from acidities, from acrimonious bile, or an increafed and depraved fecretion of the pancreatic juice, is greatly relieved by the ufe of Columbo-root, in conjunction with aromatics, chalybeates, or the teftaceous powders. But this difeafe often arifes, when fuch a caufe is leaft fufpected, from an affection of the kidneys. Under fuch circumftances, demulcents, and gentle diuretics, are the moft fuccefsful remedies; though I have frequently obferved temporary relief procured by a light infufion of this root in mint water.

SUCH an infufion fucceeds better than any other medicine I have tried, in the naufea and vomiting occafioned by PREGNANCY. But it is fometimes neceffary to premife venæfection, and always expedient to keep the patient's body moderately open with magnefia.

I COULD illuftrate the truth of thefe obfervations, by a variety of cafes; but to enter into fo minute a detail would be equally unneceffary and uninterefting. I fhall confine myfelf therefore to the relation of a few hiftories, which exemplify the peculiar, or, if the expreffion be allowable, fpecific qualities of the Columbo-root.

CASE I. T. H. of Newton-lane near Manchefter, in the month of Auguft 1770, from
expofure

expofure to cold, when overheated with hard labour, was attacked with a fevere purging and vomiting, accompanied with violent pain in his ftomach and bowels. He continued in this miferable condition twenty-four hours before I faw him, and his ftrength was then nearly exhaufted. I directed two fcruples of the powder of Columboroot, to be given every three or four hours in pepper-mint water. This remedy afforded almoft immediate relief; but the patient returning too foon to his occupation, had a relapfe, and was again reftored to health by the fame medicine.

Case II. *(b)* W. W. Auguft 31, 1770, had been feized with a loofenefs three days before, which had gradually increafed, and for the laft four hours, been moft violent, attended with frequent vomiting, and cramps in his extremities. He was directed to take a fcruple of the powder of Columbo every two hours, and had neither vomiting, nor purging after the firft dofe. Nine dofes reftored him to perfect health.

Case III. *(c)* April, 1771. Mrs. P———, about the beginning of the third week of her confinement in child-bed, began to complain of great pain, fullnefs, and uneafinefs in the bowels, accompanied with frequent and copious evacuations by ftool. What was difcharged had the colour and confiftence of

(b) Communicated by Dr. Haygarth.
(c) Communicated by Dr. Dobfon.

cream

cream. The pulfe was from 100 to 115. The tongue had a whitifh fur; and the fkin was often dry and hot. The evacuations by ftool, and the other fymptoms were always much more confiderable during the night, than in the day. Ipecacuanha as an emetic, opiates, elixir of vitriol, and other cooling reftringents, afforded no relief. A ftrong infufion of the Columbo-root in cinnamon tea, was then given with the defired effect. After every tea-cup full of the infufion, the patient found herfelf better; the painful fenfations were relieved, and the evacuations diminifhed. In about five days fhe was entirely cured.

CASE IV. R. N. Efq. aged 26, the latter end of June 1771, when the weather was extremely hot, was feized with the ufual fymptoms of a fever. An emetic and gentle cathartic were adminiftered, and faline draughts were directed to be taken at proper intervals. He perfifted in this courfe two or three days, without any fenfible relief. A continual naufea, and frequent vomitings of green bile now came on. The fkin was hot and dry; the pulfe beat an hundred and twenty ftrokes in a minute; the tongue was foul; the belly not fufficiently foluble, notwithftanding the free ufe of ftrawberries, and other fruit was enjoined; and he complained of great pain in his head and back, attended with univerfal laffitude.

A clyfter

A clyfter was immediately injected; and two fcruples of vitriolated tartar were given every four hours, in three fpoonfuls of the infufion of Columbo. The firft dofe almoft inftantly alleviated the naufea and ficknefs, and the continuance of the fame remedy entirely prevented their return; whilft the gentle *diarrhœa,* produced by the neutral falt, mitigated all the febrile fymptoms. On the eleventh day he had two bloody ftools, and as his conftitution was feeble and relaxed, the Peruvian bark, combined with aftringents, was adminiftered without delay: The hæmorrhage was foon checked, and the patient gradually recovered his ufual health and ftrength.

CASE V. June 2, 1771. Mr. W.'s fon, aged two, with other fymptoms of dentition, had fevere purging and vomiting, which continuing three days, reduced him to the loweft degree of weaknefs. I directed five grains of Columbo-root, and three grains of *pulv. e chel. c. c.* to be taken every two hours. The vomiting was ftopped by the firft dofe; the loofenefs was foon after checked; and in two days the child recovered his ufual ftrength.

I SHALL now proceed to relate the experiments which I have made on the Columbo-root.

EXPERIMENT I. Two drachms of Columbo-root, powdered, were infufed, without heat, in four ounces of each of the following *menftrua.* 1. Rectified fpirit of wine. 2. French brandy. 3. Madeira wine. 4. White wine. 5. Diftilled water. 6. White wine vinegar. 7. Hard fpring water. After twenty-four hours digeftion, the tinctures, &c. were filtered through paper, and equal quantities of each, and of their refpective *menftrua* were weighed with great exactnefs, and compared together. The tincture made with rectified fpirit of wine, appeared, by its tafte, colour, and fuperior fpecific gravity to the fimple fpirit, to be confiderably ftronger than the reft; whofe degree of impregnation feemed, by thefe tefts, to be exactly in the order in which I have enumerated the feveral *menftrua* employed in their preparation: It fhould be remarked, that the watery infufion of Columbo-root is more perifhable than that of other bitters. In twenty-four hours a copious precipitation takes place in it, and in two days it becomes ropy, and even mufty.

EXPERIMENT II. The addition of orange-peel renders the infufion of Columbo-root lefs ungrateful to the palate. An ounce of the powdered root, half an ounce of orange-peel, two ounces of French brandy, and fourteen ounces of water, macerated twelve hours without heat, and then filtered through paper, afforded a fufficiently ftrong, and tolerably pleafant infufion.

EXPERIMENT III. Twelve ounces of Columbo-root, in grofs powder, were digefted four

days

days, in three pints of rectified spirit of wine. The tincture was then filtered, and the *refiduum* boiled repeatedly in a sufficient quantity of water, till it yielded no taste to the liquor. The decoctions, having been carefully percolated, were evaporated over a gentle fire, in the common method, till about three quarts only remained. The evaporation was then continued in the vapour bath, and when nearly finished, the tincture, from which a part of the spirit had been previously drawn by the alembic, was gradually added, and the whole reduced to a pilular confistence, retaining the entire flavour of the Columbo, free from the least degree of *empyreuma*, and weighing eight ounces and two drachms. The spirit, distilled from the tincture, was neither impregnated with the taste nor odour of the root; which is a proof that no volatile parts were diffipated by this procefs. This experiment was made, at my requeft, by Mr. Henry, an ingenious and accurate Apothecary in Manchester. I have frequently used the extract of Columbo, and find it equal, if not fuperior, in efficacy to the powder.

Experiment IV. Equal weights, viz. about two drachms of beef, cut into small pieces, were macerated feparately in an ounce of a cold infusion of the Peruvian bark, and of Columbo-root, filtered and prepared in a manner exactly fimilar. The experiment was made in the month

T 2   of

of July; the weather was uncommonly warm; and the bottles were placed in a window which had a fouthern afpect. In forty-eight hours the beef in the infufion of Columbo-root had acquired a flightly putrid fœtor, whilft that in the infufion of bark remained perfectly fweet, and continued fo ten hours longer. Two drachms of beef, macerated in cold water, and intended for a ftandard, became putrid in twenty-four hours, under the circumftances above defcribed.

EXPERIMENT V. The putrid beef, employed as a ftandard in the laft experiment, was divided into two equal parts, to one of which was added an ounce of the infufion of Columbo-root; to the other the fame quantity of the infufion of Peruvian bark. After fix hours maceration, the pieces of flefh had loft much of their putrid fœtor; but that in the infufion of Columbo-root, was more offenfive than the other.

EXPERIMENT VI. To feveral phials, each containing three drachms of putrid ox gall, and two drachms of faliva, were added equal quantities, viz. an ounce of, 1. the infufion of Columbo root; 2. the infufion of Peruvian bark; 3. the infufion of chamomile flowers; 4. fpring water: the laft was intended as a ftandard. The phials were placed in a water bath, heated to about one hundred degrees of Fahrenheit's thermometer. When the infufion of bark was mixed with

with the putrid gall and faliva, it inftantly produced a coagulation of the gall, and confiderably
increafed the fœtor of it. Whereas the infufion
of Columbo united perfectly with it, and very
powerfully corrected its offenfive fmell. The
infufion of chamomile occafioned no change in
the bile, either with refpect to its fœtor or flui-
dity. After three hours digeftion, the putrid
fmell of the gall was much abated, in all the
phials but the ftandard, and even in that was lefs
perceptible than at firft. In fix hours, no fœtor
could be perceived, except in the ftandard; and
the mixture with the bark had acquired a vinous
fmell, and emitted many air bubbles. In twelve
hours, the odour of the gall was fenfible, but
not offenfive, in the mixtures with Columbo and
chamomile: The bark now fermented lefs, and
had loft fomewhat of its vinous fmell. In twenty-
four hours, the ftandard became extremely putrid;
the mixture with bark was four; the Columbo
and chamomile were ftill fweet; but in thirty
hours they became putrid; and in forty hours they
were highly offenfive.

THE inftantaneous effect of the infufion of
Columbo, in correcting the putridity of the ox
gall, ferves in fome meafure to explain its action
in the *cholera morbus,* and other difeafes, attended
with a redundance and depravation of the bile:
And at the fame time it obviates all objection

T 3   to

to the use of this remedy, previous to any artificial evacuations, in the first stage of such disorders, as they occur in hot climates; a practice which, indeed, is justified by its success. The coagulation and increased fœtor of the gall, which the infusion of bark occasioned, very well account for the disagreement of that medicine with the stomach, in the yellow fever of the West-Indies. Doctor Hillary laments that, though strongly indicated, it cannot be retained, even under the pleasantest form. Is it not probable that the Columbo-root, which so readily unites with, and so quickly sweetens putrid bile, would prove very salutary in this dangerous and malignant disease?

EXPERIMENT VII. Equal quantities viz. an ounce, of water, of the infusions of Columbo-root, Peruvian bark, and chamomile flowers, were added to four phials, each containing three drachms of fresh ox gall, and two drachms of saliva. The bottles were then placed at such a distance from the fire, as to be kept blood-warm. In six hours, all the mixtures, except the standard, were in fermentation. The infusion of bark emitted most, and that of Columbo the fewest air bubbles: The former also had acquired a vinous smell. In twenty-four hours, the standard became putrid. In forty-eight hours, the infusion of bark was sour, that of chamomile slightly putrid; but that of Columbo-root was perfectly

sweet,

fweet, and continued fo many hours afterwards, when the phials were fet afide.

N. B. The infufion of bark, when mixed with the recent gall, produced a coagulation, but not in fo great a degree as when combined with putrid bile.

Sir John Pringle found that chamomile flowers refift the putrefaction of animal flefh, more powerfully than Jefuit's bark; and from one of the preceding experiments, it appears that, in this refpect, bark is more antifeptic than Columbo-root. But as a prefervative of the *bile* from putridity, this root furpaffes *chamomile flowers*, without producing, like the bark, any changes in it by fermentation. Hence may be juftly inferred the utility of Columbo-root in diforders of a putrid tendency, and in an impaired digeftion, from corrupted bile, or vitiated and unfound faliva.

Experiment VIII. To determine the comparative action of Columbo-root on the fermentation of food in the ftomach, I digefted, in the water bath, three alimentary mixtures, prepared of two drachms of the crumb of bread; the fame quantity of roafted mutton, chopped very fmall; and an ounce of the infufions of Columbo-root, chamomile flowers, and muftard feed. The ingredients of each mixture were well united by triture, in a mortar; and a fourth phial was pro-

T 4 vided

vided as a ftandard, which contained the proportions before mentioned of bread and mutton, with
half an ounce of water, and the fame quantity of
faliva.   In twelve hours, the ftandard began to
ferment; in thirty hours, an inteftine motion was
perceptible in the other mixtures, but appeared
to be leaft in the phial which contained the
Columbo-root. In forty-eight hours, the ftandard
became four.   The third day, the mixture with
the infufion of chamomile was alfo four.   The
two remaining phials, viz. the infufions of Columbo and of muftard, were now placed by the fire,
where they continued ten days, without fhewing
the leaft figns either of acidity, or of putrefaction.

THE refemblance between the tafte of muftard
and of Columbo-root induced me to try their
comparative action on alimentary fermentation.
And it appears they concur in moderating, without fufpending, the procefs of digeftion.   This
property gives Columbo-root the advantage over
other bitters, in fuch diforders of the ftomach, as
are attended with a violent fermentation of the
food, with flatulence, and great acidity.   And if
a ftimulus be wanting to excite this organ to a
quicker expulfion of its contents, fome grateful
aromatic may be combined with it: Or perhaps
muftard-feed would equally anfwer this intention,
without increafing, like the fpices, the generation of air.   This experiment proves the remark-

able

able efficacy of the Columbo in preventing
acidities; and the fucceeding one no lefs clearly
evinces its power of neutralizing them.

EXPERIMENT IX. To an ounce of the infufions of chamomile flowers, of Columbo-root,
and of Peruvian bark, were added twenty drops
of vinegar. The infufion of Columbo entirely
neutralized the acid, that of chamomile flowers in
fome meafure covered the tafte of it; but the infufion of bark was evidently four, both to the tafte
and fmell, and it required twenty drops more of
vinegar, to render the infufion of Columbo equally
acidulous with that of the bark.

EXPERIMENT X. & XI. To afcertain the action
of Columbo-root on the heart and arteries, I took
a fcruple of the powder, in a fmall glafs of fpring
water, at feven o'clock in the evening. My
ftomach was empty; I had been fitting at reft an
hour; and my pulfe then beat feventy-four ftrokes
in a minute. I continued to fit ftill half an hour
longer, and, every fifth minute, examined my
pulfe; but could perceive no variation, either in
its regularity, fullnefs, or velocity. The fucceeding evening, I repeated the fame experiment, with
the precautions I had before obferved, and increafed the dofe of Columbo to half a drachm.
At the time I fwallowed the powder, my pulfe
beat eighty ftrokes in a minute; in ten minutes it
became fuller, and flower by three ftrokes, and
continued

continued to beat the fame number, viz. feventy-feven, for three quarters of an hour.

THESE experiments fhew that the Columbo-root does not belong to the clafs of heating bitters: It may therefore be ufed with propriety and advantage in the *phthifis pulmonalis*, and in hectical cafes, to correct acrimony, and ftrengthen the organs of digeftion. The Peruvian bark often proves oppreffive to the ftomach in fuch diforders, and fometimes excites a *diarrhœa*. But the Columbo-root occafions no difturbance, and agrees very well with a milk diet, as it abates flatulence, and is indifpofed to acidity.

P. S. 1776. THE efficacy of the Columbo root, in a variety of diforders, has now been experienced by the public; and it affords me great fatisfaction, that I have been inftrumental, in exciting the attention of Phyficians to a remedy of fuch acknowledged utility. But the high price which this root bears, the general demand for it, and the fmall quantity that now remains in England, will occafion fuch adulteration, as may prove very injurious to its reputation. Befides, the

the bitternefs of the Columbo is much impaired by keeping; it is liable to rot, and to become worm eaten; and from thefe caufes it may lofe all its medicinal virtues. I have feen many fpecimens of it, which muft fail, when adminiftered, to anfwer the views of the prefcriber. Whether we are likely to obtain any fufficient fupplies of this remedy, I am uncertain. Applications have been made to the captains of feveral fhips, bound to India; but our ignorance of the natural hiftory of the root is a great obftacle to the acquifition of it. The practitioners of phyfic in the Eaft Indies cannot, without danger, profecute botanical refearches, in a climate where all nature fwarms with life. And they employ the natives of the country to collect their fimples; whofe intereft it is to conceal the manner of their production, and their places of growth. Mr. Ives, in his voyage to India, mentions the Columbo-root in the following terms, page 482. " *Radix Indica* " *Amara*. This is the root of the *Cocculus* " *Indicus*. When quite frefh it is an emetic; " when dry a cathartic." Thefe characters are fo oppofite to the known qualities of the Columbo-root, that I apprehend Mr. Ives muft be miftaken in his account. And I have defired Doctor Lind, of Haflar hofpital, who is perfonally acquainted with that gentleman, to make farther inquiries of him, concerning the *Cocculus Indicus*.

Indicus. The Doctor has executed my com-miffion, with the moft obliging and friendly at-tention. But he has not been able to obtain, either from Mr. Ives, or from Mr. Bogue, who had the charge of the naval hofpital in India, and who is lately returned from thence, any fatisfactory information.

ESSAY

E S S A Y II.

PREPARATION, CULTURE, AND USE

OF THE

ORCHIS ROOT *(a)*.

SALEP is a preparation of the root of Orchis,
or Dogftones, of which many fpecies are
enumerated by Botanical writers. The *Orchis
mafcula, Linn. fp. pl.* is the moft valued, though
the roots of fome of the palmated forts, particularly of the *Orchis latifolia,* are found to anfwer
almoft equally well. This plant flourifhes in
various parts of Europe and Afia, and grows in
our country fpontaneoufly, and in great abun-
dance. It is affiduoufly cultivated in the Eaft;
and the root of it forms a confiderable part of the
diet of the inhabitants of Turkey, Perfia, and
Syria. A dry and not very fertile foil is beft
adapted to its growth. An ingenious friend of
mine, in order to collect the feed, tranfplanted

(a) Inferted in the Georgical Effays, publifhed by
Dr. Hunter, of York.

a number of the Orchifes into a meadow, where he had prepared a bed well manured for their reception. The next fpring few of them appeared, and not one came to maturity, their roots being black and half rotten. The fame gentleman informed me, that he had never been able to raife any plant from the feed of the wild Orchis; but he afcribes his want of fuccefs to the wetnefs of the fituation, in which he refides. I have now before me a feed pod of the Orchis, the contents of which, to the naked eye, feem to be feed corrupted and turned to duft, but, when viewed through a microfcope, appear evidently to be organized, and would, I doubt not, with proper culture germinate, and produce a thriving crop of plants. The propereft time for gathering the roots is when the feed is formed, and the ftalk is ready to fall, becaufe the new bulb, of which the Salep is made, is then arrived at its full maturity, and may be diftinguifhed from the old one, by a white bud rifing from the top of it, which is the germ of the Orchis of the fucceeding year.

SEVERAL methods of preparing Salep have been propofed and practifed. Geoffroy has delivered a very judicious procefs for this purpofe, in the *Hiftoire de l'Academie Royale des Sciences* 1740; and Retzius, in the Swedifh Tranfactions 1764, has improved Geoffroy's method. But Mr. Moult, of Rochdale, has lately favoured the public with a

new

new manner of curing the Orchis root; and as I have feen many fpecimens of his Salep, at leaft equal, if not fuperior to any brought from the Levant, I can recommend the following, which is his procefs, from my own knowledge of its fuccefs. The new root is to be wafhed in water, and the fine brown fkin, which covers it, is to be feparated by means of a fmall brufh, or by dipping the root in hot water, and rubbing it with a coarfe linen cloth. When a fufficient number of roots have been thus cleaned, they are to be fpread on a tin plate, and placed in an oven, heated to the ufual degree, where they are to remain fix or ten minutes, in which time they will have loft their milky whitenefs, and acquired a tranfparency like horn, without any diminution of bulk. Being arrived at this ftate, they are to be removed, in order to dry and harden in the air, which will require feveral days to effect; or by ufing a very gentle heat, they may be finifhed in a few hours(b).

SALEP thus prepared, may be afforded in this part of England, where labour bears a high value, at about eight-pence or ten-pence per pound. And it might be fold ftill cheaper, if the Orchis were to be cured, without feparating from it the brown fkin which covers it; a troublefome part

(b) See a Letter from Mr. John Moult to the Author, containing a new method of preparing Salep; inferted in the LIX. vol. of the Phil. Tranfactions.

of

of the procefs, and which does not contribute to
render the root, either more palatable or falutary.
Whereas the foreign Salep is now fold at five or
fix fhillings per pound.

THE culture of the Orchis, therefore, is an object highly deferving of encouragement, from all
the lovers of agriculture. And as the root, if
introduced into common ufe, would furnifh a
cheap, wholefome, and moft nutritious article of
diet, the growth of it might be fufficiently profitable to the farmer.

SALEP is faid to contain the greateft quantity
of vegetable nourifhment, in the fmalleft bulk.
Hence a very judicious writer, to prevent the
dreadful calamity of famine at fea, has lately propofed that the powder of it fhould conftitute part
of the provifions of every fhip's company. This
powder and portable foup, diffolved in boiling
water, form a rich thick jelly, capable of fupporting
life for a confiderable length of time. An ounce
of each of thefe articles, with two quarts of boiling water, will be fufficient fubfiftence for a man,
in a day *(c)*; and as being a mixture of animal
and vegetable food, muft prove more nourifhing

(c) Portable foup is fold at half a crown per pound;
Salep, if cultivated in our own country, might be afforded at ten pence per pound; the day's fubfiftence
would, therefore, amount only to two-pence halfpenny.

than

than double the quantity of rice cake, made by boiling rice in water : This laft, however, failors are often obliged folely to fubfift upon for feveral months, efpecially in voyages to Guinea, when the bread and flour are exhaufted, and the beef and pork, having been falted in hot countries, are become unfit for ufe *(d)*.

BUT as a wholefome nourifhment, rice is much inferior to Salep. I digefted feveral alimentary mixtures prepared of mutton and water, beat up with bread, fea bifcuit, Salep, rice flour, fago powder, potatoe, old cheefe, &c. in a heat equal to that of the human body. In forty-eight hours they had all acquired a vinous fmell, and were in brifk fermentation, except the mixture with rice, which did not emit many air bubbles, and was but little changed. The third day, feveral of the mixtures were fweet, and continued to ferment; others had loft their inteftine motion, and were four; but the one which contained the rice was become putrid. From this experiment it appears that rice, as an aliment, is flow of fermentation, and a very weak corrector of putrefaction. It is therefore an improper diet for hofpital patients: but more particularly for failors, in long voyages, becaufe it is incapable of preventing, and will not contribute much to check the progrefs of that

(d) Vid. Dr. Lind's Appendix to his Effay on the Difeafes of Hot Climates.

fatal difeafe, the fea fcurvy. Under certain circumftances, rice feems difpofed of itfelf, without
mixture, to become putrid. For by long keeping
it fometimes acquires an offenfive fœtor. Nor
can it be confidered as a very nutritive kind of
food, on account of its difficult folubility in the
ftomach. Experience confirms the truth of this
conclufion; for it is obferved by the planters in
the Weft-Indies, that the negroes grow thin,
and are lefs able to work, whilft they fubfift
upon rice.

SALEP has the fingular property of concealing
the tafte of falt water (e); a circumftance of the
higheft importance at fea, when there is a fcar-
city of frefh water. I diffolved a drachm and a
half of common falt in a pint of the mucilage of
Salep, fo liquid as to be potable, and the fame
quantity in a pint of fpring water. The Salep
was by no means difagreeable to the tafte, but
the water was rendered extremely unpalatable.

THIS experiment fuggefted to me the trial of
the Orchis root, as a correɗor of acidity, a property which would render it a very ufeful diet
for children. But the folution of it, when mixed
with vinegar, feemed only to dilute, like an equal
proportion of water, and not to cover its fharpnefs.

SALEP however appears, by my experiments,
to retard the acetous fermentation of milk, and

(e) Vid. Dr. Lind's Appendix.

consequently

confequently would be a good lithing for milk pottage, efpecially in large towns, where the cattle being fed upon four draff, muft yield acefcent milk.

Salep, in a certain proportion, which I have not yet been able to afcertain, would be a very ufeful and profitable addition to bread. I directed one ounce of the powder to be diffolved in a quart of water, and the mucilage to be mixed with a fufficient quantity of flour, falt, and yeaft. The flour amounted to two pounds, the yeaft to two ounces, and the falt to eighty grains. The loaf, when baked, was remarkably well fermented, and weighed three pounds, two ounces. Another loaf, made with the fame quantity of flour, &c. weighed two pounds and twelve ounces; from which it appears, that the Salep, though ufed in fo fmall a proportion, increafed the gravity of the loaf fix ounces, by abforbing and retaining more water than the flour alone was capable of. Half a pound of flour, and an ounce of Salep were mixed together, and the water added according to the ufual method of preparing bread. The loaf, when baked, weighed thirteen ounces and a half; and would probably have been heavier, if the Salep had been previoufly diffolved in about a pint of water. But it fhould be remarked, that the quantity of flour ufed in this trial was not fufficient to conceal the peculiar tafte of the Salep.

The

The reſtorative, mucilaginous, and demulcent qualities of the Orchis root render it of confiderable uſe in various diſeaſes. In the ſea ſcurvy, it powerfully obtunds the acrimony of the fluids, and at the ſame time is eaſily aſſimilated into a mild and nutritious chyle. In diarrhœas and the dyſentery, it is highly ſerviceable, by ſheathing the internal coat of the inteſtines, by abating irritation, and gently correcting putrefaction. In the ſymptomatic fever, which ariſes from the abſorption of pus, from ulcers in the lungs, from wounds, or from amputation, Salep, uſed plentifully, is an admirable demulcent, and well adapted to reſiſt that diſſolution of the *craſis* of the blood, which is ſo evident in theſe caſes. And by the ſame mucilaginous quality, it is equally efficacious in the ſtrangury, and dyſury; eſpecially in the latter, when ariſing from a venereal cauſe; as the diſcharge of urine is then attended with the moſt exquiſite pain, from the ulcerations about the neck of the bladder, and through the courſe of the *urethra*. I have found it alſo an uſeful aliment for patients who labour under the ſtone or gravel *(f)*.

FROM

(f) THE ancient chemiſts ſeem to have entertained a very high opinion of the virtues of the Orchis root, of which the following quotation from the SECRETA SE-CRETORUM of Raymund Lully, affords a diverting proof. The work is dated 1565 ; and is here copied, I believe, *verbatim*.

SEXTA

FROM thefe obfervations, fhort and imperfect
as they are, I hope it will fufficiently appear that
the culture of the Orchis root is an object of confiderable importance to the public, and highly worthy of encouragement from all the patrons of agriculture.   That tafte for experiment, which cha-
racterizes the prefent age, and which has fo
amazingly enlarged the boundaries of fcience,
now animates the RATIONAL FARMER, who fears
not to deviate from the beaten track, whenever
improvements are fuggefted, or ufeful projects
are pointed out to him.   Much has been already
done for the advancement of agriculture; but

SEXTA HERBA,

SATIRION.

" SATIRION herba eft pluribus nota, hujus radicis
collecta ad pondus lib. 4. die 20 menfis Januarij, con-
tunde fortiter & maffam contufam pone in ollam de
aurichalcum habente in cooperculo 20 foramina minuta
ficut athomi, & pone intus cù prædicta meffa lactis vac-
cini calidi ficut mulgetur de vacca ℔. 3. & mellis libram 1. vini aromatici ℔. 2. & repone per dies 20. ad
folem & conferua & utere."

" Iftius itaq; dofis ad pondus 3. 4. & hora diei deci-
ma exhibita mulieri poft ipfius menftrua eadem nocte
còcipiet fi vir cum ea agat."

U 3   the

the earth ſtill teems with treaſures, which remain
to be explored. The bounties of nature are in-
exhauſtible, and will for ever employ the art,
and reward the induſtry of man *(g)*.

(g) In 1773 the Society for the Encouragement of
Arts, Manufactures, and Commerce was, I believe, in-
duced by it to offer a premium for the culture of the
Orchis root, and the preparation of Salep.

E S S A Y

E S S A Y III.

EXPERIMENTS AND OBSERVATIONS ON THE

W A T E R S

OF

BUXTON AND MATLOCK,

IN DERBYSHIRE *(b)*.

SECTION I.

ON BUXTON WATER.

THE water of St. Ann's well at BUXTON is found, by analyfis, to contain calcareous earth, foffil alkali, and fea falt; but in very fmall proportions. For a gallon of the water, when evaporated, yields only twenty three or twenty-four grains of fediment. It ftrikes a flight green colour with fyrup of violets; fuffers no change from an infufion of galls, from the fixed vegetable alkali, or from the mineral acids; becomes milky with the volatile alkali, and with *faccharum faturni*; and lets fall a precipitate, on the addition

(b) Inferted in the Philof. Tranf. vol. LXII. p. 455.

U 4   of

of a few drops of a folution of filver, in the nitrous acid. The fpecific gravity of this water is precifely equal to that of rain water, when their temperatures are the fame; but it weighs four grains in a pint lighter, when firft taken from the fpring. The temperature of the bath is about 82 degrees of Fahrenheit's thermometer; that of St. Ann's well, as it is a fmaller body of water, and expofed to the open air, is fomewhat lefs. The water is tranfparent, fparkling, and highly grateful to the palate *(i)*.

In October 1769, I paffed a few days at Buxton; and, during my ftay there, amufed myfelf with the following experiments on the effects of the water of St. Ann's well on my pulfe.

EXPERIMENT I. October 12th. Eight o'clock in the morning. The day cold and moift. My pulfe beat 84 ftrokes in a minute. I drank at the well a third of a pint of water, and ufing every neceffary precaution, examined my pulfe at certain intervals of time. In five minutes, pulfe 80. In ten minutes, pulfe 80, fuller and harder. In twenty minutes, pulfe 85. In half an hour, pulfe 90.

EXPERIMENT II. Eleven o'clock *a. m.* Two hours after breakfaft. The air warm and ferene.

(i) I am indebted to the information of Dr. Bullock, the phyfician who attends at Buxton, for fome of thefe facts.

Pulfe

Pulfe 90. I repeated the draught of water. In feven minutes, pulfe 109. In fifteen minutes, pulfe 103. In thirty minutes, pulfe 100. Head ach. In an hour and a half, pulfe 95. Head ach abated.

EXPERIMENT III. October 13th. Eight o'clock in the morning. The day cold. Pulfe 92. I drank the quantity of water above mentioned. In five minutes, pulfe 86. In fifteen minutes, pulfe 86, full and hard. In twenty minutes, pulfe 100. In half an hour, pulfe 92.

FROM the firft and third experiments, it appears that the coldnefs of the morning counteracted, for a time, the effects of the Buxton water, and reduced the vibrations of my pulfe from 84 to 80, and from 92 to 86. But the ftimulus of the water foon became fuperior to the fedative powers of the cold, to which I was expofed; for within the fpace of half an hour, my pulfe rofe to 90 in the firft, and to 100 ftrokes in the fecond trial. At eleven o'clock before noon, when the air was warm and ferene, the water in a much fhorter time exerted its full force, increafing the velocity of my pulfe from 90 to 109 vibrations in a minute.

THESE experiments evince the heating quality of Buxton water, and fuggeft to us the precautions to be obferved in the ufe of it. Small quantities only fhould be drunk at once, and

frequently

frequently repeated; the bowels fhould be kept foluble with lenitive electuary, or any other mild purgative; and at the beginning of the courfe, the patient may be directed to fuffer the water to remain a few feconds in the glafs, before he fwallows it. For this celebrated fpring abounds with a mineral fpirit, in which its ftimulus, and indeed its efficacy refides, and which is quickly diffipated by expofure to the air.

THE Honble. and ingenious Mr. Cavendifh has fhewn, by his Experiments on Rathbone-place water, Philof. Tranfact. vol. LVII. that calcareous earths may be rendered foluble in water, by furnifhing them with more than their natural proportion of fixed air. And it has lately been difcovered that iron, alfo, may be fufpended by this principle, in the fame *menftruum (k)*. It appeared, therefore, highly probable to me, that a chalybeate impregnation might, with great facility, be communicated to the Buxton water, when frefh drawn from the fpring; a quality which in many cafes would add greatly to its medicinal efficacy. I fuggefted the trial to Mr. Buxton, a worthy and fenfible Apothecary near the wells, who has lately, at my requeft, made the following experiment.

(k) Vid. Mr. Lane's Experiments, Phil. Tranf. vol. LIX.

EXPERIMENT

EXPERIMENT IV. A quart bottle, containing two drachms of iron filings, was filled by immersion, with the water of St. Ann's well, corked and agitated briskly under the surface of the water. It was then suffered to remain in the well till the filings had subsided, when the water was carefully decanted into a half pint glass. To this were added three drops of the tincture of galls, which immediately occasioned a deep purple colour; and the transparency was presently restored by a few drops of the acid of vitriol; evident proofs that the solution of the iron was effected in a few minutes. The water also, without the tincture of galls, had a chalybeate taste, and left an agreeable astringency upon the palate.

By this experiment it appears that a warm chalybeate, abounding with a mineral spirit, and grateful to the taste, may with very little trouble be obtained. And this method of impregnating the Buxton water with iron must increase its tonic powers, and in many cases improve its medicinal virtues. It is a common practice to join the use of a chalybeate spring, in the neighbourhood of St. Ann's well, with that of the Buxton water. But the superiority of this artificial mineral water must be apparent, if we consider its agreeable warmth, volatility, levity, and gratefulness to the palate.

BUXTON

Buxton bath is very frequently employed as a temperate cold bath. For as the heat of the water is fixteen or eighteen degrees below that of the human body, a gentle fhock is produced on the firft immerfion, the heart and arteries are made to contract more powerfully, and the whole fyftem is braced and invigorated. But this falutary operation muft be greatly diminifhed, often indeed more than counterbalanced, by the relaxing vapours which copioufly exhale from the bath, to which the patients are expofed during the time of dreffing and undreffing. A feparate room is indeed provided for the ladies; but the gentlemen have no other accommodations than what the vault affords in which the bath is contained, and are therefore liable to all the inconveniences which arife from warmth and moifture.

June 12, 1772. THE mercury in Fahrenheit's thermometer ftood in the fhade at 65; but in this vault quickly rofe to 78 degrees.

SECTION

SECTION II.

O N

MATLOCK WATER.

EXPERIMENT I. A Thermometer, made by Dollond, and graduated according to Fahrenheit's fcale, was expofed for a fufficient length of time to the ftream of water, as it gufhes out of the rock, and alfo immerfed in the bafon which receives it. The mercury rofe to 66 degrees.

EXPERIMENT II. Six drops of *fp. fal. ammon. vol.* were poured into a glafs of the fpring water, which contained about the fixth of a pint; a very flight cloudinefs immediately enfued; but no precipitation was afterwards obfervable.

EXPERIMENT III. Six drops of a folution of falt of tartar occafioned a cloudinefs juft perceptible, in the fame quantity of water. No precipitation enfued.

EXPERIMENT IV. Six drops of a folution of *faccharum faturni* immediately produced a milkinefs in the water, but no fenfible precipitation.

EXPERIMENT V. Six drops of a folution of filver in the nitrous acid inftantly occafioned
a milkinefs

a milkinefs in the water: And after ftanding an hour, a grey powder was obfervable at the bottom of the glafs.

EXPERIMENT VI.   Ten drops of the infufion of galls neither produced any change of colour in the water, at the time they were added, nor was the flighteft purple hue perceptible two hours afterwards.

EXPERIMENT VII.   A piece of paper, befmeared with frefh fyrup of violets, was dipped into a glafs full of water.   No change of colour enfued.

EXPERIMENT VIII.   Another piece of paper, moiftened in the fame manner with the fyrup, was placed over a glafs of water, as foon as it was taken from the fpring.   The paper fuffered no change of colour, although it remained an hour upon the glafs.

EXPERIMENT IX.   My pulfe beat 84 ftrokes in a minute, at the time when I drank a half pint glafs of the Matlock water.   In twenty minutes my pulfe rofe to 88.   In half an hour they funk to 82; and continued to vibrate the fame number of times for an hour, which was as long as I thought it neceffary to examine them.

EXPERIMENT X.   The mercury in Fahrenheit's thermometer, when immerfed in each of the baths, ftood at 68; in the river Derwent, which flows through the valley of Matlock, at 52.

These

Thefe experiments were made on the 12th of June 1772, and the weather was warm.

EXPERIMENT XI. A four ounce phial, after being accurately counterpoifed in a very nice balance, was filled to the brim with diftilled water, which weighed three ounces, four drachms, forty-five grains and a half. The fame phial, exactly balanced as before, was then filled to the brim with Matlock water, of the fame temperature with the diftilled water, which weighed three ounces, four drachms, and forty-fix grains.

MATLOCK water is grateful to the palate, and of an agreeable warmth, but exhibits no marks of mineral fpirit, either by its tafte, fparkling appearance in the glafs, or by the chemical teft employed in experiment VIII. The fecond and third experiments fhew, that it is very flightly impregnated with felenites or other earthy falts; and of this its comparative levity affords alfo a further proof. For it weighs twenty-fix grains in a pint lighter than the Manchefter pump water; and only four grains heavier than diftilled water. The precipitation of a grey powder, by the addition of a folution of filver in *aqua fortis* to the water, renders it probable that a fmall portion of fea falt is contained in it. For the powder is found to confift of the particles of filver combined with the muriatic acid, which is feparated from the foffil alkali by the fuperior affinity the nitrous

acid

acid bears to it; and thus a double elective attraction takes place in this experiment.

THIS water has been said to contain iron. But the affertion is at leaft rendered doubtful by the fixth experiment, which was made with the utmoft accuracy; and I am inclined to think that it is entirely without foundation. The fpring is juftly celebrated for its efficacy in hæmoptoes; and hence it may have been too haftily concluded that it poffeffes fome flight degree of ftypticity, by means of a chalybeate impregnation.

THE ninth experiment affords a prefumption, that the water is not poffeffed of any ftimulating powers. For the fmall increafe of quicknefs in my pulfe, on drinking half a pint of it, may be afcribed more to the quantity received into the ftomach, than to the heating quality of the water.

THE Briftol and Matlock waters appear to refemble each other, both in their chemical and medicinal qualities. I have examined and compared them together by the tefts mentioned above; and fo far as fuch trials may be deemed conclufive, there feems to be no other than the following flight difference between them. The Briftol water becomes a little more milky, on the addition of a folution of fixed alkali, and of *faccharum faturni*, than that of Matlock. The former, alfo, weighs near a grain in a pint heavier than the latter. Is it not to be lamented, therefore,

that

that fo little attention is paid to Matlock, even by the phyſicians who reſide in the neighbourhood of it? In hectic caſes, hæmoptoes, the diabetes, and other diſorders, in which the circulation of the blood is rapid and irregular, Matlock water, on ſome accounts, claims the preference to that of Briſtol. For as it is not ſenſibly impregnated with any mineral ſpirit, it ſhould ſeem to be leſs diſpoſed to quicken the pulſe, and may therefore be drunk in larger quantities. But it muſt be acknowledged that the climate of Briſtol is ſuperior to that of Matlock; a circumſtance of the higheſt importance to conſumptive patients. In this deep, though delightful valley, ſurrounded by very high mountains, the ſun diſappears earlier in the evening, the fogs are longer in diſperſing, and it may be preſumed that rain falls here more frequently and copiouſly, than in other places. For at Chatſworth, which is encompaſſed alſo with hills, and is about ten miles diſtant, in 1764, 1765, 1767, and 1768, about thirty-three inches of rain, at a medium, fell each year.

THE following Table exhibits a comparative view of the different temperatures of Bath, Buxton, Briſtol, and Matlock waters, meaſured by Fahrenheit's thermometer.

B A T H *(f).*

King's Bath Pump - -	112°.
Hot Bath Pump - - -	114½.
Crofs Bath Pump - - -	110.

B R I S T O L *(f).*

Hot Well Pump - - -	76.

B U X T O N.

Bath - - -	82.
St. Ann's Well - - -	81×.

M A T L O C K.

Baths - - - -	68.
Spring - - - -	66.

(f) Vid. Mr. Canton's Experiments, Philofophical Tranfactions, vol. LVII. p. 203.

ESSAY

E S S A Y IV.

MEDICINAL USES

ŏ F

F I X E D A I R *(a)*.

IN a courſe of Experiments, which is yet un-
finiſhed, I have had frequent opportunities of
obſerving that FIXED AIR may, in no inconſiderable
quantity, be breathed without danger or uneaſineſs.
And it is a confirmation of this concluſion, that
at Bath, where the waters copiouſly exhale a
mineral ſpirit *(b)*, the bathers inſpire it with impunity. At Buxton alſo, where the bath is in
a cloſe vault, the effects of ſuch *effluvia*, if noxious,
muſt certainly be perceived.

ENCOURAGED by theſe conſiderations, and ſtill
more by the teſtimony of a very judicious phyſician

(a) INSERTED in the Appendix to Dr. Prieſtley's Experiments and Obſervations on Air, vol. I. p. 300.

(b) SEE Dr. Falconer's very uſeful and ingenious
Treatiſe on the Bath Water, ſecond edit. p, 313.

X 2   at

at Stafford, in favour of this powerful antiseptic
remedy, I have administered fixed air, in a considerable number of cases of the PHTHISIS PUL-
MONALIS, by directing my patients to inspire the
steams of an effervescing mixture of chalk and
vinegar; or, which I have lately preferred, of vinegar and pot-ash. The hectic fever has, in several
instances, been greatly abated; and the matter ex-
pectorated has become less offensive, and better
digested. I have not yet, however, been so fortunate, in any one case, as to effect a cure; although the use of mephitic air has been accompanied with proper internal medicines. But Dr.
Withering, the gentleman referred to above, informs me that he has been more successful. One
phthisical patient under his care has, by a similar
course, entirely recovered; another was rendered
much better; and a third, whose case was truly
deplorable, seemed to be kept alive by it more
than two months *(c)*. It may be proper to
observe

(c) IN a Treatise on the FOXGLOVE, published in
1785, Dr. WITHERING has inserted the following
note. " Many years ago, I communicated to my
" friend, Dr. Percival, an account of some trials of
" breathing FIXED AIR, in CONSUMPTIVE CASES.
" The results were published by him, in the second
" volume of his Essays Medical and Experimental, and
" have since been copied into other publications. I
" take this opportunity of acknowledging, that I sus-
" pect myself to have been mistaken, in the nature of
" the disease, there mentioned to have been cured.
" I believe

obſerve that fixed air ſeems only to be indicated
in the latter ſtages of the *phthiſis pulmonalis*, when
a purulent expeɓoration takes place. After the
rupture and diſcharge of a VOMICA alſo, ſuch
a remedy promiſes to be a powerful palliative.
Antiſeptic fumigations and vapours have been
long employed, and much extolled in caſes of this
kind. I made the following experiment, to
determine whether their efficacy, in any degree,
depends on the ſeparation of fixed air from their
ſubſtance.

ONE end of a bent tube was fixed in a phial
full of lime water; the other end in a bottle of the
tinɓure of myrrh. The junɓures were carefully
luted, and the phial, containing the tinɓure of
myrrh, was placed in water heated almoſt to the
boiling point, by the lamp of a tea-kettle. A
number of air bubbles were ſeparated but probably not of the mephitic kind: For no precipitation enſued in the lime-water. This experiment
was repeated with the *Tinɓt. Tolutana*, *Ph. Ed.*
and with *Sp. Vinos. Camph.* and the reſult was
entirely the ſame. The medicinal aɓion, there-

" I believe it was a caſe of *Vomica*, and not a true
" *Phthiſis*, that was cured. The *Vomica* is almoſt always
" curable. The fixed air correɓs the ſmell of the matter,
" and very ſhortly removes the heɓic fever. My pati-
" ents not only inſpire it, but I keep large jars of the
" effervefcing mixture conſtantly at work, in their
" chambers." See Withering on the Foxglove, p. 205.

fore

fore, of the vapours raifed from fuch tinctures, cannot be afcribed to the extrication of fixed air; of which it is probable bodies are deprived by *chemical folution*, as well as by *mixture*.

IF mephitic air be thus capable of correcting purulent matter in the lungs, we may reafonably infer it will be equally ufeful, when applied externally to foul ULCERS. And experience confirms the conclufion. Even the fanies of a CANCER, when the carrot poultice failed, has been fweetened by it, the pain mitigated, and a better digeftion produced. The cafes I refer to are now in the Manchefter infirmary, under the direction of my friend Mr. White, whofe fkill as a furgeon, and abilities as a writer are well known to the public.

Two months have elapfed fince thefe obfervations were written *(d)*, and the fame remedy, during that period, has been affiduoufly applied, but without any further fuccefs. The progrefs of the cancers feems to be checked by the fixed air; but it is to be feared that a cure will not be effected. A palliative remedy, however, in a difeafe fo defperate and loathfome, may be confidered as a very valuable acquifition. Perhaps NITROUS AIR might be ftill more efficacious. This fpecies of factitious air is obtained from all the metals except zinc, by means of nitrous acid;

(d) May, 1772.

and

and Dr. Prieftley informs me, that, as a fweetener and antifeptic, it far furpaffes fixed air. He put two mice into a quantity of it, one juft killed, the other offenfively putrid. After twenty-five days, they were both perfectly fweet.

In the ULCEROUS SORE THROAT, much advantage has been experienced from the vapours of effervefcing mixtures drawn into the *fauces*. But this remedy fhould not fuperfede the ufe of other antifeptic applications.

A PHYSICIAN, who had a painful APTHOUS ULCER at the point of his tongue, found great relief, when other remedies failed, from the application of fixed air to the part affected. He held his tongue over an effervefcing mixture of pot-afh and vinegar; and as the pain was always mitigated, and generally removed by this vaporization, he repeated it, whenever the anguifh arifing from the ulcer was more than ufually fevere. He tried a combination of pot-afh and oil of vitriol, well diluted with water; but this proved ftimulant, and increafed his pain; probably owing to fome particles of the acid thrown upon the tongue, by the violence of the effervefcence. For a paper, ftained with the purple juice of radifhes, when held at an equal diftance over two veffels, the one containing pot-afh and vinegar, the other the fame alkali and *Spiritus Vitrioli tenuis*, was unchanged by the former,

X 4 but

but was fpotted with red, in various parts, by the latter.

IN MALIGNANT FEVERS, wines abounding with fixed air may be adminiftered, to check the feptic ferment, and fweeten the putrid *colluvies* in the *primæ viæ*. If the laxative quality of fuch liquors be thought an objection to the ufe of them, wines of a greater age may be given, impregnated with mephitic air, by a fimple, but ingenious contrivance of Dr. Prieftley *(e)*.

THE patient's common drink might alfo be medicated in the fame way. A putrid DIARRHOEA frequently occurs, in the latter ftages of fuch diforders; and it is a moft alarming and dangerous fymptom. If the difcharge be ftopped by aftringents, a putrid *fomes* is retained in the body, which aggravates the delirium, and increafes the fever. On the contrary, if it be fuffered to take its courfe, the ftrength of the patient, muft foon be exhaufted, and death unavoidably enfue. The injection of mephitic air into the inteftines, under thefe circumftances, bids fair to be highly ferviceable. And a cafe, of this deplorable kind, has lately been communicated to me, in which the vapour of chalk and oil of vitriol, conveyed into the body by the

---

(e) Directions for impregnating water with fixed air, in order to communicate to it the peculiar fpirit and virtues of Pyrmont water, and other mineral waters of a fimilar nature.

machine

machine employed for tobacco clyfters, quickly reftrained the *diarrhœa*, corrected the heat and fœtor of the ftools, and in two days removed every fymptom of danger *. A fimilar inftance of the falutary effects of mephitic air, thus adminiftered, has occurred, alfo, in my own practice, the hiftory of which I fhall briefly lay before the reader. May we not prefume that the fame remedy would be equally ufeful in the DYSENTERY? The experiment is at leaft worthy of trial.

ELIZABETH GRUNDY, aged feventeen, was attacked on the 10th of December 1772, with the ufual fymptoms of a continued fever. The common method of cure was purfued; but the difeafe increafed, and foon affumed a putrid type.

On the 23d, I found her in a conftant delirium, with a *fubfultus tendinum*. Her fkin was hot and dry, her tongue black, her thirft immoderate, and her ftools frequent, extremely offenfive, and for the moft part involuntary. Her pulfe beat 130 ftrokes in a minute; fhe dozed much; and was very deaf. I directed wine to be adminiftered freely; a blifter to be applied to her back; the *pediluvium* to be ufed feveral times in the day; and mephitic air to be injected, under the form of a clyfter every two hours. The next day, her ftools were lefs frequent, had loft their fœtor, and

---

* See a cafe by Mr. Hey of Leeds, in the Appendix to Dr. Prieftley's Obfervations on Air, vol. I.

were no longer difcharged involuntarily; her pulfe was reduced to 110 ftrokes in the minute; and her delirium was much abated. Directions were given to repeat the clyfters, and to fupply the patient liberally with wine. Thefe means were affiduoufly purfued feveral days; and the young woman was fo recruited by the 28th, that the injections were difcontinued. She was now quite rational, and not averfe to medicine. A decoction of Peruvian bark was, therefore, prefcribed, by the ufe of which fhe fpeedily recovered her health.

I might add another hiftory of a putrid difeafe, in which the mephitic air is now under trial, and which affords the ftrongeft proof both of the *antifeptic*, and of the *tonic* powers of this remedy; but as the iffue of the cafe remains yet undetermined, (though it is highly probable, alas! that it will be fatal) I fhall relate only a few particulars of it. Mafter D. a boy of about twelve years of age, endowed with an uncommon capacity, and with the moft amiable difpofitions, has laboured many months under a hectic fever, the confequence of feveral tumours in different parts of his body. Two of thefe tumours were laid open by Mr. White, and a large quantity of purulent matter was difcharged from them. The wounds were very properly treated by this fkilful furgeon, and every remedy, which my beft judgment could fuggeft, fuggeſt, was aſſiduouſly adminiſtered.   But the matter became ſanious, of a brown colour, and highly putrid.   A *diarrhœa* ſucceeded; the patient's ſtools were intolerably offenſive, and voided without his knowledge.   A black fur collected about his teeth; his tongue was covered with *aphthæ*; and his breath was ſo fœtid, as ſcarcely to be endured.   His ſtrength was almoſt exhauſted; a *ſubſultus tendinum* came on; and the final period of his ſufferings ſeemed to be rapidly approaching.   As a laſt, but almoſt hopeleſs effort, I adviſed the injection of clyſters of mephitic air.   Theſe ſoon corrected the fœtor of the patient's ſtools, reſtrained his *diarrhœa*, and ſeemed to recruit his ſtrength and ſpirits.   Within the ſpace of twenty-four hours, his wounds aſſumed a more favourable appearance; the matter diſcharged from them became of a better colour and conſiſtence; and was no longer ſo offenſive to the ſmell.   The uſe of this remedy has been continued ſeveral days, but is now laid aſide.   A large tumour is ſuddenly formed under the right ear; ſwallowing is rendered difficult and painful; and the patient refuſes all food and medicine. Nouriſhing clyſters are directed: But it is to be feared that theſe will renew the looſeneſs, and that this amiable youth will quickly ſink under his diſorder *(f).*

(f) He languiſhed about a week, and then died.

THE ufe of *Wort*, from its faccharine quality, and difpofition to ferment, has lately been propofed as a remedy for the SEA SCURVY. Water, or other liquors, already abounding with fixed air in a feparate ftate, fhould feem to be better adapted to this purpofe; as they will more quickly correct the putrid difpofition of the fluids, and at the fame time, by their gentle ftimulus, *(g)* increafe the powers of digeftion, and give new ftrength to the whole fyftem.

DR. PRIESTLEY, who fuggefted both the idea and the means of executing it, has, under the fanction of the College of Phyficians, propofed the fcheme to·the Lords of the Admiralty, who have ordered trial to be made of it, on board fome of his Majefty's fhips of war. Might it not, however, give additional efficacy to this remedy, if, inftead of fimple water, the infufion of malt were to be employed?

I am perfuaded fuch a medicinal drink might be prefcribed alfo, with great advantage, in SCROPHULOUS COMPLAINTS, when not attended with a hectic fever; and in other diforders, in which a general acrimony prevails, and the crafis of the blood is deftroyed. Under fuch circum-

(g) The vegetables, which are moft efficacious in the cure of the fcurvy, poffefs fome degree of ftimulating powe·.

ftances,

ftances, I have feen *vibices*, which fpread over the body, difappear in a few days from the ufe of wort.

A GENTLEMAN, who is fubjeft to a fcorbutic eruption in his face, for which he has ufed a variety of remedies with no very beneficial effeft, has lately applied the fumes of chalk and oil of vitriol to the parts affefted. The operation occafions great itching and pricking in the fkin, and fome degree of drowfinefs; but evidently abates the ferous difcharge, and diminifhes the eruption. This patient has feveral fymptoms which indicate a genuine fcorbutic DIATHESIS; and it is probable that fixed air, taken internally, would be an ufeful medicine, in this cafe.

THE faline draughts of Riverius are fuppofed to owe their antiemetic effefts to the air, which is feparated from the falt of wormwood, during the aft of effervefcence. And the tonic powers of many mineral waters feem to depend on this prin-ciple. I was lately defired to vifit a lady, who had moft fevere convulfive RETCHINGS. Various remedies had been adminiftered without effeft, before I faw her. She earneftly defired a draught of malt liquor; and was indulged with half a pint of Burton beer, in brifk effervefcence. The vo-mitings ceafed immediately, and returned no more. Fermenting liquors, it is well known, abound with fixed air. To this, and to the cor-

dial

dial quality of the beer, the favourable effect
which it produced, may juftly be afcribed. But
I fhall exceed my defign by enlarging further on
this fubject. What has been advanced, it is
hoped, will fuffice to excite the attention of phyficians to a remedy, which is capable of being applied to fo many important medicinal purpofes.

P. S. 1776. May not mephitic water prove
an active and ufeful remedy in fuch fpecies of
dropfies as originate from obftructions in the
liver, or from a general *atonia* of the folids, and
poverty of the fluids? From its ftimulant and
penetrating powers, it fhould feem well adapted
to pervade the minuteft feries of veffels; as a
ftrengthener, it will give vigour to the organs of
digeftion; and as a diuretic, will tend to carry
off, by urine, the fuperabundant ferofities. In
the *anafarca* and *afcites* the blood is generally of
a loofe texture, and the coagulable lymph is
fometimes fo much diffolved, that the whole
mafs affumes the appearance of gelly. As fixed
air has been fhewn, by Dr. Hales and Dr. Macbride, to be a bond of union to the particles of
matter, may not mephitic water contribute to
supply

supply the animal fluids with this cementing principle? Other tonic and diuretic remedies may
be combined with this grateful liquor; and if
the patient's thirst be immoderate, and his case
attended with imminent danger, he may be allowed to drink of it to satiety *(h)*. The waters
of Bath in Somersetshire, have been found to be
signally serviceable in œdematous swellings of
the legs, which have succeeded intermittents;
and also in anasarcas, when the strength has not
been too far impaired *(i)*. I have repeatedly
experienced the salutary effects of Buxton water

(h) Sanatur, indulgens fibi, dirus hydrops.
THE following passage is extracted from a letter which
I have lately received from my learned friend Dr. Baker.
   " HAVE you heard of M. Bacher? Such is said to
" have been his success in dropsies, that the French
" government has been induced, from the report made
" of the effects of his *tonic pills,* to purchase the secret
" of their composition; trials being first made under the
" eye of the court physicians. The chief ingredient in
" the pills is the black hellebore; but Bacher says,
" that without the assistance of *diluents* he could do no-
" thing. ' *Le malade buvoit a fa foif,*' is the language
" of every page. This puts me in mind of some cases,
" which I published, in the second volume of the
" Medical Transactions; and I have lately been in-
" formed from Vienna, that Dr Colin has more suc-
" cess than others with the same medicines, probably
" because his patients are allowed to drink *ad libitum.*"

(i) See Falconer on the Bath waters.

in

in similar cases: And as these celebrated springs
owe their virtues, in part, to the mineral spirit
which they contain, their efficacy in dropsies
affords sufficient encouragement to the trial of
mephitic water, in the same disorders.

FIXED AIR, conveyed by a proper tube into
the nostrils, seems likely to prove the best topical application in the OZÆNA; whether the dif-
ease be seated in the *antrum Highmorianum*, or in
the frontal sinuses. It will be easy to guard the
patient against drawing into his lungs too large
a quantity of this air, by directing him to breathe
with his mouth open, during the operation.

ESSAY

E S S A Y V.

ANTISEPTIC AND SWEETENING POWERS,

AND ON THE VARIETIES OF

FACTITIOUS AIR.

THOUGH the fact has lately been controverted by an ingenious writer, I am fully convinced with Dr. Macbride, from the evidence of repeated experiments, that fixed air has the property both of retarding and of correcting putrefaction. It may afford matter of amusement, to confider in what manner thefe effects are produced.

THAT fixed air may reftrain, and even prevent putrefaction, without poffeffing any inherent antifeptic quality, is not difficult to conceive. For by furrounding the putrefcent fubftance with that kind of air, which it yields by putrefaction, and which requires fome vehicle to difcharge or carry it off, the feparation of it is prevented, and the body thus retained in its original ftate. This may be illuftrated by a wet fponge or cloth, which will never become dry in an atmofphere faturated with moifture : Or ftill more appofitely by putting a mixture of fulphur and iron filings in a confined place, or into air in which candles have burned out. Under thefe circumftances, no heat, effervefcence, or fume can be generated; whereas the fame mixture in frefh air prefently grows hot, fmokes copioufly, and fmells very offenfively *(a)*. The fame obfervation will account for the curious fact, mentioned by Dr. Alexander, that the *effluvia* of putrid fubftances retard putrefaction in the bodies expofed to them. Perhaps, however, the generation of a volatile alkali may have fome fhare in producing this effect.

But fuppofing the foregoing hypothefis to be well founded, which I advance only as conjecture, how are we to explain the fweetening powers of fixed air? An eminent philofopher feems to hint that fixed air may act as a *menftruum* for the putrid *effluvium*, and thus imbibe or difcharge it from the feptic body. The fame idea fuggefted itfelf to Mr. Henry, in confequence of the following experiment, to which I was a witnefs. A piece of putrid flefh was fufpended twelve hours, in a three pint bottle clofely corked, and filled

(a) See Dr. Prieftley's moft ingenious papers on factitious air, which will probably be publifhed in the LXII. vol. of the Philof Tranf.

with

with fixed air, which had been feparated from chalk by the vitriolic acid. The beef was confiderably fweetened, but the air in the bottle was rendered intolerably offenfive. Now it affords a natural folution of this fact, if we admit that fixed air, by the laws of chemical affinity, abftracts from the feptic body, and holds fufpended or diffolved the putrid particles which it emits. And fuch an affinity feems probable, from their ready combination, as well as from their difpofition to fly off together from putrefying fubftances. But how is the putrefactive procefs checked, and the frefh generation of *effluvia* reftrained, under fuch circumftances? A piece of the fame flefh, which was employed in the foregoing experiment, was left all night in the external air, by the circulation of which the *effluvia* could not fail to be carried off, as they were formed; yet the offenfive odour of the flefh was not diminifhed. Has not the reafon of this difference, between the expofure of a putrid fubftance to common air, and to mephitic air, been before affigned, when it was fuggefted that the latter may perhaps reftrain the flight of that principle in bodies, the feparation of which conftitutes an effential part of the procefs of putrefaction? Animal flefh will neither become putrid in *vacuo*, nor when clofely confined from the accefs of common air. In both cafes a vehicle is wanting for the efcape

of

of the mephitic air. In like manner red hot wood ceafes to burn in inflammable air, becaufe fuch air is already faturated with phlogifton.

I HAVE advanced the preceding conjectures, concerning the manner in which fixed air may retard and correct putrefaction, not as affording me full conviction, or to indulge the fpirit of hypothefis, but to promote the further inveftigation of a fubject fo curious and interefting.

EXPERIMENT I.   It is a fact lately afcertained by a very accurate philofopher, that putrefaction generates air fimilar to that which animals have breathed.   But this and the fucceeding experiment fhew that there is fome little diverfity in their properties and effects.   Air was blown forcibly from the lungs, for a fufficient length of time, into a phial containing diftilled water and iron filings.   The water was then filtered, and a few drops of the infufion of galls were added to it.   A dark red colour, inclining to purple, was inftantly produced.

EXPERIMENT II *(b)*.   Eight ounces of ox-gall were poured into a bottle, which had a tube communicating with another phial, containing half an ounce of iron filings, and four ounces of diftilled water.   After ftanding two days, part of the water was filtered, and fuffered no change of

(b) Communicated by Dr. Falconer of Bath.

colour ·

colour from the addition of an aftringent tincture.
But the next day, when the fermentation in the
gall was more evident, another filtered portion
of the water ftruck, with the fame tincture, a deep
rofy red.   On the fifth and fixth days, when the
gall became intolerably putrid, though the vapour ftill corroded the iron filings, it feemed to
have loft the power of diffolving them.   For the
aftringent tincture no longer produced any change
of colour in the water, and the iron was evidently precipitated.

EXPERIMENT III *(c)*.   Solutions of iron in water, obtained by different kinds of fixed air, vary
in the colours which they ftrike with an infufion
of galls.   When the vitriolic acid and foffil alkali
are employed, a black tinge is produced; when
magnefia, or calcareous earths and the fame acid
are ufed, a purple hue is ftruck; and when the
air is fupplied by fermentation, the artificial chalybeate is changed, by galls, into a rofy red.

EXPERIMENT IV.   Air, difcharged from chalk
by the vitriolic acid, readily and perfectly combines with water; but when feparated by the
nitrous acid, the union is more difficult to be
effected, and much lefs complete.   And the
artificial mineral water, made by the latter, is

(c) By the fame.

Y 3   more

more pungent and fparkling than by the former acid.

EXPERIMENT V. Factitious air, feparated from fteel filings by the vitriolic acid, neither occafioned any precipitation in lime water, nor rendered the cauftic fixed alkali mild. Whereas the air, fet free from chalk and magnefia by the fame acid, inftantly produced a milkinefs in lime water, and reftored to the cauftic alkali the power of effervefcence.

EXPERIMENT VI. A piece of putrid mutton, which had been employed as a ftandard in fome other experiments, was divided into two equal parts: One of thefe was fufpended by a thread in a phial, containing an effervefcing mixture of chalk and dilute fpirit of vitriol; the other in a fimilar phial, with a mixture of iron filings and the fame acid. The mouths of the phials were flightly ftopped with folded paper; and a brifk fermentation took place in each of them. After being expofed fixteen hours to the air detached from thefe fubftances, the bits of mutton were taken out, and examined. They were both confiderably firmer in their texture; and the one, which had been fufpended over the effervefcing mixture of chalk and oil of vitriol, was entirely fweetened; but the putrid fetor of the other was not in the leaft degree corrected.

EXPERIMENT

EXPERIMENT VII.   A piece of putrid flesh was suspended about half an hour, over a mixture of iron filings and nitrous acid, and was perfectly sweetened.   It had acquired a pungent and slightly acid smell, but remained firm and free from fetor, when this odour was washed off.   The water, in which the flesh was washed, did not effervesce with *lixivium tartari*; nor did the vapour, arising from the spirit of nitre and iron filings, produce any change of colour in a paper covered with syrup of violets; presumptive proofs that the sweetness of the flesh was not restored by any acid fumes.

THE fixed air of metals seems, by some of these experiments, to be of a kind different from that which is contained in alkalis and calcareous earths.   And consequently the action of these substances, as *fluxes*, cannot be explained on the principle of their restoring the air which had been lost by calcination.   Indeed there are other proofs that the resuscitation of calces does not depend on this cause.   I have been assured by an able chemist, that he has repeatedly restored *minium* to its metalline state, by the caustic alkali, assisted by a proper degree of heat; and that several of the metals may be revived by the force of fire alone. It is true that a mild calcareous earth, employed as a flux, is always rendered caustic by the opera-tion.   But this may be owing to the action of the

Y 4   fire,

fire, and not to the lofs of its air by elective attraction. Perhaps the operation of alkalis and calcareous earths, as fluxes, may depend on their abforbing the matter, which feems to be added to metallic fubftances, by the procefs of calcination, and which furnifhes fuch an amazing increafe of weight *(d)*. Inflammable bodies may produce the fame effect, by volatilizing and carrying it off.

(d) ANTIMONY, when calcined, gains one eleventh part of its original weight; zinc one tenth; tin one fixth; and lead, when converted into minium, one fourth.

ESSAY

E S S A Y VI (a).

ON THE

NOXIOUS VAPOURS

OF

CHARCOAL.

THE accurate and ingenious Dr. Hales has
proved, by a great variety of experiments,
that air enters in a very confiderable proportion
into the compofition of all bodies; that air,
thus combined, is in a fixed ftate, and contributes
to form the union and firm connection of the
conftituent parts of bodies; and that on their de-

(a) This effay was communicated in 1772, by the
late learned and much refpected Dr. Dobfon; who then
refided at Liverpool, but afterwards removed to Bath.
The few philofophical errors it contains muft be imputed to the imperfect knowledge of factitious air, which
fubfifted at the time when it was written. I again infert
it, with peculiar pleafure, as a memorial of reciprocal
efteem and friendfhip. January 1, 1788.

ftruction

ftruction or decompofition, this fixed air is again reftored to its ftate of elafticity.

FIXED AIR, whether procured by fire, fermentation, or chemical refolution, has been fuppofed to be a body *fui generis*; and to poffefs properties, by which it is always diftinctly characterized. It is more conformable however to the fimplicity which is conftantly obferved in the operations of nature, to conclude, that as it is common atmofpheric air which enters into the compofition of bodies, it is likewife the fame air which is again detached, on their decompofition or deftruction; that its varieties depend on adventitious matter; and that it has different degrees of mixture and compofition, accordingly as it is obtained from different fubftances, or by a different procefs.

THAT by degrees however, it is decompounded; returns to its original fimplicity; is reftored to the common magazine from which it was taken; and that the atmofphere is thus conftantly gaining, by one procefs, what it lofes by another.

FACTITIOUS or FIXED AIR is the general term, by which this fubject is diftinguifhed; and when it produces any noxious effects, either in confequence of the procefs by which it is procured, or the manner in which it is applied, it may then be properly called MEPHITIC AIR.

MUCH has been done, by fome very ingenious modern writers, to illuftrate this fubject; and
much

much ftill remains to be done, to compleat the chemical and medical hiftory of fixed air. The prefent commentary chiefly refpects the factitious air of charcoal; or the mephitic vapours which arife from this fubftance, in the ftate of ignition. And the following hiftory points out both the noxious qualities of thefe vapours, and their mode of action on the animal œconomy.

OCTOBER 5, 1769. A fervant to a gentleman's family in Liverpool, fhut himfelf up in a fmall room to clean plate. In this room there was a chafing-difh of burning charcoal, and the door and window were clofed. He foon felt himfelf *very ill*, as he expreffed it; was chilly, fickifh, and had fhooting pains in the head. He continued to be affected in this manner for upwards of an hour and a half, during which time he had been twice called out, but returned again to the fame fitutation in a few minutes. The chills, ficknefs, and pain in the head became more fevere, and were increafed by fits; he retched, but could not vomit. Thefe were the only fenfations he could recollect; and on my afking him, whether he did not feel an oppreffion at his breaft, or a fenfe of fuffocation, he anfwered in the negative.

HE remembered that he heard the clock ftrike eleven, which was an hour and a half from his firft going into the room; and ftill finding him-

felf

felf very ill, but having no fufpicion of the caufe, he leaned forwards, refted his head upon his hands, and from that time had no further know-ledge of what paffed.

ABOUT half an hour after this, fome of the family going near the door, were alarmed by his groans. The door was forced open, and he was found extended on the ground; his eyes fixed and ftaring; his hands clenched; his arms, legs, and whole body rigid; and his countenance, which was naturally pale, had now a death-like appear-ance.

HE was immediately carried into the open air; but it was with difficulty that his limbs were fo bent that he could be feated in a chair. He continued to groan, and on the application of hartf-horn drops to his nofe, exerted a kind of motion, as if offended. Cold water thrown upon his face, had a more powerful effect to roufe him. After ten minutes, he came to himfelf; and in about twenty minutes, he was able to walk.

AT this time I firft faw him. He complained of pain in his head, coldnefs and ficknefs; was hot to the touch; his pulfe, fmall and frequent, 120 in a minute. While I was examining him, I obferved his voice faultered; his eyes became fixed; he ftaggered forwards, and would have fallen, had he not been fupported. He was placed in a chair, and remained in a ftate of

infenfibility

infenfibility near a minute; there was no rigidity; the colour of the countenance did not change; but the pulfe was extremely fmall, frequent, and irregular. On coming to himfelf, he complained much of pain in his head, was fick, retched, trembled, and was cold and hot by fits; a confiderable degree of fever remained for two days, and then gradually left him.

WE have here a fair opportunity of obferving the effects of thefe noxious vapours. The patient was near two hours ftruggling with the poifon; and the whole progrefs of the fymptoms clearly points out an immediate affection of the brain and nervous fyftem, not of the lungs.

IT is the common apprehenfion, that thofe who are killed by the effluvia of burning charcoal, are *fuffocated*; and this apprehenfion is fupported by the authorities of fome very diftinguifhed practical writers.

MORGAGNI, in his excellent work *de Sedibus et Caufis Morborum*, afferts, that thofe who die from the *fteams of charcoal*, the fteams of the fermenting grape, in the Grotto di Cani, and in the cavern of Pyrmont, are *fuffocated (b)*.

HOFFMAN, in his Differtation *de fumo carbonum noxio*, fays, that thefe vapours being received into the breaft, diftend the lungs, prevent the ad-

(b) Epift. 19. § 40.

miffion

miſſion of air, and thus *ſuffocate (c)*.   The mode
of operation is expreſſed in very ſtrong terms.
*Eadem enim horum operandi ratio eſt, ac ſi aſperam
arteriam filo conſtringas ; nam utroque horum aeris
ſufficiens introitus impeditur (d).*

DOCTOR HALES concludes, that the ſteams of
the Grotto di Cani, and ſeveral other noxious
vapours, deſtroy the elaſticity of the air, occaſion
the veſicles of the lungs to collapſe, and thus
ſuffocate, and cauſe ſudden death *(e)*.

SUCH are the reſpectable authorities which give
weight to the common opinion, that thoſe who are
killed by theſe noxious effluvia, are ſuffocated.
The following experiments, hiſtories, and obſervations, tend however to eſtabliſh a different
doctrine.

WE learn from the experiments of the celebrated
Greenwood, that the air of a well, in which the
men who went down periſhed, and in which a
lighted torch was inſtantly extinguiſhed, did not
differ from common air, either in gravity, hu-
midity, or elaſticity *(f)*.

THE ſame is found to be true of the Grotto
di Cani.   In this, the height of the mercury in
the barometer was not altered by the deadly

(c) Hoffman, tom. IV. p. 697. 22.
(d) Ib.
(e) Hales's Statics, p. 260, 261.
(f) Saggio delle Tranſar. tom. V. p. 2.

vapours *(g)*. And we have the fame proof of the
ftate. of the air in the cavern of Pyrmont *(h)*
It appears likewife from the experiments of the
learned Leonardo Capuano, that thofe animals
which do *not breathe*, are deftroyed in the Grotto
di Cani, though flowly and with more difficulty *(i)*.

DR. HALES indeed proves, that the fumes of
burning fulphur, and the exhalations from the
lungs of animals, bring into a fixed ftate part of the
air through which they are difperfed, and confequently diminifh its elafticity. That this circumftance however is not the caufe of death, is hence
evident; in high winds and ftorms, and on
afcending very high mountains, a greater diminution of elafticity takes place, without fuch fatal
effects *(k)*.

ALL thefe noxious vapous, whether arifing from
burning charcoal, the fermenting grape, the
Grotto di Cani, or the cavern of Pyrmont, operate nearly in the fame manner. When accumulated and confined, their effects are often
inftantaneous; they immediately deftroy the ac-

(g) Mead de Venenis, tent. 6.
(h) Commerc. litter. A. 1737. Heb. 8.
(i) Delle Mofette, Lez. 1.
(k) Veratti Com. Acad. Bonon. tom. II. part II.
p. 271, 276. And Element. Phyfiolog. Haller. vol. III.
p. 208.

tion

tion of the brain and nerves, and in a moment arreft the vital motions. When more diffufed, their effects are flower, but ftill evidently mark out a direct affection of the nervous fyftem.

THOSE who are expofed to the vapours of the fermenting grape, are as inftantly deftroyed, as they would be by the ftrongeft electrical fhock. A ftate of infenfibility is the immediate effect upon thofe animals, which are thruft into the Grotto di Cani, or the cavern of Pyrmont; the animal is deprived of motion, lies as if dead, and if not quickly returned into the frefh air, is irrecoverable. And if we attend to the hiftories of thofe who have fuffered from the vapours of burning charcoal, we fhall in like manner find that the brain and moving powers. are the parts primarily affected.

A COOK, who had been accuftomed to make ufe of lighted charcoal more than his bufinefs required, and to ftand with his head over thefe fires, complained for a year of very acute pain in the head; and after this, was feized with a paralytic affection of the lower limbs, and a flow fever (l).

A PERSON was left reading in bed, with a pan of charcoal in a corner of the room. On being vifited early the next morning, he was found with his eyes fhut, his book open and laid on

(l) Morgagni. Epift. 64. § 15.

one

one fide, his candle extinguifhed and to appearance like one in a deep fleep. Stimulants and cupping glaffes gave no relief; but he was foon recovered by the free accefs of frefh air *(m)*.

Four prifoners, in order to make their efcape, attempted to deftroy the iron work of their windows, by the means of burning charcoal. As foon as they commenced their operations, the fumes of the charcoal being confined by the clofenefs of the prifon, one of them was ftruck dead; another was found pale, fpeechlefs, and without motion; afterwards he fpoke incoherently, was feized with a fever, and died. The other two were with great difficulty recovered *(n)*.

Two boys went to warm themfelves in a ftove, heated with charcoal. In the morning they were found deftitute of fenfe and motion, with countenances as compofed as in a placid fleep. There were fome remains of pulfe, but they died in a fhort time *(o)*.

A fisherman depofited a large quantity of charcoal in a deep cellar. Some time afterwards, his fon, a healthy ftrong man, went down into the cellar with a pan of burning charcoal and a light in his hand. He had fcarcely defcended to the bottom, when his candle went out. He

(m) Chefneou, 696.
(n) Donatus. Epift. 694.   *(o)* Id. 695.

returned, lighted his candle, and again defcended. Soon after he called aloud for affiftance. His mother, brother, and a fervant hafted to give him relief, but none of them returned. Two others of the village fhared the fame fate. It was then determined to throw large quantities of water into the cellar; and after two or three days, they had accefs to the dead bodies. *(p)*

CÆLIUS AURELIANUS fays, that thofe who are injured by the fumes of charcoal, become cataleptic. *(q)* And Hoffman himfelf, in another part of his works, enumerates a train of fymptoms which, in no refpect, correfpond with his idea of fuffocation. Thofe who fuffer from the fumes of burning charcoal, fays he, have fevere pains in the head, great debility, faintnefs, ftupor and lethargy. *(r)*

IT appears, from the above hiftories and obfervations, that thefe vapours exert their noxious effects on the brain and nerves. Sometimes they occafion fudden death; at other times, the various fymptoms of a debilitated nervous fyftem, according as the poifon is more or lefs concentrated. The olfactory nerves are firft and principally affected, and the brain and nervous fyftem

(p) Hiftoire de l' Academié de Science, Ann. 1710.

(q) De morbis acutis, lib. II. c. x.

(r) Tom. I. p. 229. § 5.

by

by fympathy or confent of parts. It is well
known, that there is a ftrong and ready confent
between the olfactory nerves and many other parts
of the nervous fyftem. The effluvia of flowers
and perfumes, in delicate or irritable habits,
produce a train of fymptoms, which though tranfient, are analogous to thofe which are produced
by the vapours of charcoal; viz. vertigo, ficknefs, faintnefs, and fometimes a total infenfibility.
The female malefactor, whom Dr. Mead inoculated by putting into the noftrils doffils of cotton
impregnated with variolous matter, was immediately on the introduction, afflicted with a moft
excruciating head ach, and had a conftant fever till
after the eruption.

THE vapours of burning charcoal, and other
poifonous effluvia, frequently produce their prejudicial, and even fatal effects, without being either
offenfive to the fmell, or oppreffive to the lungs.
It is a matter of importance therefore, that the
common opinion fhould be more agreeable to
truth; for where fuffocation is fuppofed to be
the effect, there will be little apprehenfion of
danger, fo long as the breaft keeps free from pain
or oppreffion.

IT may be well to remember, that the poifon
itfelf is diftinct from that grofs matter which
is offenfive to the fmell; and that this is frequently in its moft active ftate, when undiftin-

guifhed

guiſhed by the ſenſe. Were the following cautions generally attended to, they might in ſome inſtances be the happy means of preſerving life. Never to be confined with burning charcoal in a ſmall room, or where there is not a free draught of air by a chimney or ſome other way. Never to venture into any place in which air has been long pent up, or which from other circumſtances ought to be ſuſpected; unleſs ſuch ſuſpected place be either previouſly well ventilated, or put to the teſt of the lighted candle. For it is a ſingular and well known fact, that the life of flame, is in ſome circumſtances, ſooner affected and more expeditiouſly extinguiſhed by noxious vapours, than animal life. A proof of which I remember to have received from a very intelligent clergyman, who was preſent at a muſical entertainment at Oxford. The room was crouded; and during the entertainment, the candles were obſerved to burn dimly, and ſome of them went out. The audience complained only of faintneſs and languor; but had the animal effluvia been ſtill further accumulated, or longer confined, they would have been extinguiſhed as well as the candles.

THE moſt obvious, effectual, and expeditious means of relief to thoſe who have unhappily ſuf fered from this cauſe, are ſuch as will diſlodge and waſh away the poiſon; reſtore the energy of the brain and nerves; and renew the vital motions.

Let

Let the patient, therefore, be immediately carried
into the open air, and let the air be fanned back-
wards and forwards to affist its action; let cold
water be thrown on the face, and let the face,
mouth and noftrils be repeatedly wafhed; and as
foon as practicable, get the patient to drink fome
cold water.   But if the cafe be too far gone to be
thus relieved, let a healthy perfon breathe into the
mouth of the patient; and gently force air into
the mouth, throat and noftrils.   Frictions, cupping, bleeding, and blifters are likewife indicated.
And if after the inftant danger is removed a
fever be excited, the method of cure muft be
adapted to the nature and prevailing fymptoms of
the fever.

E S S A Y VII.

O N   T H E

A T R A B I L I S.

THE ancients, as appears from Galen, fup-
poſed the *atrabilis* to be derived either from
the dregs of the blood, or from yellow bile torrefied and highly concoĉted.   A celebrated modern
anatomiſt is of opinion that it is blood, which
having lodged ſome time in the inteſtinal canal,
has acquired a blacknefs and putridity.   But is it
not more probable that, in general, it is no other
than gall, become acrid by ſtagnation in the *veſica
feilea*, and rendered viſcid by the abſorption of its
fluid parts ?   When diſcharged into the *duodenum*
in this ſtate, it occaſions univerſal diſturbance and
diſorder, till evacuated either by vomiting or
purging.   I have lately had under my care
a young Gentleman, labouring under a *maraſmus*,
produced by exceſſive intemperance.   During
the courſe of his diſorder, which at laſt proved
fatal,

fatal, he feveral times voided both by ftool and vomiting, a confiderable quantity of black, tenacious, and moft offenfive bile. The fymptoms preceding the difcharge, and which ceafed foon afterwards, were a quick pulfe, head-ach, delirium, hiccup, intenfe thirft, inward heat, and an uncommon fœtor in his breath. A lady aged thirty, unhappily addicted to habits which have a peculiarly pernicious effect upon the liver, after a conftipation of the belly during fix days, was feized with a violent and inceffant vomiting of black and vifcid bile. The *infufum fenæ limoniatum,* warmed with the tincture of Columbo foon checked her retchings, and operating by ftool, prevented the return of her vomiting. The matter difcharged in both thefe cafes bore not the leaft refemblance to grumous blood. I have feveral times obferved the febrile fymptoms in children, which are afcribed to dentition, relieved by thefe pitchy ftools. And I recollect three cafes of the *acute afthma,* as Dr. Millar names it, the paroxyfms of which feemed to be critically terminated by a fimilar evacuation. Whether, in thefe inftances, the black bile was the caufe or the effect of the difeafe, cannot, with certainty, be determined; but the former appears to be the more probable opinion.

E S S A Y

E S S A Y VIII.

ON THE

SEPTIC QUALITY

OF

SEA SALT,

&c. &c.

SIR JOHN PRINGLE has ſhewn, that one drachm of ſea ſalt preſerves two drachms of freſh beef, in two ounces of water, above thirty hours uncorrupted, in a heat equal to that of the human body, that is, twenty hours longer than water alone; but that half a drachm of ſalt does not preſerve it above two hours longer than pure water; that twenty-five grains have little or no antiſeptic virtue; and that ten grains both heighten and haſten the corruption of the fleſh (a). The reſult of this experiment is ſo curious and un-expected, that I wiſhed to inveſtigate the cauſe of it.

(a) Pringle's Diſeaſes of the Army, Appendix, p. 38.

EXPERIMENT

EXPERIMENT I. May 15, 1772. Equal parts, viz. two drachms, of the lean of mutton, chopped very fmall, were feparately put into five wide mouthed phials, and to each were added two ounces of pump water. Ten grains of fea falt were diffolved in the firft; the fame quantity of brown bay falt in the fecond; of *fal catharticus amarus* in the third; and of true Glauber's falt in the fourth. The fifth contained only flefh and water, and was intended for a ftandard. The bottles were flightly corked, and after a gentle agitation placed in a window, expofed to the weftern fun. The mercury in Fahrenheit's thermometer then ftood in the fhade at 65 degrees.

IN twenty-nine hours the mixture which contained the *fal catharticus amarus* had acquired fomewhat of a putrid taint.

IN forty hours the ftandard was flightly offenfive. The mixture with fea falt was putrid, and that with the cathartic falt was yet more putrid.

IN fifty hours the ftandard and the two mixtures above-mentioned were equally putrid. The two others were fweet.

IN fixty-two hours the ftandard was become much more offenfively putrid than the two mixtures with fea falt, and cathartic falt, in which the putrefactive procefs appeared not to have advanced any further. The flefh, with the brown
bay

bay falt, was now flightly tainted; but that with the true Glauber's falt was ftill fweet.

In feventy-five hours the mixture with brown bay falt was become putrid, and that with the true Glauber's falt a little offenfive. And in twelve hours longer the latter mixture was alfo putrid.

From this experiment it appears that common falt, in the quantity of ten grains, promotes putrefaction; and that the *fal catharticus amarus*, in the fame proportion, is yet more feptic; but that bay falt, in this quantity, refifts putrefaction; and that true glauber's falt exceeds, in this refpect, even bay falt. The feptic and antifeptic qualities of thefe falts, when ufed in fo fmall a quantity, are therefore evidently dependent on, and proportioned to their degrees of purity. Alimentary falt, it is well known, contains in its cryftals an earthy falt, fimilar to that of Epfom; which is a powerful ferment, almoft equally capable in a fmall as in a large quantity, of exciting the putrefactive procefs in fubftances difpofed to it Whereas the pure neutral itfelf, which confifts of the muriatic acid and the foffil alkali, can only exert its antifeptic powers when ufed in a proportion adequate to the action of the bitter falt it is combined with, and fuperior to the putrid
tendency

tendency of the animal flesh, it is employed to preserve (b).

EXPERIMENT II. May 21. Six days from the commencement of the experiment, the pieces of flesh in the solutions of common salt, and of *sal catharticus amarus*, were not more offensive than on the third day; and the mixtures emitted no air bubbles. But the standard, at this time, was intolerably putrid, very frothy, and the bits of mutton had risen to the surface of the water.

THIS experiment shews that both sea salt and the bitter purging salt, though they quicken putrefaction, prevent the progress of it beyond a certain degree. A quality which must increase the usefulness of the former, as a seasoning to our food.

A LATE eminent and learned writer has related the history of a violent scurvy, produced by drinking sea water. A young lady, aged sixteen, tall, thin, and of a delicate constitution, though in tolerably good health, was advised to use sea water on account of a strumous swelling and inflammation of the upper lip. She drank a pint of it every morning, ten days successively; which

(b) SIR JOHN PRINGLE informs me, he has long suspected, but never ascertained the fact by experiment, that the septic quality of sea salt is owing to some heterogeneous substance joined to it.

did

did not pafs off freely by the ufual evacuations. At the end of this period, fhe was fuddenly feized with a profufe difcharge of the *catamenia*, was perpetually fpitting blood from the gums, and had innumerable petechial fpots on different parts of her body. Her pulfe was quick, though full; her face pale and fomewhat bloated; and her flefh foft and tender. She was often faint, but foon recovered her fpirits. The flux from the *uterus* at length abated; but that from the gums in-creafed to fuch a degree, that her apothecary took a little blood from her arm. From the orifice blood continually oozed for feveral days.. At laft an hæmorrhage from the nofe came on, attended with frequent faintings, in which fhe at length expired, choaked as it were with her own blood. Before fhe died, her right arm was mortified from the elbow to the wrift. And it is further to be remarked, that though blood let from her, fome weeks before fhe began the ufe of fea water, was fufficiently denfe; yet that drawn in her laft ficknefs was mere putrid, and diffolved gore (*c*).

DR. HUXHAM explains the diffolvent action of fea water, in this inftance, by fuppofing an accumulation of the marine falt in the mafs of blood, which running into *moleculæ*, too large

(*c*) Vide Philof. Tranfact. vol. LIII. p. 6.

to

to pafs the minuteft veffels, occafioned ftagnations; and by irritating the capillaries, produced ruptures of them, extravafations, blotches, and livid fpots. But do not the preceding experiments fuggeft a better folution of the fact? Sea water abounds with the cathartic falt, which conftitutes the bittern of it; and this has been proved to be a powerful feptic.

A PHYSICIAN, who often takes magnefia, to correct an acidity in his ftomach, arifing from indigeftion, invariably obferves that the difcharges which it produces are peculiarly putrid and offenfive. Hence it is probable that this earth, combined with an acid of the vegetable, as well as of the mineral clafs, promotes putrefaction. Should we not, therefore, employ the *fal catharticus amarus* and *magnefia alba* with caution, in difeafes of a putrid tendency?

I CANNOT omit this opportunity of recommending the calcination of magnefia, as a great improvement of that medicine. The lofs of its fixed air, which by this procefs appears to conftitute feven twelfths of its weight, obviates the flatulence which it produces in the *primæ viæ*, without diminifhing its purgative or abforbent qualities. Care, however, fhould be taken that the magnefia be free from any calcareous earth, otherwife the action of the fire will render this mild powder offenfively cauftic to the ftomach,

as

as I have more than once experienced. Magnesia may be calcined with very little trouble, in a common crucible, placed in a glowing fire, and kept red hot during the space of two hours. This improvement was suggested to me by a physician in London, distinguished for his knowledge of chemistry.

ESSAY

E S S A Y IX.

ON

C O F F E E.

THOUGH Coffee has been in general ufe
for more than a century paſt, has been ana-
lyſed by fire, and variouſly inveſtigated by writers of learning and reputation; yet neither chemiſtry nor experience have hitherto aſcertained
its true nature, or medicinal qualities. Of this
the contradictory teſtimonies which have been delivered concerning it, afford a painful evidence.
For it is ſurely to be lamented that an article
of diet, active in its powers, and univerſally employed, ſhould be ſo little underſtood. The following experiments may perhaps lead to farther
inquiries on this uſeful ſubject.

EXPERIMENT I.   Thirty berries of roaſted,
and the ſame number of unroaſted Coffee were
each digeſted, forty-eight hours, in two ounces of
rectified ſpirit of wine. The former tincture was
ſtrongly impregnated with the peculiar taſte and

odour

odour of the Coffee; the latter had acquired little or no fenfible flavour.

EXPERIMENT II. Ten drops of a folution of green vitriol, were added to a tea fpoonful of each of the above-mentioned tinctures, diluted with an ounce of water. Both affumed a purple colour; but the change was greateft in the tincture prepared with unroafted Coffee. A fimilar difference was obfervable in the infufions of roafted and unroafted Coffee, prepared with water, allowance being made for the dark hue communicated to the *menftruum* by the roafted Coffee.

THESE facts evince the action of fire in diminifhing aftringency; and furnifh an additional proof of the impropriety of employing heat in preparations of the bark, and other vegetables of a like quality.

EXPERIMENT III. Two drachms of roafted mutton, chopped very fmall, were digefted in an ounce of pump water, and in the fame quantity of a ftrong infufion of roafted Coffee. The phials which contained the mixtures, were placed at a moderate diftance from the fire, fo as to be kept nearly blood warm. In thirty hours the mutton and water became putrid; but the infufion of Coffee continued fweet twelve hours longer.

EXPERIMENT

EXPERIMENT IV. To illuftrate the action of Coffee on the digeftion of food in the ftomach, I prepared three alimentary mixtures, confifting of equal parts, viz. two drachms, of roafted mutton, of the crumb of bread, and of faliva, beat into a pulp, and feverally combined with an ounce of the infufions of coffee, of green tea, and the fame quantity of pump water. The bottles were placed, as in the former experiment, at a proper diftance from the fire, and every now and then carefully examined. A fermentation was firft perceived in the ftandard, i. e. the mixture with pump water, which became four in about forty-eight hours. The infufion of Coffee emitted few air bubbles, and continued near four days without fhewing any figns of acidity. By an accident, the phial, which contained the tea, was broken at the beginning of the experiment.

EXPERIMENT V. March 29, 1772. I awoke at five o'clock in the morning with the head-ach. My pulfe was hard and full, and beat 92 ftrokes in a minute. I drank four difhes of ftrong Coffee. In half an hour the pain in my head was relieved; yet my pulfe ftill continued to vibrate the fame number of times, but was fofter and lefs full. In an hour it funk to 70. In an hour and a half it rofe again to 76; and in two hours to 80, which is the ftandard of its frequency in health. I was in a recumbent pofture during the whole time of this experiment, which I have fince repeated feveral times, under different circumftances, with no material variation in the refult.

FROM thefe obfervations we may infer, that Coffee is flightly aftringent, and antifeptic; that it moderates alimentary fermentation; and that it is powerfully fedative. Its action on the nervous fyftem probably depends on the oil it contains; which receives its flavour, and is rendered mildly empyreumatic by the procefs of roafting. Neumann obtained, by diftillation, from one pound of Coffee, five ounces, five drachms and a half of water; fix ounces and half a drachm of thick fœtid oil, and four ounces and two drachms of a *caput mortuum*. And it is well known that rye, torrefied with a few almonds, which furnifh the neceffary proportion of oil, is now frequently employed as a fubftitute for thefe berries.

THE MEDICINAL QUALITIES of Coffee feem to be derived from the grateful fenfation which it produces in the ftomach; and from the fedative powers it exerts on the *vis vitæ*. Hence it affifts digeftion, and relieves the head-ach; and is taken in large quantities, with peculiar propriety, by the Turks and Arabians, becaufe it counteracts the narcotic effects of opium, to the ufe of which thofe nations are much addicted.

IN

In delicate habits it often occafions watchfulnefs, tremors, and many of thofe complaints which are denominated nervous. It has even been fufpected of producing palfies; and from my own obfervation I fhould apprehend, not entirely without foundation. Slare affirms that he became paralytic by the too liberal ufe of Coffee; and that his diforder was removed by abftinence from that liquor.

Coffee berries are faid to be remarkably difpofed to imbibe exhalations from other bodies, and thereby to acquire an adventitious and difagreeable flavour. A bottle of rum, placed at fome diftance from a canifter of Coffee, fo impregnated the berries, in a fhort time, as to injure their flavour. Some years fince a few bags of pepper were conveyed, in a Coffee-fhip from India, the effluvia of which being abforbed by the Coffee, the whole cargo was fpoiled *(a)*.

P. S. 1776. A phyfician* was affected with a fevere head-ach, October 19, 1774, in confequence of having been difturbed in the night. At two o'clock in the afternoon he took eighteen

(a) Miller's Gardener's Dictionary, eighth edit. Article, Coffee.

* The author of thefe Obfervations.

drops

drops of laudanum; and immediately afterwards, three difhes of very ftrong Coffee. He lay down, and endeavoured to compofe himfelf to fleep. His pain abated in half an hour; and in an hour was entirely removed: but he felt not the leaft difpofition to fleep, though he is often drowfy after dinner, and fometimes indulges himfelf in fleeping at that time.

November 1. HE repeated, on a fimilar occafion, the ufe of laudanum and Coffee, in the like quantity as before. The effects were pre-cifely the fame; eafe from pain, but no difpo-fition to fleep.

November 16. HE took eighteen drops of laudanum, when fuffering under the head-ach, but without Coffee. The opiate compofed him to fleep in an hour; but did not entirely remove the pain in his head. Thefe facts confirm a remark which I have before made, that Coffee is taken, with peculiar propriety, by the Turks and Arabians, becaufe it counteracts the narcotic effects of opium.

A VERY ftrong infufion of Coffee affords moft relief, in pains of the head, when taken cold. And, in this form, it is an ufeful and agreeable vehicle to *Sp. Æther. Sp. Vol. Aromat. Elixir Paregor.* and other antifpafmodic remedies. In the delirium of fevers, efpecially if the patient be comatofe, Coffee is an excellent auxiliary to the

usual

ufual means employed. The odour of it is peculiarly grateful; and if inhaled a fufficient length of time, proves powerfully fedative. Mr. Pope is faid to have derived great benefit from it, under the fevere head-achs, to which he was liable; and I have feen many inftances of its efficacy.

A DECOCTION of raw Coffee berries fweetened with honey, has been recommended in the gravel. I have no experience of the falutary effects of Coffee in this diforder; but I know that both roafted and raw it is an active diuretic; and I have frequently prefcribed it with fome fuccefs in dropfies, efpecially when originating from hepatic obftructions.

THE following curious and important obfervation is extracted from a letter, with which I was favoured by Sir John Pringle, in April 1773. " On reading your fection concerning Coffee, " one quality occurred to me which I had.ob- " ferved of that liquor, confirming what you have " faid of its fedative virtues. It is the beft abater " of the paroxyfms-of the periodic afthma, that " I have feen. The Coffee ought to be of the " beft Mocco, newly burnt, and made very " ftrong immediately after grinding it. I have " commonly ordered an ounce for one difh; which " is to be repeated frefh after the interval of a " quarter, or half an hour; and which I direct to

" be

" be taken without milk or fugar. The medi-
" cine in general is mentioned by Mufgrave,
" in his Treatife *de Arthritide anomala* ; but I
" firſt heard of it from a phyſician of this place,
" who having once practiſed at Lichfield, had
" been informed by the old people of that place,
" that Sir John Floyer, during the latter years of
" his life, kept free from, or at leaſt lived eafy
" under his afthma, from the uſe of very ſtrong
" Coffee. This difcovery, it feems, he made
" after the publication of his book upon that
" diſeaſe." Since the receipt of this letter, I
have frequently directed Coffee in the afthma
with great fuccefs.

A REVIEW OF THE MOST IMPORTANT CONCLU-
SIONS DEDUCED FROM THE PRECEDING EXPE-
RIMENTS.

1, COLUMBO-ROOT yields its virtues
moſt perfectly to rectified ſpirit of wine ;
and to other *menſtrua*, in the following order.
1. to French brandy.   2. to Madeira wine.
3. to white wine.   4. to diſtilled water.   5. to
white wine vinegar.   6. to hard pump water.

2. THE

2. THE watery infusion of Columbo-root is more perishable than that of other bitters. In twenty-four hours a copious precipitation takes place in it; and in two days it becomes ropy, and even musty.

3. THE addition of orange peel renders the infusion of Columbo-root less ungrateful to the palate.

4. TWELVE ounces of Columbo-root yield eight ounces and two drachms of extract, which retains the entire flavour of the root, and is equal, if not superior in efficacy to the powder.

5. PERUVIAN BARK resists the putrefaction of animal flesh more powerfully than the Columbo-root; but as a preservative of the bile from putridity, this root exceeds the cortex.

6. PERUVIAN BARK, mixed with putrid gall, instantly produces a coagulation, and considerably increases the fœtor of it. Whereas the infusion of Columbo-root unites perfectly with it, and very powerfully corrects its offensive smell. This serves, in some measure, to explain the action of this remedy in the *cholera morbus*, and other diseases attended with a redundance and depravation of the bile.

7. COLUMBO-ROOT moderates, without suspending the fermentation of alimentary mixtures; prevents them from growing four; and neutra-

lizes

lizes acidities when formed, much more completely than Peruvian bark, or chamomile flowers.

8. Columbo-root does not increase the quickness of the pulse; and may therefore be used with propriety in the *phthisis pulmonalis*, and in hectical cases, to correct acrimony, and to strengthen the organs of digestion.

9. The Columbo-root is an useful remedy in the *cholera morbus*; in diarrhœas; in the dysentery; in bilious fevers; in a languid state of the stomach, attended with want of appetite, nausea, and indigestion; and in habitual vomitings, when they proceed from a weakness or irritability of the stomach, from an irregular gout, from acidities, or from acrimonious bile.

10. The Orchis-root might be cultivated to great advantage in England, and salep, which is a preparation of it, might be afforded at eightpence or ten-pence *per* pound. Whereas foreign salep is now sold at five or six shillings *per* pound.

11. Rice, as an aliment, is inferior to Salep, being slow of fermentation, and a very weak corrector of putrefaction. It is therefore an improper diet for hospital patients; and more particularly for sailors, in long voyages; because it seems incapable of preventing, and will not contribute much to check the progress of that fatal disease, the sea scurvy.

12. Cheese,

12. CHEESE, when mellowed by age, ferments readily with flesh and water; but separates a rancid oil, which appears to be incapable of any further change, and must, as a septic, be pernicious in the scurvy. The same objection may be urged, with still greater propriety, against the use of cheese in hospitals; because convalescents are so liable to relapses, that the slightest error of diet may occasion them.

13. SALEP has the singular property of concealing the taste of salt water; a circumstance of the highest importance at sea, when there is a scarcity of fresh water.

14. SALEP retards the acetous fermentation of milk; and consequently would be a good lithing for milk pottage, especially in large towns, where the cattle, being fed upon sour draft, must yield ascescent milk.

15. SALEP, in a certain proportion, would be an useful and profitable addition to bread. For by absorbing and retaining more water than flour alone is capable of, it occasions a considerable increase of weight.

16. BUXTON WATER is found, by analysis, to contain calcareous earth, fossil alkali, and sea salt; but in very small proportions: For a gallon of the water, when evaporated, yields only twenty-four grains of sediment.

17. THE

17. The temperature of Buxton bath, is 82 degrees of Fahrenheit's thermometer; that of St. Ann's well somewhat lefs.

18. Buxton water, when drunk, quickens the pulfe very confiderably, and fometimes occafions the head-ach. By the mineral fpirit which it contains, it readily diffolves iron; and fuch an impregnation muft, in many cafes, improve its medicinal virtues.

19. Matlock water is grateful to the palate, and of an agreeable warmth, but exhibits no marks of any mineral fpirit. It is very flightly impregnated with *felenites*, and contains a fmall portion of fea falt. Some have fuppofed that it is a chalybeate, but without foundation.

20. The Briftol and Matlock waters appear to refemble each other, both in their chemical and medicinal qualities.

21. Matlock bath raifes Fahrenheit's thermometer to the 68th; the fpring to the 66th degree.

22. Fixed air may, in no confiderable quantity, be breathed without danger or uneafinefs. And in feveral cafes of the *phthifis pulmonalis*, the fteams of an effervefcing mixture of chalk and vinegar, have been infpired with great advantage. Antifeptic fumigations and vapours have been long employed and much extolled in fuch diforders. But their efficacy does not appear to
depend

depend on the extrication of fixed air from their substance.

23. THERE appears to be a diversity in the properties, and effects of different species of factitious air.

24. THE fixed air of metals seems to be of a kind different from what is contained in alkalis and calcareous earth: And consequently the action of these substances as *fluxes* cannot be explained on the principle of their restoring the air, which had been lost by calcination.

25. COMMON SALT, in the quantity of ten grains, promotes putrefaction; the *sal catharticus amarus*, in the same proportion, is yet more septic; but BAY SALT in this quantity resists putrefaction; and GLAUBER'S SALT exceeds, in this respect, even BAY SALT. The septic and antiseptic qualities of these salts, when used in so minute a quantity, is therefore evidently dependent on, and proportionate to their degrees of purity.

26. SEA SALT, and the bitter purging salt, though they quicken putrefaction, prevent the progress of it beyond a certain degree a quality which must increase the usefulness of the former, as a seasoning to our food.

27. COFFEE is slightly astringent, and antiseptic; moderates alimentary fermentation; is

diuretic

diuretic; and powerfully fedative. Its action on the nervous fyftem probably depends on the oil it contains; which receives a new flavour, and is rendered mildly empyreumatic by the procefs of roafting *(b)*.

(b) Studious, literary men, and thofe confined by their occupations or profeffions to a fedentary courfe of life, are peculiarly incident to head-ach, indigeftion, acidity, flatulence, a painful diftenfion of the ftomach. To fuch I recommend the daily ufe of a few grains of rhubarb, immediately before dinner; and two or three difhes of very ftrong coffee, about an hour after it.

SELECT

SELECT HISTORIES

OF

DISEASES,

WITH REMARKS.

Longum iter per precepta; breve et efficax per exempla.
SENECA.

─────────────

(a) THE HISTORY AND CURE OF A DIFFICULTY IN DEGLUTITION, OF LONG CONTINUANCE, ARISING FROM A SPASMODIC AFFECTION OF THE OESOPHAGUS.

MISS L——r, aged thirteen, a fprightly girl, of a delicate and irritable habit of body, during feveral years had a difficulty of fwallowing; which occafionally left her for a month or two, and then fuddenly returned without any apparent caufe. September 3, 1768, I was defired to vifit her. She had then laboured under her diforder fix or eight months without any intermiffion, and was reduced almoft to a fkeleton,

(a) THIS Cafe was read before the College of Phyficians, Auguft 9, 1769, and is publifhed in the Medical Tranfactions, vol. II.

though

though she still retained her natural vivacity.
When she attempted to swallow solids, they
passed down readily as far as the upper orifice of
the stomach; but when arrived there, they were
instantly, and with a strong convulsive motion,
thrown up again. Liquids sipped slowly, and
swallowed leisurely, met with no resistance; but
if hastily drunk, or in too large a quantity,
they were quickly regurgitated. Warm liquors
were swallowed with more ease than cold ones;
and in the evening, the difficulty in deglutition
generally abated. She complained of no other
pain but an uneasy craving in her stomach; nor
was there any external swelling, or inward soreness, through the whole passage of the *œsophagus*.
When she was in her ninth year the *catamenia*
appeared, and had recurred once or twice since
that time, without any regularity. Her belly
was costive; her pulse was quick and small; and
her feet were usually cold. She was neither of
a strumous nor scorbutic habit of body; and
her friends could give me no satisfactory account
of the origin or cause of her disorder.

I APPREHENDED her case to be spasmodic,
complicated with a slight thickening of the
œsophagus about the part affected, the consequence
of a contraction so long continued. The following medicines were therefore prescribed.

R. *Elixir.*

R. *Elixir. myrrhæ comp. tinct. valerian. vol. aa.*
ʒiv. M. dentur guttæ viginti in thea pulegii
bis die.

R. *Ol. amygdal. ʒj. sp. sal. ammon. cum calce*
viva ʒvj. camphoræ oleo solutæ ʒij. ol. succin.
ʒiss. M. f. linimentum, quo bene fricetur spina
dorsi, a prima cervicis vertebra usque ad duo-
decimam dorsalem, mane & vesperi quotidie.

R. *Merc. dulcis sexies sublimat. gr. ss. mucilag.*
gum. Arab. ℈ij. sp. nitri dulcis ℈ij. vin. an-
timon. gutt. vj. Aq. fontan. ʒss. Sacchari alb.
℈j. M. f. haust. hora decubitus quotidie su-
mendus, vini antimonialis dosin sensim augendo.

R. *Extract. cort. Peruvian. mollis. castor. Russic.*
galban. colat. aa. partes æquales, camphoræ sp.
vin. rect. trit. ʒj. ol. succini. ℈j. balsam. Pe
ruvian. q. s. M. f. emplastrum scrobiculo cordis
applicandum, & semel in septimana renovandum.

DIRECTIONS were given that her feet and legs
ſhould be kept warm; that her drinks ſhould
not be taken cold; that her diet ſhould conſiſt of
broth, mutton, or beef tea, as it is called, panada
vermicelli, ſago, rice, milk, chocolate, cocoa,
ſalep, &c. that a little wine ſhould be occaſionally
allowed; that ſhe ſhould abſtain from tea and
coffee; that moderate exerciſe ſhould be daily
uſed; and that a nouriſhing clyſter, prepared of
milk, broth, &c. ſhould be injected every morning and noon; to obviate the looſening effect
of

of which, a few red rose leaves were ordered to be boiled in it, or a little starch to be added to it.

SEPTEMBER 22. The liniment, calomel draught, and clyster, had been neglected. But the plaster had been applied; she had taken the drops with regularity, and had carefully observed the regimen prescribed to her. The difficulty in deglutition was sensibly abated, her appetite was mended, and she had recovered flesh and strength.

October 1. The mercurial draught had purged her. To prevent this effect, fifteen or twenty drops of *elixir paregoricum* were added. But a few days afterwards it occasioned a soreness in her gums, and a slight salivation. The use of it was therefore discontinued.

October 21. She could now swallow solid food without any difficulty. Her appetite was good, her belly regular, her pulse fuller and slower, her flesh and strength recruited, and her health, in every other respect, was perfectly re-established. I directed her to continue the use of her medicines, and to persevere in her regimen a month or two longer; and she has ever since been entirely free from her disorder.

I SHALL beg leave to make some general observations on obstructed deglutition, without confining myself to the particular consideration of the case which has been related.

I. A DIFFICULTY

I. A DIFFICULTY in fwallowing may proceed from fuch a variety of caufes, not eafy to be diftinguifhed, and yet each requiring a particular method of cure, that the phyfician's practice in fuch cafes muft be uncertain and perplexed. And what adds confiderably to this embarraffment is, that the effect often co-operates with the original caufe, and confirms the difeafe. Thus a con-ftriction of the *æfophagus*, arifing from a fpafmodic affection, will, if it continue long, produce either an enlargement of the glands, or a thickening of the fubftance of the gullet, about the part affected. On the contrary, if the ftricture proceed from a glandular tumour, from fchirrofities, or fungous excrefcences, it will at the fame time be com-plicated with fome degree of fpafm; of which, amongft feveral inftances that have fallen under my obfervation, I fhall mention the following. A farmer's wife, aged fifty, of a ftrumous habit, perceived an impediment in her throat to the paffage of folid food, fome months before fhe applied for advice. Her diforder had increafed by degrees, and fhe was then unable to fwallow any thing but liquids. A furgeon examined the gullet with a probe, and found the two glands, which are fituated about the fifth vertebra of the back, confiderably enlarged. Æther was then a fafhionable remedy in this part of the country; and fhe was induced, by the fame of its effects,

VOL. I.   B b   to to wish a trial might be made of it. A dose, properly diluted, was given her, and about half an hour afterwards she had the power of swallowing, without much difficulty, a morsel of solid food. But the relief was only temporary. She relapsed in an hour or two, and had again recourse to the same remedy, which after a few trials lost all its efficacy; and the poor woman having languished about six months, died literally famished. From this and other instances, I should apprehend that the use of antispasmodics would assist the operation of the mercurial course, so judiciously recommended by Dr. Munckley in the first volume of the Medical Transactions; and would quicken, as well as render more certain the cure of this deplorable disease.

II. In spasmodic affections of the *œsophagus*, external applications to the spine are likely to be very serviceable, from the contiguity of that tube to the *vertebræ*. And, perhaps, nothing would be more effectual in such cases than a blister, applied either to the neck, or between the shoulders. That epispastics are powerful antispasmodics, experience hath fully ascertained; and when the disorder is attended with an enlargement of the substance, or a fullness of the glands of the gullet, they would have additional efficacy, by producing a copious discharge of serous humours,

and

and by that mean unloading the veffels of the part affected.

VOLATILE and antifpafmodic liniments are alfo highly ufeful, as the cafe above recited fufficiently evinces. It is indeed to be lamented that external applications of this kind are not more frequently employed in practice; for there is juft reafon to apprehend that powerful effects might be expected from them in various difeafes. In the hooping cough particularly, I have obferved confiderable benefit to accrue from the ufe of a liniment, fimilar to the one prefcribed above.

III. WHEN conftrictions of the *œfophagus*, arifing from fpafm, have been of long continuance, and do not yield to medicine, electricity furnifhes us with no improbable means of relief. The public indeed have been much difappointed in the medical effects of electricity. But this hath, in part, proceeded from the mifapplication of fo powerful a remedy. It appears to me, and I am confirmed in this opinion by the obfervation of a very eminent phyfician, that the electric fhock bids fair to do much more good in difeafes from rigidity, than in thofe from laxity. Amongft many other proofs of this, may be adduced the cure of an univerfal *tetanus*, the hiftory of which is publifhed by Dr. Watfon, in one of the late volumes of the Philofophical Tranfactions.

B b 2 IV. STIMU-

IV. STIMULATING vapours conveyed into the *pharynx* have a tendency to remove spasms, even when seated deep in the *œsophagus*. A few years ago, an elderly gentlewoman, after eating pease, felt an uneasy sensation as if one of them stuck low down in her throat, and suddenly found herself deprived of the power of deglutition. Notwithstanding the use of a variety of remedies, her inability to swallow continued five or six days. She was directed to fumigate her throat with *assafœtida*, dissolved in a strong infusion of the aromatic herbs: and drawing in the vapours very forcibly, the spasm was instantly resolved; nor has she ever since suffered the least return of it.

V. WHEN this dreadful disease is so confirmed as to be deemed incurable, the patient's life may be prolonged by the daily injection of nutritive clysters, and by bathing his feet, hands, and arms, and occasionally his whole body, in new milk, broth, decoctions of salep, sago, or vermicelli, &c. The absorption by the lymphatics of the skin is very considerable. It has been found by experiment that the hand, after being well chafed, will imbibe, in a quarter of an hour, nearly an ounce and a half of warm water. And allowing that the surface of the hand is to that of the body as one to sixty, the absorption of the whole, in the same space of time, would amount to upwards of seven pounds. The

copious

copious discharge of urine in the *diabetes,* so much exceeding in quantity the patient's drink, confirms in some measure this calculation. And the curious fact related by Dr. Chalmers, at the same time that it affords a further proof of the great absorption by the pores of the skin, points out to us the valuable purposes to which it may be applied, in the disorder under consideration. A negro man, who had eaten or drunk but little before he was gibbeted, in March, 1759, at Charles Town in South Carolina, and had nothing given him afterwards, regularly voided every morning a large quantity of urine, but discharged no more till about the same hour the next day. The dews of the evening, imbibed by the body, supplied in this case a superabundance of fluids in the night, and a sufficient quantity to support perspiration in the day. Had these fluids been of a nutritious quality, it is not improbable that, even under such circumstances, the poor negro might have been kept alive for a considerable length of time.

Prosper Alpinus relates that the Egyptian women, in order to become fat, use every day a tepid bath; and whilst they continue in it, receive nourishing clysters, and a variety of the richest foods. By these means the females of that country, particularly the Hebrew women who reside there, are for the most part immoderately

B b 3   corpulent.

corpulent. *Illarum plurimæ perinde ac sues cernun-*
tur pinguissimæ humi recumbentes, maximeque Hebreæ,
quibus istud vitii aliis familiarius observatur.

I HAVE not enlarged upon the necessity of conveying aliment into the body by clysters, in obstructions of the *æsophagus*, because this must be
obvious to every practitioner. The other method of nutrition, if not less known, is certainly
less attended to, and in general is altogether neglected. It may perhaps be thought an omission,
that no notice has been taken of the administra-
tion of medicines under the form of clysters, in
these deplorable cases. But I apprehend, however useful they might be in many respects, they
would, in general, too much interfere with the
nourishment of the patient.

CASES

C A S E S

of

D R O P S I E S.

C<small>ASE</small> I. MRS. P———N, aged 33, a
woman of a very delicate con-
ftitution, and fubject to a *profluvium menfium*,
which had greatly impaired her ftrength, perceived, about two years ago, an indolent, moveable tumour in the lower part and left fide of her
belly, which gradually though flowly increafed.
Before it acquired any confiderable bulk, her
right leg began to fwell, her urine was voided
in fmall quantity; the fymptoms of thirft and
inward heat enfued; the *abdomen* became enlarged; a fluctuation was foon perceptible; and
a complete *afcites* was formed.

T<small>HE</small> tumour in the lower part of her belly,
which from its fituation I apprehend was an incyfted dropfy of the left *ovarium*, now began to
be extremely painful, the fwelling of the *abdomen*

B b 4

increafed,

increafed, a general *anafarca* was coming on,
and her cafe became every day more and more
deplorable. Such was the ftate of the diforder,
when the patient, as fhe arofe out of bed in the
morning, (February 2, 1771,) was feized with
a naufea, without any apparent caufe, fucceeded
by a violent vomiting. At three o'clock in the
afternoon I was firft called to her affiftance, and
found her quite exhaufted with inceffant retchings.
Her pulfe was fo feeble as to be fcarcely perceptible, her extremities were cold, and her legs and
thighs were affected with a moft painful fpafm.
She had difcharged near ten pints of water, and
this evacuation had entirely removed the anafarcous fwellings, and greatly diminifhed the fullnefs and tenfion of the belly. The tumour of
the left *ovarium*, though much decreafed in bulk,
was evident to the touch, and appeared to be
ftill moveable under the fingers. Gentle cordials
were directed to fupport the patient's ftrength;
warm fomentations were applied to her legs and
thighs; and an opiate was adminiftered, to procure for her a fhort interval of reft and eafe. She
enjoyed a few hours refrefhing fleep; the vomiting then recurred, and continued five or fix
days, with intermiffions, which gradually became
longer and longer. Her thirft, during thefe
evacuations, was almoft infupportable; but fhe
refrained with great refolution from all liquids,
except

except a little red Port wine, diluted with mint
water. Oranges too were freely allowed, and
were highly grateful to her. All her dropfical
fwellings were now removed; and the tumour
of the *ovarium* itfelf was no longer perceptible.
When the vomiting ceafed, a gentle *diarrhœa*
fucceeded. An infufion of the bark, with the
fp. nitr. dulcis, and *tinct. mart. in fp. falis* wa-
given. Her thirft abated, her appetite returned,
and in a few weeks fhe recovered a tolerable degree of health and ftrength; and ftill continues
free from any of her former ailments, though it is
now four months from the time when her vomitings commenced. The quantity of water fhe
difcharged, exclufive of her evacuations by ftool
and urine, amounted to about three gallons.

THE cafe, before us, affords a ftriking proof
of the efforts which nature exerts to relieve herfelf. By what fecret inftruments this falutary
change was produced in the prefent inftance, we
may conjecture, but cannot afcertain. It is
not to be fuppofed that the extravafated fluids
paffed, by percolation, through the coats of the
ftomach or inteftines, and were then difcharged
by vomiting; becaufe thefe coats in the living body are inpervious to water, and tranfmit it only when the circulation ceafes, when
their veffels fhrink, and the *mucus*, lining the
internal cavity, is dried or abraded. Nor is it
eafy to conceive, how the hydropic cyft of the

ovarium

ovarium fhould thus empty itfelf into the ventricle; or fo large a quantity of water tranfude, with fuch rapidity, through the interftices of its fibres. For that the ftomach was not ruptured is evident from the fpeedy recovery of the patient. The effect therefore muft be afcribed, not to a mechanical caufe, but to that vital energy which, by imperceptible means, regulates the motions, and corrects the diforders of the animal frame; though fometimes with a degree of violence dangerous to, and even deftructive of life. In the prefent cafe, it appears probable, that a fudden change took place in the courfe of circulation; the lymphatics recovered their power of abforption, and performed their office with renewed vigour; the vafcular fyftem became overloaded, and the exhalant arteries of the ftomach and inteftines poured forth the fuperfluous fluids, reftoring thus the equilibrium.

INSTANCES of a fudden, and partially increafed action of the veffels frequently occur; as in the *diarrhœa*, *cholera morbus*, hyfteric difeafe, *profluvium urinæ*, &c. &c. But the following hiftory, related by Doctor Simfon, admirably illuftrates, and at the fame time confirms, what I have advanced. *Cum homo adolefcens, febri correptus, cui acceffcrat diarrhœa, cum extremo ftupore fenfuum, nihil plane ore haurire vellet (quamquam immoderato æftu totus torrefceret) quo humectaretur,*

jubeo

jubeo in aquam egelidam immergi pedes; quo facto,
protinus aquæ mirum cerno in vafe decrementum,
deinde ejufdem vixdum coloratæ, e veftigio impetuo-
fam, more cataractæ, per anum effufionem (a).

SEVERAL inftances are recorded of anafarcas,
and fome few even of the afcites, which have
been cured by vomiting. But I believe it has
rarely if ever happened, at leaft I do not recollect
fuch a cafe either in books or in practice, that a
dropfy of the *ovarium* has been removed by the
fpontaneous efforts of nature. Deductions from
fingular and folitary facts, though contrary to the
rules of philofophizing, are not always to be rejected; but may be allowed, with proper caution
and referve, when the nature of the fubject admits
not of better evidence. The hiftory before us
furnifhes, I apprehend, an exception to the general laws of reafoning by induction; and one inftance, well authenticated, of the cure of a difeafe,
which the moft eminent phyficians have confidered as irremediable, may juftly lead us, in
fimilar circumftances, to imitate by art the operations of nature; and to excite thofe efforts, which
when fpontaneous, have proved fo falutary. In
the incipient ftate of a dropfy of the *ovarium,*
emetics, repeatedly adminiftered, would be likely
means of promoting the abforption or difcharge

(a) Simfon de Re Medica, p. 183.

of

of the incyfted fluid. They produce the ftrongeft contractions in the abdominal mufcles, agitate all the vifcera of the lower belly, quicken the circulation of the blood, and by their general action on the whole fyftem, remove obftructions in the minuteft and moft remote feries of veffels. Hence the powerful effects of Turpeth vomits, in white fwellings of the joints; in which the glands are at leaft equally difeafed, and the extravafated fluid as much out of the courfe of circulation, as in the fpecies of dropfy we are now confidering. But unfortunately this diforder is fo infidious in its attack, and fo little alarming in its progrefs, that it becomes almoft incurable before the patient is apprehenfive of any degree of danger. However, in its more advanced ftages, emetics may be adminiftered with fafety, and fometimes perhaps with advantage. If the *morfus diaboli* adhere to the enlarged *ovarium*, and the fallopian tubes be not totally obftructed, the action of vomiting may force a paffage for the fluid, and thus procure at leaft fome temporary relief. I have now under my care a lady, who has long been afflicted with a dropfy of this kind, and who has frequent difcharges of bloody water from the womb, fucceeded always by a diminution of bulk. A troublefome *hernia* forbids the exhibition of an emetic, which otherwife I fhould not hefitate to direct. Befides we may poffibly be fo fortunate as to co-

operate

operate with nature at the moſt favourable conjuncture; and by affiſting her efforts, of themſelves perhaps too languid, may effect a cure. Such inſtances do not unfrequently occur, in almoſt every ſpecies of diſeaſe; and it is upon this principle alone, that we can explain the amazing ſucceſs which has attended the exhibition of remedies, by no means adequate to the effects produced by them. Mr. W. a hard drinker, when paſt the meridian of life, had a jaundice which was ſucceeded by an *aſcites*, a dropſy of the *thorax*, and an *anaſarca*. The prognoſtic was in this caſe extremely unfavourable, and I ſcarcely indulged the leaſt hope of his recovery. Diuretics, purgatives, &c. under various forms, were affiduouſly adminiſtered, but with no very advantageous effects. Amongſt other medicines, he had pills compoſed of *extract. jalap. pulv. ſcillar. ſiccat.* and *merc. dulcis*, and was directed to increaſe the doſe of theſe *pro re nata*. Finding the uſual quantity inſufficient to procure the neceſſary diſcharges, he took, if I recollect aright, two pills extraordinary, the conſequence of which was an *hypercatharſis*, which greatly reduced his ſtrength, but carried off all his dropſical ſwellings, and by the aid of cordials and corroborants, produced a perfect cure. The following curious caſe, communicated to me by a phyſician of eminence in a neighbouring town, further illuſtrates the
                                obſervation

observation advanced above; and at the same time shews the resources which medicine affords to a sagacious practitioner, in the most desperate stages of this disorder.

CASE II. Miss H. of Namptwich in Cheshire, aged upwards of forty, had laboured for some time under an *ascites*, when she was removed to Liverpool in February 1769, for the benefit of medical advice. Two physicians and a surgeon were consulted; and after a gentle evacuation by stool, and the exhibition of a few cardiacs, it was agreed that she should be tapped without delay. Eighteen pints of water were drawn off, and two large schirrous tumours, one nearly the size of an infant's head, the other not much less in bulk, were discovered. These she had perceived for many years, and they had succeeded a fever, imperfect in its crisis. The operation had almost proved fatal to her; her mouth was covered with *aphthæ*, and so many alarming symptoms came on, that death was hourly expected. However in a fortnight she was tolerably recovered, and in a month the *paracentesis* was again repeated. She bore it better, but soon filled again; and was obliged to submit to the operation every third week. Tired with the frequency of this painful palliative, after the fifteenth repetition of it, she requested one of her physicians, in a most pressing manner, to prescribe some medicine,

which

which might at leaft protract the period of tap-
ping. It was now the latter end of Auguft; the
weather was favourable, and he directed her to be
confined to her bed for three days; to be affiduoufly rubbed morning and evening with dry
cloths, impregnated with the fumes of camphor;
and to take internally the *julepum e camphora*,
prepared with only two thirds of a pint of water, and warmed with the addition of one
ounce of *aqua juniperi compofita*. Under this
form fhe took a drachm of camphor daily, for
the fpace of a fortnight. A continued gentle
diaphorefis was the happy confequence; every
day fhe decreafed in bulk; and the abatement
of her fwellings encouraged her refolutely to per-
fevere in the ufe of her medicine. She recovered
her health; and remained near two years free
from any dropfical complaints. But in the
fummer of 1771, her diforder recurred; and on
the 16th of July fhe was again tapped. On the
8th of October following, fhe voided by the *anus*
near twelve pints of a mucilaginous liquor, in
colour refembling *pus*, but without any offenfive
fmell. After this remarkable difcharge, fhe was
better for a fhort time; but a violent and very
painful aphthous complaint, attended with a profufe fpitting of vifcid phlegm and faliva, enfued;
by which her ftrength was exhaufted, and fhe
died on the 9th of November, quite emaciated.

O<small>N</small>

On the fame day, her body was opened in the prefence of two phyficians, and other gentlemen of the faculty; and I am favoured by Mr. Wickfted, a very ingenious furgeon at Nampt-wich, who attended the patient during her laft illnefs, with the following account of the appearances on diffection.

" On opening the abdomen, a large hard tu-
" mour prefented itfelf, which on examination
" feemed to be the right *ovarium* very much
" enlarged, and fchirrous. It was in figure like an
" impregnated *uterus*, filling the lower fpace of
" the abdomen, and rifing feveral inches above
" the brim of the *pelvis*. This fubftance was
" found attached to the *uterus*, and weighed three
" pounds and feven ounces. By its preffure the
" *uterus* and bladder were forced down into the
" lower part of the *pelvis*; and when divided, it
" refembled a piece of boiled udder, in colour and
" firmnefs.

" The left *ovarium* was very hard, and en-
" larged to the fize of a goofe egg. The body
" of the *uterus*, which with the bladder had been
" preffed by the weight of the tumour out of
" its ufual fituation, was hardly to be diftinguifhed
" from the left *ovarium*, which was nearly of the
" fame fize and firmly united with it, and feemed
" to be a little difeafed. The fallopian tubes
" were

" were almoſt obliterated. The bladder and
" ureters were found.

" The hydropic cyſt (which extended to the
" margin of the ribs, and appeared to be formed
" either from the diſtended peritonæal coats of the
" *ovaria*, or the duplicatures of the *peritonæum*)
" contained three quarters of a pint of a fluid,
" ſimilar to that which had been evacuated by
" ſtool.

" The ſtomach and inteſtines were in a found
" ſtate, and no where adhered to the above-
" mentioned cyſt. But at the bottom of the
" *pelvis* the cyſt had a *firm attachment to the*
" *rectum*, of the compaſs of half a crown; yet
" there was no viſible perforation, by which ſo
" large a quantity of fluids could eſcape. The
" *omentum* was waſted to a membranous ex-
" panſion. The kidnies, ſpleen, pancreas, and
" meſenteric glands were found. The ſubſtance
" of the liver was not at all diſeaſed, but its
" whole convex ſurface was fixed, by ſtrong
" adheſions, to the *diaphragm*. Both lobes of the
" lungs were found adhering to the *pleura*; their
" internal ſtructure, however, ſeemed to be per-
" fect. The heart was in a good ſtate; and
" the *pericardium* contained about two ounces of
" limpid water."

Case III. Mr. G. H. of Oldham, near Mancheſter, aged upwards of fifty, low of ſtature, cor

pulent, and habitually addicted to intemperance, in April, 1770, was afflicted with a dry cough, *dyspnœa, ascites;* and swelled legs. By the use of pills composed of *sapo venet. gum. ammoniac.* and *pulv. scillar.* and a mercurial cathartic, which I directed to be repeated at such intervals as not to debilitate his strength, he recovered his former state of health. But on the second of January, 1771, I was again called to his assistance: He had been suddenly seized, a few days before, with a difficulty of breathing, which increased rapidly, and was then attended with a cough and frothy expectoration: His pulse was languid and oppressed, his heat natural, his face bloated, and his legs were slightly œdematous: The *abdomen* was not fuller than usual, nor had he, previous to his attack, any symptoms of water in the cavity of the chest. A brisk purgative, *radix Senekæ, oxymel scillit.* blisters to the legs, *camphor, sal. volatile,* venesection, &c. &c. were tried, but without effect. Respiration became more and more laborious; and in two days the patient was freed from his sufferings by death.

IT appears probable that an *anasarca,* or infarction of the cellular membrane of the lungs, was the proximate cause of the *orthopnœa,* which in so short a time proved fatal to the patient. This disorder may, like other dropsies, arise from a general laxity of the solids, tenuity of the
fluids,

fluids, or obftructed circulation of the blood; but in fuch inftances the prefumption is, that it will be flowly and gradually produced. How then are we to account for its fudden and rapid formation in the cafe I have juft related? The ancient phyficians, who had no opportunities of diffecting human bodies, obferved in brutes, particularly in oxen, fheep, and fwine, large hydatids in the lungs; and to the rupture of thefe, Hippocrates and Galen, reafoning from analogy, afcribed the *hydrops pectoris* in the human fpecies. Willis and Morgagni have adopted their opinion, and confirmed the teftimony of the father of phyfic, and his learned commentators. Morgagni fays, *In fue autem, cæteroquin fano, ut cætera ejufmodi hic omittam, a me in beftiis, hominibufque confpecta, hydatidem vidiffe memini, quæ minorem fui partem in pulmonis fuperficie oftendens, interius adeo fe amplificabat, ut aquæ limpidæ uncias aliquot contineret (b).* And another laborious anatomift (*Bonetus in Sepulch. Anatom. Obf.* 33 and 36,) informs us that the lungs of a man were found full of bladders which, when opened, difcharged either water, or a clear liquor, refembling the white of an egg. Thefe obfervations, I think, point out the caufe, and at the fame time account

(b) Morgagni de caufis & fedibus Morb. epift. 16. Art. 36.

for

for the rapid progrefs, and fatal termination of the pulmonary *œdema*, under which my patient laboured. Some hydatids, contained in the cellular membrane of the lungs, were probably ruptured internally; and in a habit abounding with the *colluvies ferofa*, the extravafated fluids would be every inftant accumulating, and the bronchial veficles becoming more and more compreffed, fuffocation inevitably enfued.

THE diagnoftics of the *hydrops pectoris*, whether the water be contained in the cellular membrane of the lungs, or in the cavity of the cheft, are fometimes very obfcure. Doctor Hoadly relates that he was prefent at the diffection of a dropfical man, from the fymptoms of whofe difeafe it was with fuch certainty concluded, that water was contained in one fide of the breaft, that the only motive for examination was to determine into which cavity the fluid was extravafated. On opening his body, however, they difcovered not a fingle drop of water, but found an almoft total adhefion of the external coat of the lungs to the pleura; together with an inflammation, and numberlefs fmall ulcers in one lobe.

A SENSIBLE fluctuation of water in the breaft is a fymptom which rarely occurs; and it appears from Morgagni's obfervations, that it is not unufual for patients, labouring under this diforder, to bear with eafe a recumbent pofture.

But

But an *œdema*, or dropfy of the cellular membrane of the lungs, when its attack is fudden, may often be diftinguifhed by the following figns, though it muft be acknowledged that they fometimes prove equivocal. The difficulty in refpiration is conftant, and increafed by the leaft motion, yet not much varied by different attitudes of the body; the patient complains of great anxiety about the *præcordia*, and when he attempts to take a deep infpiration, he finds it impoffible to dilate his cheft, and his breath feems to be fuddenly ftopped. The pulfe is fmall, languid, and opprefled; the face pale and bloated; the legs ufually fwelled; and the whole habit is, for the moft part, leucophlegmatic.

A DISEASE fo urgent in its fymptoms, fo quick in its progrefs, and fo often fatal in its termination, requires a method of cure of adequate expedition and efficacy. A brifk mercurial cathartic, which will not only unload the inteftinal canal, but promote abforption, by ftimulating and increafing the action of the whole vafcular fyftem, fhould be adminiftered without delay. I have lately feen furprizing relief, in a very alarming cafe, almoft inftantly procured by fuch a remedy *(c)*. Blifters to the legs have, alfo, fometimes a good

(c) A fimilar cafe is recorded by Dr. Simfon, in the Edin. Med. Effays, vol. VI. p. 126.

effect;

effect; for by deftroying the cuticle, and *rete mucofum*, they difcharge the water from the cellular membrane of a depending part, and thus in fome degree produce a general depletion. Punctures, made with a fmall lancet, or with fuch an inftrument as Dr. Fothergill has lately recommended, will anfwer the fame end; and be lefs liable to produce pain and inflammation. Diuretics, fudorifics, and expectorants, as they increafe the more fluid excretions, are indicated in this difeafe. And if the moft powerful medicines of one clafs fail, recourfe fhould immediately be had to another. Seneka root, in liberal dofes, fometimes anfwers every intention, and operates powerfully by the fkin, the kidneys, and the bronchial glands, to the great relief of the patient. But if the moft active medicines prove ineffectual, and the aggravation of all the fymptoms threaten almoft inftant diffolution, might not the *paracentefis* of the lungs be attempted, with fafety and advantage? *Melius eft anceps remedium quam nullum*, is an eftablifhed maxim in phyfic, and certainly in this inftance would juftify the trial of an operation, which is neither very painful, nor likely to be attended with any dangerous confequences. Many cafes have been recorded of wounds in the lungs, which have been healed, without much difficulty. Nor have fuch accidents been fucceeded by an *emphyfema*; for it may

be

be concluded from Mr. Hewfon's ingenious experiments, that a puncture or incifion will not occafion any emiffion of air, into the cavity of the *thorax*, on account of the effufion of blood, and fubfequent inflammation, by which the divided veficles are firft filled, and afterwards entirely clofed. To produce a difcharge of air, a laceration or fuperficial abrafion of the lungs feems to be neceffary; and hence it is that fractured ribs are the moft frequent caufes of the *emphyfema*.

Should the *paracentefis* of the lungs ever be deemed expedient, the cheft may be perforated by cautioufly diffecting with a knife, as in the operation for the *empyema*. If the lungs adhere to the *pleura* where the incifion is made, they may be punctured with a lancet, and the water will thus be difcharged without falling into the cavity of the *thorax*; but a trocar will be neceffary to obviate, as much as poffible, this inconvenience, if there be no adhefion. The operation, for evident reafons, fhould firft be performed on the right fide, and if this do not afford the patient fufficient relief, another opening may be made between the feventh and eighth ribs of the left fide, in order to avoid the *pericardium*.

Case

CASE OF A PALSY, ARISING FROM THE EFFLUVIA
OF LEAD, IN WHICH ELECTRICITY WAS SUC-
CESSFULLY EMPLOYED.

ELECTRICITY, like all other active remedies, may prove injurious as well as beneficial to the human body; and it is to be re-
gretted that experience has not yet fupplied us
with any certain *criteria*, by which to determine
when it will be hurtful, when innocent, or efficacious. That analogy may deceive us is evident from many examples. A girl, about fixteen,
who had loft the ufe of her arm, which was
greatly wafted, became univerfally paralytic, after
being electrified; and remained fo above a fortnight. The general palfy was removed by proper medicines; but the difeafed arm continued as
before. Electricity was again tried, and repeated
three or four days, when the girl became a fecond
time univerfally paralytic, and even loft the ufe
of her tongue. By a courfe of medicine, fhe
was once more relieved from this additional
palfy; but the original one, which affected her
arm, remained incurable *(a)*. A gentleman,
aged forty-eight, inclined to corpulency, and
of a phlegmatic temperament, had a paralytic

(a) Vid. Philof. Tranfact. vol. XLVIII. p. 786; alfo
Prieftley's Hiftory of Electricity, p. 386.

affection

affection of the leg and thigh. Electricity was tried, but the flighteft fhocks always increafed the torpor of the limb. The fame gentleman, twelve months afterwards, was attacked with an *hemiplegia*. To gratify his inclination, and contrary to my own judgment; I confented to the ufe of electricity, a fecond time: and this remedy, which had before proved injurious, was now at leaft innocent, and even thought to be beneficial to him.

THE electrical fhock, incautioufly communicated, may be productive of dangerous and even fatal confequences. Mr. R. aged fifty, fubject to various nervous and hypochondriacal complaints, after fuffering feveral flight paralytic affections, which yielded to medicine, was at length deprived of the ufe of one fide. Electricity, and other active remedies were applied. Gentle fhocks were repeatedly given by a fkilful perfon; and the patient feemed to receive benefit from each operation. But by an unfortunate miftake in the pofition of the chain, the fhock was one day conveyed through the epigaftric region, and not along the paralytic arm, which refted upon it. A violent pain was inftantly perceived in the ftomach, which, in a few minutes, was fucceeded by a profufe vomiting of blood. The hæmorrhage continued two or three days, and fo exhaufted the

the ſtrength of the patient, as certainly to ac-
celerate, and perhaps to occaſion his death.

PALSIES frequently ſucceed the *colica piĉtonum*;
whether owing to ſome nervous ſympathy between
the bowels and the limbs, or to the tranſlation
of any morbid acrimony, cannot eaſily be determined. In ſuch caſes, the waters of Bath, in
Somerſetſhire, are highly beneficial; and electricity, it is probable, would be an uſeful auxiliary
to them. When the circumſtances of the patient
render a journey to thoſe celebrated ſprings impracticable or inconvenient, the latter remedy
may be tried alone, with ſome proſpect of ſucceſs.
Of this the following curious caſe, communicated
to me by Dr. Withering, affords a preſumptive
proof.

JOSEPH ADAMS, aged 20, was admitted into
the Stafford infirmary on the 16th of September,
1768. Some months ago he felt a numbneſs
and coldneſs in the left leg and thigh, which gradually extended all over him, his head excepted,
which is now the only part he can move. His
limbs are often ſeized with involuntary twitchings,
as in the *chorea S. Viti*. Pulſe natural. Appetite good. Coſtive. This man was formerly uſed
to work in lead mines, at which time he was
often ſenſible of a ſweet taſte in his mouth; but
for two years paſt has been employed in digging
a navigable canal, and has been much expoſed to

wet

wet and cold. An antimonial vomit, a mercurial purge, and an emulfion, with a large proportion of *ol. olivar.* were prefcribed.

On the 21ft. He could move his right arm, and his legs a little, as he lay in bed. A number of fmall electrical fhocks were paffed through both arms, and ordered to be repeated daily.

23d. Sweats after being electrified; is univerfally warmer; can ftir his left arm.

24th. Feels a tingling in his right arm. His fingers contract upon the chain, when the fhock paffes. The frequency of his pulfe is not increafed during the operation. Electrify all his limbs.

27th. Can fhut both his hands, and bring the right up to his mouth, when lying in bed; but not when raifed up.

29th. Feels the fhocks more fenfibly than he did at firft. They always excite a ftrong tingling fenfation. When raifed upon his feet, can ftand upright betwixt two affiftants.

At this time it was difcovered that he had feveral venereal fhankers, and an ulcer upon the *glans penis.* The electricity was difcontinued, and a courfe of fublimate folution, and mercurial unction entered upon; by which means all the venereal fymptoms were fubdued.

November 30th. His paralytic complaints being juft in the fame ftate as on the 29th of

September,

September, recourfe was again had to the electrical machine; and two large fpoonfuls of *ol.
olivar.* were given twice a day, to prevent coftivenefs.

December 18th. SWEATS when electrified:
has more motion in his body; feeds himfelf in
bed, but cannot when up. The fingers fometimes drawn inwards, fo as almoft to touch the
plams of his hands; his arms and legs always
benumbed, except for a fhort time after the ufe
of the machine.

28th. PALSY much the fame; for the relief,
gained at the time of electrifying, ceafes in a fhort
time after it is over. Continues very coftive.
The antimonial vomit was repeated; a drachm
of *pilul. gummos.* ordered to be taken twice in a
day, with three ounces of the decoction of Peruvian bark. Omit the electricity.

January 10, 1769. THESE medicines at firft
gave him ftools, but they have not now that
effect. The palfy in the fame ftate. Complains
of great pain in the right fhoulder, and right fide
of the neck. A blifter was applied to the neck, the
pills were continued, and the bark decoction was
changed for four ounces of paralytic infufion.
An ounce of volatile liniment was ordered to be
rubbed daily upon the fpine; iffues to be made
in the thighs; and when the blifter healed, a
feton in his neck. He continued nearly in this
method

method until the 12th of April, without any other advantage than being free from his pains. He was ordered into the warm bath, every other day, and to take as much of the frefh leaves of cuckow pint *(b)*, twice every day, as his ftomach would bear.

May 3d. THE cuckow pint creates an uncommon heat in his ftomach, but produces no other fenfible effect. Let blifters be applied to his legs, and afterwards to the lower part of the fpine.

28th. THE palfy continuing in the fame ftate, recourfe was again had to electricity.

Auguft 21ft. Has improved, though very flowly, in ftrength and motion. The mufcles of his back allow him to ftoop, and raife himfelf again: the right arm nearly as ftrong as when in health; but for more than a week paft, his palfy has continued the fame, and he complains of griping pains in his belly, which is tenfe and very coftive. The ufual medicines not giving him ftools, let him take a large fpoonful of caftor oil every morning. Continue the electricity.

September 6th. FREE from the pain in his belly; the caftor oil purges him confiderably. Has more ufe in his left arm, and fweats profufely after electrifying.

(b) Arum Maculatum, *Linnæi* Species Plantarum.

13th. STOOD

13th. STOOD himself to day.

November 10th. CAN raise himself from his chair, and stand without help.

22d. WALKS about, with the assistance of his chair.

December 17th. DURING this month was a good deal afflicted with the gravel, which gave way to the usual remedies.

27th. WALKS with one stick.

January 3, 1770. BEGINS to walk without a stick. From this time he continued mending until the 11th of May; when he was discharged perfectly cured.

THE first circumstance which strikes our attention, in the history of this disease, is the distance of time betwixt the patient's exposure to the deleterious *effluvia* of the lead mines, and the appearance of the palsy. That the palsy was occasioned by lead is most probable; as there seemed to be, through the whole of the cure, more or less of the *colica pictonum* existing. The effects of the castor oil in this disease are too evident to pass unnoticed; especially as I have heard some very ingenius and candid practitioners assert, that they have found no more purgative quality in that oil, than in an equal quantity of olive oil. The medicine they used must have been highly adulterated.

THAT

THAT electricity does not afford relief in paralytic complaints, after five days application,
has been afferted by a very ingenious philofopher;
and I am afraid it is an opinion which has been
too generally received. Dr. De Haen, in his
Ratio Medendi, produces inftances to the contrary;
but none more ftriking than the above cafe,
wherein it appears that the palfy continued in the
fame ftate, whenever the fhocks were omitted.
Patients are frequently difcouraged by the painful
fenfation which large fhocks excite, from perfe-
vering in an electrical courfe; and it is not uncommon to find, that any given degree of fhock
will occafion more pain in a difeafed, and even
in a paralytic limb, than in a found one: I cannot omit adding, that I have never met with
a cafe which refifted the power of fmall and repeated fhocks, that would yield to great and terrify-
ing ones. Like other active and ufeful remedies,
electricity may be given in too large a dofe, and
may then produce confiderable mifchief. Nor
are there wanting feveral well authenticated facts,
to fupport this opinion. The largeft fhock I
have ever found ufeful, has been from an eight
ounce phial, coated in the common manner;
and even this, in many irritable habits, is confiderably too ftrong. For there is an amazing
difference in the fenfibility of different conftitutions to the electrical ftimulus. Quick, lively
people

people feel the moſt from it; thoſe the leaſt, who are dull and ſlow of apprehenſion.

WHEN the gout leaves the extremities, and invades other parts of the body, ſinapiſms, bliſters, and volatile epithems, are often applied to the wriſts or to the feet, to recall the diſorder to its uſual and natural ſeat. The ſame remedies are alſo employed to ſolicit the gout to the extremities, when it has yet made only irregular attacks on the ſyſtem. Might not ſlight, or even ſevere ſhocks of electricity, be highly ſerviceable on ſuch occaſions? The ſtimulating applications, above mentioned, chiefly affect the ſkin; whereas the electrical ſtroke inſtantly pervades the tendons, articulations, and other internal parts, ſuppoſed to be the ſeat of this diſorder.

IN palſies, proceeding from the receſſion of the gout, we ſhould be leſs liable to diſappoint-ment in our expectations from electricity, when thus partially applied, than by the general ſhocks ſo indiſcriminately given.

CASES

C A S E S

O F

OBSTINATE   COLICS,

CURED BY THE USE OF ALUM.

A DUTCH writer of confiderable merit, but not generally known in England, has re-commended the ufe of alum in the *Colica pictonum*, and in other obftinate and painful affections of the bowels; and has favoured the public with feveral well authenticated hiftories of its beneficial effects *(a)*.

I HAVE

(a) DE Colica Pictonum Tentamen, & Appendix, auctore, Joanne Grafhuis, M. D.

" CURATIONIS methodus (colicæ fcilicet Pictonum)
" quatuor indicationibus abfolvitur. Expoftulat 1. leni-
" men doloris, nulla habita ad caufam fpecialem ratione.
" 2. Caufæ proximæ vel ablationem vel extinctionem.
" 3. Partium affectarum in integram, quantum fieri
" poffit, reftitutionem. 4. Alvi interea temporis, diffi-
" cillime in plerifque conftipatæ, toto curationis decurfu
" exfolutionem. Prima indicatio anodyna expofcit;
" fecunda demulcentia; tertia roborantia. Sine his,
" levatio morbi duabus prioribus indicationibus impe-
" trata, raro tuta fidaque eft, hifce folis aliquando cura-

VOL. I.   D d   " tio

I HAVE adminiftered this remedy in about
fifteen cafes, with a degree of fuccefs which confirms his teftimony, and induces me to propofe it
to the trial of other phyficians. The dofe, in
which I have given it, has ufually been from ten
to twenty grains, mixed with an equal proportion
of fugar. When there was reafon to apprehend
that it might be too rough and auftere in its
action, I have directed it to be combined with
gum arabic or *fperma ceti*: And in cafes of
flatulence, when a warm opiate was indicated,
half a fcruple of the *philonium Londinenfe* made an
ufeful addition to it. Fifteen grains of alum,
given every fourth, fifth, or fixth hour, for the
moft part prove gently aperient; and when the
fymptoms are not very fevere, the fecond or third
dofe feldom fails to mitigate the pain; and fometimes entirely removes it. This remedy, when

" tio integre abfolvitur abfque ùllo aliorum extradictis
" jam indicationibus præfidio. Siquidem hand raro
" vidi morbum anodynis & demulcentibus, feorfum et
" per fe, vel combinatis, fat magnâ copiâ & fatis diu
" affumptis, vinci non potuiffe: in quibus cafibus omni
" fpe fanationis impetrandæ abjecta, roborantibus fortio-
" ribus non calidis, ut inteftinorum tonus relaxatus
" emendaretur, adhibitis, invincibilem ut videbatur
" hoftem profligari feliciter. Quare hæc methodus a me
" tentata, deinceps mihi maxime commendabilis fuit;
" eoque felicior quo medicamentorum adftrictoria poten-
" tia major, eorumque propinatio liberalior diutur-
" niorque." De Colica Pictonum, p. 48.

continued

continued for a fufficient length of time, feems to abate flatulence, to obviate fpafm, to improve the appetite, and to ftrengthen the organs of digeftion. On thefe tonic powers the virtues of alum muft chiefly depend; though they may, in part, arife from its obtunding the morbid fenfibility of the inteftines, by an immediate action on their nerves. To thefe it is applied more quickly, forcibly, and through a larger extent than moft other aftringents, from its ready folubility, great ftypticity, and unchangeable nature. But without difcuffing the mode of its operation, I fhall briefly relate the two following hiftories, felected from feveral others, bf its falutary effects.

CASE I. January 28th, 1772. Mr. G. aged thirty, a temperate and active man, had been fub-ject more than twelve months, to a violent pain in the right *hypogaftrium*, which often recurred periodically, and continued two or three days, leaving a yellownefs of the countenance, and great forenefs of the *abdomen*. His belly was moderately foluble, and his pulfe regular in the fhort intervals of his fits. For as he lived at a diftance from Manchefter, I had no opportunity of feeing him in the paroxyfms of his diforder. The diagnoftics of this cafe were obfcure; but from a fufpicion that his pain might be in the courfe of the ureter, I directed the following medicines.

R. *Pulv.*

R. *Pulv. Uvæ Urſæ ʒj. Aluminis uſti ʒſs. M. f.*
pulvis in doſes 24 *æquales dividendus*; *quarum capiat*
unam ter die, ex unciis tribus decoɛ̌ti ſequentis.

R. *Rad. Petroſelini. Paſſular. ſolis. exacinat. aa*
ʒj. *Semin. & ſummît. Dauci ſylv. Herb. parietar.*
aa ʒ ſs. *aq. fontanæ* ℔iij. *coque ad* ℔ij. *colaturæ*, &
adde ſp. Nitri dulcis ʒj. *aq. Junip. com. ʒiij. M.*

THESE remedies were continued three weeks,
and, during the uſe of them, the patient ſuffered
no return of his diſorder. The medicines proved
diuretic; but he diſcharged no gravel, nor did
his urine at this time aſſume any remarkable
appearance.

MR. G. now conſidered himſelf as cured, and
therefore negleɛted the repetition of his powders.
In leſs than a month his colic recurred with great
violence; and, April 27, 1772, he again applied
to me for advice. I preſcribed fifteen grains of
burnt alum, and the ſame quantity of ſugar, to
be taken twice every day, in any agreeable vehicle, during the ſpace of ſeven or eight weeks.
And by ſteadily perſevering in this courſe, he
has remained ſix months entirely free from his
diſorder.

CASE II. September 21, 1772, E. P. a houſe-
painter, aged 28, had complained ſeveral days
of a violent pain in the region of the navel, attended with a ſlight nauſea, and frequent cramps
in the extremities. Sixteen hours before I ſaw
him,

him, he had taken two doſes of caſtor oil, which had yet procured no ſtool, nor afforded any relief. He was now afflicted, during the ſhort remiſſions of his colic, with very ſevere pains in his arms and ſhoulders. His countenance was yellow; his pulſe beat about ſeventy-five ſtrokes in a minute; and his feet were cold. I directed him to go into the warm bath in the evening; and to take the following bolus every ſixth hour.

R. *Spermatis Ceti. Aluminis rup. aa* ℈j. *Syr. ſimplicis q. s. M. f. bolus.*

The pain was much abated by the uſe of this medicine, before he tried the warm bath.

April 27th. He had taken ſeven doſes of alum, and was entirely free from pain; but remained extremely coſtive. The bolus was therefore omitted; and a ſolution of the cathartic ſalt in barley-water was ordered to be given at proper intervals, till ſeveral ſtools were procured. The ſucceeding day he continued eaſy: But to prevent a relapſe, I preſcribed a ſcruple of alum, mixed with an equal quantity of ſugar, to be ſwallowed twice every day, during the following week or fortnight. The patient ſoon recovered his health and ſtrength, and I have reaſon to believe has remained ever ſince free from his diſorder.

Since

Since the preceding account of the virtues of alum, in obstinate colics, was written, I have had long and full experience of the efficacy of this remedy, in various painful affections of the bowels, of the chronic kind, and not attended with inflammatory symptoms.

C   A   S   E   S

W   A   R   M   B   A   T   H

WAS SUCCESSFULLY EMPLOYED.

THE ufe of WARM BATHING is of great an-
tiquity. Hippocrates recommends it in
the ftrongeft terms. *Calidum, feu Therma cutim
emollit, attenuat, dolores tollit, rigores, convulfiones,
nervorum diftenfiones mitigat, capitis gravitatem
folvit (a)*. Ariftotle, Pliny, Galen, and Celfus
have given their teftimony in its favour. The
Romans derived this practice from the Greeks,
and regarded it both as an efficacious remedy,
and as one of the higheft enjoyments of luxury.
But under the reign of Auguftus Cæfar, who
was cured of a lingering and dangerous malady,
by the ufe of cold bathing, the warm bath fell,
for a fhort time, into difrepute. This appears
from Horace :

> Sane Myrteta relinqui,
> *Dictaque ceffantem nervis elidere morbum
> Sulfura contemni vicus gemit, invidus ægris*

(a) Hippoc. Aph. 22. fect. 5.

D d 4   *Qui*

*Qui caput & stomachum supponere fontibus audent
Clusinis, Gabiosque petunt, & frigida rura.*

Hor. Lib. I. Ep. xv.

VAPOUR bathing, as I am well informed, is an universal practice amongst the native Indians of North America. When afflicted with the rheumatism, a disease to which, from their climate, mode of life, and rigid fibres, they are peculiarly incident, they shut themselves in a close place; and pouring water upon a large stone, heated to a sufficient degree, they expose themselves for a considerable time to the steams which arise from it. Covered with a profuse sweat, they then plunge into the cold bath; and afterwards receive the hot vapours as before, repeating, for the most part twice or thrice, these severe operations. A similar practice prevails in Russia and Siberia; and every person in those countries, from the sovereign, to the meanest peasant, uses twice in a day such artificial hot baths. The Abbé Chappe d'Auteroche, who travelled into Siberia in the year 1761, by order of the king of France, informs us that the heat of these baths is raised to 148, and occasionally even to 168 degrees of Fahrenheit's thermometer. In this intense heat the Russians sometimes remain two hours, pouring hot water frequently over their bodies; and then rush into the open air, dissolved in sweat, to roll themselves in the snow, during

the

the moſt piercing froſt, when the thermometer ſtands ten degrees below o. Many chronic diſ-eaſes are cured by this method of bathing; and the rheumatiſm is ſaid to be almoſt unknowrt in Ruſſia.

Prosper Alpinus relates that warm baths are uſed by the Egyptians, in all fevers, except thoſe of the peſtilential kind; and in a variety of other diſorders. They are employed alſo by the females of that country, eſpecially by the Hebrew women, to render them more corpulent. *Quod ut obtineant, multis diebus, dulcibus tepidis Balneis indulgent, in ijſque diu morantes, comedunt, potant, clyſteribuſque ibi ex variis pinguedinibus, ac adipibus paratis utuntur, multaque etiam medicamenta per os aſſumunt.*

In England, warm bathing is rarely employed in private practice, notwithſtanding ſeveral modern writers of reputation have ſtrongly recommended it, and the experience of ages hath evinced its utility. To excite more attention to a remedy, which though well known is too much neglected, I ſhall briefly relate a few caſes, in which it proved eminently ſuccefsful.

Case I. January 14, 1770. A young gen-tleman of an irritable habit, after drinking freely, and ſwallowing a large quantity of Cayenne pep-per, was ſeized with an inflammatory *angina.* The fever, ſwelling of the *fauces,* laborious re-ſpiration,

spiration, difficult deglutition, and a violent pain in the head, were succeeded by a delirium; and although these symptoms were in some degree ·mitigated by venæsection, cathartics, blisters, leeches applied to the throat, *pediluvia*, and by nitrous and antimonial medicines, yet they continued with great severity; and the patient passed six days and nights, without enjoying the least slumber. Under these circumstances, (January 20th) the warm bath was prescribed, and the young gentleman directed to sit in it half an hour. The delirium soon abated; he fell into a profound and refreshing sleep, in which he continued thirteen hours; and then awoke entirely free from fever or delirium. And in a short time he recovered his usual health and strength.

CASE II. Master S. P. aged two years, healthy but of a delicate make, and with a head larger than is natural, was seized August 13, 1771, at one o'clock in the morning, with severe convulsions. He had been slightly indisposed a day or two before, and the preceding evening a few eruptions were observed on his face and neck. His sister had just recovered from the small pox, and he had not been separated from her during her illness; so that there remained no doubt concerning the cause of these symptoms. An emetic was administered, and a laxative clyster afterwards injected. But the fits continued

with

with great violence, recurring at shorter and shorter intervals, notwithstanding the application of a blister to the back, an antispasmodic liniment to the spine, and the assiduous use of paregoric elixir, foetid *sal volatile*, musk, camphor, the *pediluvium*, &c. The child's strength was now almost exhausted, his respiration became laborious, his extremities cold, his pulse trembling, quick and languid, and his face was alternately flushed, and of a cadaverous paleness. The variolous eruption neither increased nor receded.

SUCH was the situation of my little patient at eleven o'clock at night, when I directed him to be immersed, as high as the chin, in warm water. The relief this afforded was almost instantaneous. Every convulsive motion ceased; his breathing became free and regular; he took notice of those around him; and seemed sensible of the present ease enjoyed. He remained in the bath about ten minutes, and was much refreshed by it, but had a fit not long afterwards: This however was very slight, and yielded immediately to a clyster prepared of a strong infusion of Valerian root and assafoetida, with a few drops of *tinct. Thebaica*, which was in readiness, and should have been injected on his coming out of the water. He retained the clyster only a few minutes; but passed the rest of the night in a composed and comfortable sleep, and the next morning the
eruption

eruption was univerfal. The puftules were diftinct; but fo flow in fuppurating, that they died
away without coming to any degree of maturity,
although a cordial diet was enjoined, the bark
prefcribed, and fmall dofes of fulphur, mixed with
fyrup of poppies, were frequently adminiftered.

CASE III. Mrs. H. aged thirty-five, a lady
of a tender conftitution, fubject to fcorbutic eruptions, and enfeebled by frequent child bearing,
received, in the beginning of January 1770, a
fevere fhock by the untimely death of an infant
at the breaft, which occafioned a mifcarriage, and
profufe uterine hæmorrhage. A variety of hyfterical fymptoms fucceeded, and gradually increafed. February 18th, my affiftance was defired. She was then afflicted with great languor
of body, and dejection of mind, with flatulence,
want of appetite, and a violent fenfe of fuffocation in her throat. Every morning a *delirium*
came on, attended with fevere convulfions. Her
pulfe was quick, fluttering, and irregular; her
fkin was dry, and fince her mifcarriage, free from
any eruption; and fhe complained of an oppreffion about the *præcordia*. A blifter to the head
was directed; a cordial and nourifhing diet recommended; and the frequent ufe of the *pediluvium* enjoined. The following medicines were
alfo prefcribed.

℞. *Affafœtidæ*

℞. *Assafœtidæ electæ gr. xv. Pulv. Ipecac: Extract. Thebaic. aa gr. j. Ol. Menthæ gutt. ij. Syr. simp. q. s. M. f. pilulæ mediocres, omni nocte hora somni sumendæ.*

℞. *Pulv. Cort. Peruvian. ʒj. Rasur. Ligni Guaiac. Sasafrag. Cort. Winteran. Rad. Glycyrrhiz. aa ʒij. Aq. Font. bullient ℔j. Infunde vase clauso per sex horas, deinde cola.*

℞. *Colaturæ præscriptæ ʒiss. Tinct. Valerian. vol. Tinct. Castor. aa ʒj. M. f. Haustus ter die sumendus.*

By these remedies she was much relieved, and continued better till the 12th of March; when she relapsed into all her former complaints, which recurred with an increased degree of dejection and anxiety of mind. Without my knowledge she had tried the cold bath, and had been sensibly injured by it. No eruption yet appeared on her skin; and the delirium, which was more violent than before, now invaded her always in the evening. Troches of sulphur, and the compound lime water, with the pills mentioned above; were at this time prescribed; and the patient was directed to use the warm bath every night, previous to the accession of the delirium.

March 13th. THE delirium recurred with much less violence, and was of shorter continu-

ance

ance; and after bathing the patient fell into a found and composed sleep.

March 16th. THE warm bath was omitted, and the delirium was much more violent, and lasted longer. The following draught was directed to be taken an hour before its accession, the succeeding evening, and the use of the bath to be repeated.

R. *Sagapeni, Mosch. aa gr. x. Camphoræ gr. ij. Mucilag. Gum. Arab. q. s. simul tritis gradatim adde Aquæ Menth. vulg. simp. ʒiſs. Tinȼt. Valer. simp. ʒij. Syr. è Cort. Aurant. ʒj. M. f. Hauſtus.*

BY these means, assiduously pursued, the patient recovered her health before the end of March. Whenever the warm bath was omitted, which happened twice or thrice, she suffered sensibly by the neglect. Her delirium was more severe, and of longer duration; her sleep was shorter and less refreshing; and the succeeding day she was more troubled with anxiety of mind, oppression about the *præcordia*, and other nervous symptoms.

CASE IV. A Clergyman, who resides about forty miles from Manchester, consulted me, by letter, in the beginning of March 1769. He had been several years afflicted with a variety of hypochondriacal complaints, which had succeeded the sudden repulsion of an eruption on his foot, by means of an astringent bath; and he was then
under

under a continual anxiety and diftraction of mind.
He had one prevailing idea conftantly in his head,
and one diftreffing image before his eyes. Thefe
fymptoms of his diforder he afcribed to a violent
commotion of mind, at a time when he was under great depreffion of fpirits, and which occafioned a fudden ftart, or convulfive motion, in
one part of his head. In this part he felt a conftant and forcible fpafm, which he fuppofed extended itfelf to his breaft and bowels, as he generally perceived a fenfe of contraction in thofe
parts, attended with an inward heat. His eyes
were particularly affected, being drawn, as it were,
out of their fockets, and endued with an unna-
tural fenfibility. In a fecond letter, dated March
11th, he informed me that he perceived every
night, when he lay in bed, a continual motion
from his forehead upwards, and about his tem-
ples, like the undulation of waves. The uneafinefs and pain in his head was fo extreme, that he
could not bear even the preffure of his hat. But
all this bodily pain was trifling in degree, when
compared to the diftrefs of his mind, arifing from
the irrefiftible force with which external objects
diftracted his eyes and imagination.

UNDER thefe unhappy circumftances, he had
confulted feveral phyficians of great eminence, and
had tried a variety of medicines, the detail of
which, as well as of thofe which I prefcribed to
him,

him, would be equally tedious and unneceſſary. Nothing had afforded him ſo much relief, as the warm *pediluvium*, and the extract of opium, of which he had habituated himſelf to take ten or twelve grains every day. Medicine proving ſo ineffectual, I adviſed the gradual diſcontinuance of his opiates; recommended the frequent uſe of the warm bath; and directed hot water to be poured in a ſtream, upon the part of his head which was moſt affected. The following paſſages, extracted from his letters, ſhew the beneficial conſequences of this courſe. " My days begin to be eaſier, and " I have not had ſuch bad nights ſince I went " into the warm bath, which is near two months " ago. It has wonderfully ſoftened and compoſed " my head, and enabled me to ſleep ſooner and " ſounder than I uſed to do. I have made ſeve- " ral attempts to uſe the cold bath along with it, " but I am always obliged to deſiſt, as it immedi- " ately alters me for the worſe, greatly increaſes " the diſtreſs in my head, and renders my ſleep " more diſturbed. I am however attempting it " again; and I hope with a better proſpect of " ſucceſs. I ſhould be much encouraged by " finding myſelf able to bear it; as I am perſuaded " it would have a happy effect in ſtrengthening " and reſtoring me."—" I find myſelf daily ad- " vancing towards a more perfect ſtate of health. " I have brought myſelf at length to bear the
" cold

" cold bath very well. I ufe it every other day,
" and find a very happy effect from it, in reftoring
" my fpirits, and ftrengthening my whole frame.
" But it would not do without the affiftance of the
" warm bath, which is my conftant antidote
" againft any difagreeable effects from the other,
" and gives me never-failing relief and reft at
" night. The pouring warm water, in a conftant
" ftream, upon that part of my head, where my
" complaint lies, has, I apprehend, been of fingu-
" lar fervice in foftening and opening it, and
" contributed greatly to that happy change which
" I find in myfelf: I have been gradually wean-
" ing myfelf from opium; and have reduced the
" dofe from three pills to one."

THIS gentleman foon recovered his health, and
has been ever fince free from any returns of his
diforder.

I HAVE recommended warm bathing in a variety of other complaints, and for the moft part
with the happieft fuccefs. Like other remedies,
however, it has fometimes difappointed my ex
pectations; and in two inftances its operation
proved in fome degree unfavourable. The one
cafe was a violent pain refembling the fciatica, but
which I believe proceeded from an affection of
the kidney. The other was a moft troublefome
fenfe of motion in the *uterus*, from one fide of the
pelvis to the other, which occurred at the end of

every fortnight, in the intervals between the *catamenia*, and lasted generally three or four days.
The patient was free from this complaint when in
a sitting posture; and it was most uneasy to her
when she was walking.   The warm bath aggravated the pain in the former instance; and seemed
to protract the disorder a day or two in the latter.

MISCELLA-

MISCELLANEOUS

C   A   S   E   S

AND

O B S E R V A T I O N S.

I. IT is highly probable that Palfies frequently
arife from difeafes of the *vifcera*, without
any previous fault in the brain or fpinal marrow.
And confiderable errors may be committed in
practice, by a want of precifion in diftinguifhing
the caufes from which they proceed.   Large
evacuations are often indifcriminately directed
in thefe diforders, from a fuppofition that they
arife from plenitude; and thus irreparable mifchief
is done in thofe cafes of weaknefs or irritability,
which are now moft numerous.

I HAVE feen feveral *hemiplegias* which derived
their origin from affections of the liver; others
from an *atonia* of the ftomach and bowels; and
three inftances have occurred to me of palfies
from pregnancy. The following hiftory is of
this kind.

E e 2   MRS.

Mrs. D. of Rochdale, aged 21, whose *menses* had always recurred with regularity, but attended with great pain and general disorder, in the spring of 1771 had a miscarriage. The following August, the *catamenia* did not appear at the usual period. She had a violent pain in the loins and about the *os sacrum*, which continued several hours, and was then succeeded by a pain equally acute in her head. Soon afterwards, she lost all power of speech, and the use of her right side. Her habit was not plethoric; but an experienced and sensible apothecary, before my arrival, had taken from her arm half a pound of blood; had applied a blister to her back; and a volatile liniment to the side affected. By these means she recovered, in about sixteen hours, the use of her side; but still complained of a *torpor* in it, and of a dull pain and confusion in her head. Her pulse was soft and natural; and her blood of a proper texture. I considered the palsy as arising from an uterine affection; and directed a gentle purgative of rhubarb and magnesia, every other night, and an infusion of Peruvian bark and Valerian, to strengthen the habit of the patient, and to abate irritability. Venæsection was also recommended a few days before the next period of the *catamenia*. At the return of this period she had a second paralytic stroke, of the same kind as before, and preceded by the like symptoms. Venæsection

had

had been omitted, and fhe had negle&ed her medicines. She was now evidently in a ftate of pregnancy. I advifed a repetition of the remedies before prefcribed; and recommended the ufe of a temperately cold bath. She complied with thefe injun&ions, and had no return of her diforder.

II. Fuller, in his *Medicina Gymnaftica*, ftrongly recommends Coltsfoot, in confump-tive diforders. It appears to be anodyne, and a corre&or of acrimony; but only exerts thefe powers when taken in a large quantity. I gave a ftrong infufion of it to a young woman, who had various running fores, he&ic heats, a colli-quative *diarrhœa*, and wandering pains all over her body. It produced a better digeftion in the ulcers; alleviated her pains; and abated the vio-lence of the *diarrhœa*. Cicuta, and Peruvian bark were before adminiftered with good effe&; but had been for fome time difcontinued, on ac-count of their expenfivenefs. I thought the *tuffi-lago* afforded more relief to the patient than either of them.

III. Large dofes of opium have been fre-quently adminiftered, in painful and fpafmodic difeafes, not only with fafety, but with the hap-pieft fuccefs. Dr. Vaughan, of Leicefter, informs me, that he lately gave to a lady, in the fifth month of her pregnancy, who had an acute pain in her bowels which threatened an abortion, twenty-two grains of the extract of opium, and three hundred drops of laudanum, in the space of thirty-six hours. And by these means, and these alone, she perfectly recovered. But the nervous system, especially in spasmodic disorders, is subject to great and sudden changes, which must sometimes render the doses of medicines, powerful in their operation, uncertain and liable to produce the most dangerous effects. The following case, communicated to me by a young physician, who is likely to be an ornament to his profession, affords a striking confirmation of the truth of this observation.

A youth, who was admitted into the hospital at —— on account of a violent spasmodic disease, which recurred periodically in the evening, after trying a variety of remedies, was directed to take the *extractum Thebaicum*, in such a quantity as might prove sufficient to mitigate the violence of the paroxysms. The dose amounted to twenty-two grains, and was repeated every night, during the space of a week, without producing any soporific effects. On the eighth night it was observed that he had no return of the spasm; and in the morning he was found dead. It is probable that a sudden alteration had taken place in the nervous system of this patient, and that the opium, in consequence of it, exerted, with full force, its usual powers on the body.

IV. I have

IV. I have lately received, from a clergyman of great learning and humanity, a fmall quantity of feed, which is brought from the coaft of Malabar, and is celebrated in the Eaft Indies as a powerful remedy for the colic. It is called by the Portuguefe AJAVA. " Captain B. formerly " commander of the Prince Henry Indiaman, " procured fome of it from the Jefuit's College at " Goa, brought it over with him to England, and " diftributed it amongft fuch of his neighbours and " acquaintance as were troubled with the colic, " who found great benefit from the ufe of it. Be-" ing himfelf exceedingly afflicted at times with the " windy gout, and having in one of his fits applied " feveral things in vain, he made trial of the *ajava* "*feed*, and found it fo very efficacious in expelling " the wind, and removing the gout from the fto-" mach and head, that he has ever fince taken it " on the like occafions. The moft ufual effect of " it is to procure a plentiful difcharge of wind, " and fometimes it relieves the diforder by a ftool " or two," From the fenfible qualities of this feed, I fhould judge it to be an active remedy: But I have yet had no experience of its efficacy, and mention it only to promote an inquiry into its medicinal virtues.

V. A LADY, aged 40, was fubject feveral years to an exceffive degree of acidity in her ftomach and bowels, which medicines fometimes palliated,

but

but never cured. By degrees the acidity abated,
and at length entirely ceafed; but fhe became
fubject to frequent diarrhœas, to a *profluvium
menfium*, and to copious and fudden difcharges
of urine. She complained of great feeblenefs, of
wearinefs in her legs, and of a conftant pain in her
loins. Her pulfe was languid and flow, her fkin
cold, of a dark hue, and covered with freckles.
She had often a putrid tafte in her mouth, at
which time the faliva was tinged with blood;
and in the intervals of her *menfes*, fhe had a continual difcharge of brown, fœtid water from the
uterus.

THESE fymptoms are characteriftics of a true
fcurvy or diffolution of the blood; which, in this
inftance, feems to have been produced by the
long continuance of an acid acrimony in the firft
paffages. Dr. Gaubius has well defcribed the
effects of fuch an acrimony. *Acor primis maxime
viis infeftus, tempore & fanguinem humorefque inde
deductos fubiens, nafcitur ex ufu diuturno acidorum
aut acefcentium, quæ viribus corporis non fubiguntur;
aut quia ex fe indomabilia funt naturæ humanæ, aut
ob virtutis coctricis impotentiam. Debilitas igitur
folidorum univerfalis, aut privata vifcerum primæ
digeftionis; irritabilitas regulares horum motus
turbans; inertia defectufve fuccorum præparantium;
circulationis & caloris naturalis languor; neglectus
motus animalis, eo difponunt, ut pateat, cui maxime
ætati,*

ætati, fexui, vitæ generi, hoc acre frequentius eveniat (a).

To determine the comparative nutritive powers of different foods, a few years ago, a phyfician, of diftinguifhed abilities, made a variety of experiments, to which he at length fell an unfortunate facrifice. I have been well informed that he lived a month upon bread and water only, by which he daily diminifhed in his weight. At the end of that time, he added fugar to his bread and water, and confined himfelf a fortnight longer to this diet. His breath then became offenfive, his gums bled, putrid floughs appeared in his mouth, and *vibices* fpread themfelves over different parts of his body. Thefe fymptoms were removed by a return to animal diet, and by the ufe of the bark.

It is contrary to the prevailing THEORY, that vegetable food fhould give rife to putrefaction in the animal fyftem; but there are many proofs of the truth of it. Dr. Biffet relates feveral cafes of highly putrid fevers, quick in their progrefs and fatal in their termination, wherein the feptic ferment evidently began in the *primæ viæ*, after eating heartily of acefcent food. Calves, alfo, put to graze in a rich pafture, towards the clofe of autumn, are fometimes affected with a putrid difeafe, which deftroys them in thirty hours.

(a) Gaubij Pathologia, fect. 307.

The

The farmers call it the *quarter felon*, becaufe one hind quarter becomes putrid and emphyfe-matous; and as foon as the *emphyfema* extends to the fpine, the animal expires: It is moft incident to calves that are healthy. Juices, which are perfectly animalized or affimilated, are lefs prone to putrefy than fuch as are crude, or blended with a great proportion of acefcent chyle. The meat of bullocks and of fheep, which have been kept fafting a fufficient length of time before they are killed, that is till the recent chyle be completely affimilated, is firmer and continues fweet much longer, than the flefh of fuch as are flaughtered foon after taking them from their paftures *(b)*.

The learned writer, whom I have quoted above, obferves : *Dulciaria, faccharata, mellita, hifque fimilia, ufu immodico, per occultam acrimoniam den-tibus inimica funt; pro vi fua fermentante, acidum ingenerant, et quæ ex hoc profluunt mala; præterea folvunt tenuantque humores; horum minuta denfitate et firmas partes relaxant; non uno hinc nomine generi nervofo infefta, infantibus, fexui fequiori, debilibus, hyftericis, hypochondriacis, obfunt (c).*

From the ufeful and accurate experiments of Sir John Pringle, it appears that bread, water, and frefh gall, when fermented together, firft

(b) Vid. Biffet's Medical Obfervations, p. 85.

(c) Gaubij Pathologia, fect. 470.

turned

turned four, then putrid. And Dr. Bryan Robinson found that perspiration is diminished by fruit, and garden vegetables. Perhaps these facts may reflect some light on the preceding observations.

VI. Mr. WILLIAM WHITE of York, the ingenious author of an Essay on the Diseases of the Bile, has lately communicated to me some curious experiments on the solution of those calculous concretions, which are called gall stones. He has discovered that *alcohol*, saturated with *oleum terebinthinæ æthereum*, quickly and totally dissolves them. And induced by the powerful action of this *menstruum* out of the body, he has administered it internally with some degree of success; and is desirous of recommending it to the trial of others. Such a remedy, if it prove effectual, must be regarded as a valuable addition to the *materia medica*. But if we consider the peculiar œconomy observed by nature, in the circulation of the blood through the liver; the long stagnation of the bile in the gall bladder; and the quickness with which *alcohol* and oil of turpentine pass off by urine and perspiration, it is to be feared that such a *menstruum*, powerful as it may be, will scarcely reach the solvend. To this objection, also, we may add, that the diagnostics of the disease are often obscure and uncertain. The same gentleman informs me, that
he

he was not long since present at the dissection of a
woman, who had laboured several months under
an obstinate jaundice, attended with violent and
periodical pains in the region of the liver, with
costiveness, white stools, and other symptoms of
biliary concretions. No such cause however was
found; but a large schirrus extended itself from
the *pylorus* along the *duodenum*, so as to close
the orifice of the *ductus communis*, and thus prevent the passage of the bile into the intestines.

PROPOSALS FOR ESTABLISHING MORE ACCURATE,
AND COMPREHENSIVE BILLS OF MORTALITY, IN
MANCHESTER,

THE establishment of a judicious and accurate register of the births and burials, in
every town and parish, would be attended with
the most important advantages, medical, political,
and moral. By such an institution, the increase
or decrease of certain diseases; the comparative
healthiness of different situations, climates, and
seasons; the influence of particular trades and
manufactures on longevity; with many other curious circumstances, not more interesting to phyficians, than beneficial to mankind, would be ascertained

certained with tolerable precifion. In a political view, exact regifters of human mortality are of ftill greater confequence, as the number of people and the progrefs of population in the kingdom, may, in the moft eafy and unexceptionable manner, be deduced from them. They are the foundation likewife of all calculations concerning the values of affurances on lives, reverfionary payments, and of every fcheme for providing annuities for widows, and perfons in old age. In a moral light, alfo, fuch *tables* are of evident utility, as the increafe of vice or virtue may be determined, by obferving the proportion which the difeafes, arifing from luxury, intemperance, and other fimilar caufes, bear to the reft; and in what particular places diftempers of this clafs are found to be moft fatal.

A FEW examples may perhaps confirm and illuftrate thefe obfervations. In the Pais de Vaud, a diftrict of the province of Bern in Switzerland, and in a country parifh in Brandenburgh, 1 in 45 of the inhabitants dies annually; and at Stoke Damarell in Devonfhire, 1 in 54; whereas in Vienna, and Edinburgh, the yearly mortality appears to be 1 in 20; in London 1 in 21; in Amfterdam and Rome 1 in 22; in Northampton 1 in 26; and in the parifh of Holy Crofs, near Shrewfbury, 1 in 33. In the Pais de Vaud, the proportion of inhabitants, who attain the age of eighty, is 1 in 21$\frac{1}{2}$; in Brandenburgh 1 in 22$\frac{1}{2}$; in Norwich 1 in 27;

in

in Manchefter 1 in 30; in London 1 in 40; and in Edinburgh 1 in 42. Thefe facts afford a ftriking but melancholy proof, of the unfavourable influence of large towns on the duration of life. From the moft accurate computation, London is found to contain 601750 inhabitants; and from 1759 to 1768, the burials have exceeded the chriftenings every year upwards of 7000; which is the recruit the metropolis requires annually from the country, to fupport the prefent number of its people. In 1757, a furvey was made of Manchefter and Sal-ford. The number of inhabitants then amounted to 19839; and the burials, exclufive of thofe amongft Diffenters, were 778. But fince that time the populoufnefs of Manchefter has confider-ably increafed. Half of all that are born in this town die under five years old. The ifland of Ma-deira is fo remarkably healthy, that two thirds of all who are born in it live to be married. Au-tumn is the moft healthy, and fummer the moft fickly feafon there. The mortality of fpring and fummer is to that of autumn and winter, as 115 to 100. In Manchefter, difeafes are moft frequent and fatal in the months of January, February, and March; and leaft fo in July, Auguft, and September. The mortality of thefe two feafons is as 11 to 8; and of the firft fix months of the year, compared with the laft fix months, as 7 to 6. M. Muret, Secretary to the Œconomical

Society at Bern, informs us, that he had the curiofity to examine the regifter of mortality in one town, and to mark thofe whofe deaths might be imputed to intemperance. And he found the number fo great, as to incline him to believe that drunkennefs is more deftructive to mankind than pleurifies, fevers, or the moft malignant diftempers *(d)*. Such are the important ufes, to which Tables of Human Mortality have been applied.

THE following plan of a more exact and comprehenfive regifter, than has hitherto been kept, is fubmitted to the confideration and correction of thofe who undertake the charge of the BILLS of MORTALITY in *Manchefter.*

I. LET a table of *chriftenings, marriages,* and *burials* be kept in every church, chapel, and place of religious worfhip in the town, and delivered at certain ftated times, to the Clerk of the parifh church, to be formed into one general BILL, and quarterly or annually publifhed. It is of importance that the *ftill-born* children, and thofe who die before *baptifm,* fhould alfo be regiftered : and the midwives fhould be defired to deliver an

(d) See a very valuable Treatife on Reverfionary Payments, by the Rev. Dr. Price; the Bern Obfervations for the year 1766 ; Philofophical Tranfactions, vol. LVII. and LIX ; and Dr. Short's new Obfervations.

account

account of them. Perhaps the Sextons may aſſiſt
in aſcertaining their number, as they are uſually
interred in church yards, or other public burial
grounds.

II. LET the table of *chriſtenings* ſpecify the
males and *females* who are baptized; and the table
of *deaths* expreſs the *males* who die, under the
ſeveral denominations of children, bachelors, married men, and widowers; the *females* who die
under the correſponding denominations of children, maidens, married women, and widows.
An obſervance of theſe diſtinctions will determine
the comparative number of *males* and *females*
who are born; the difference between the ſexes
in the expectation of life; and the proportion·
which the annual births, deaths, and marriages
bear to each other. Thus by the BILLS of MOR-
TALITY which have been keept at Vienna, Breſlaw,
Dreſden, Leipſic, Ratiſbon, and other towns in
Germany, it appears that the proportion of *males*
to the *females* who are born is as 19 to 18 : But
the proportion of *boys* to *girls*, who die under ten
years of age, is as 7 to 6; and of *married men*
to *married women*, in Breſlaw, as 5 to 3; in Dreſden, as 4 to 1. At Vevey, in Switzerland, for
twenty years, ending in 1764, there died in the
firſt month 135 *males* to 89 *females*; and in the
firſt year 225, to 162. The ſame accounts ſhew
likewiſe that, both at Vevey and Berlin, the *ſtill-*
born

born males are to the *still-born females*, as 30 to 21. In the parifh of Holy Crofs, Salop, an account was taken by the Vicar, A. D. 1760, of the number of *males* and *females* of the age of feventy and upwards: The latter amounted to *thirty-five*, the former only to *eight*. At Paris, and in Sweden, it has been obferved, that *women* not only live longer than *men*, but that *married women* live longer than *fingle women*. And in Switzerland it appears particularly, from the calculations of M. Muret, that of equal numbers of *fingle* and *married* women, between the age of 15 and 25, more of the former died than of the latter, in the proportion of 2 to 1 *(e)*.

LET the ages under *five*, be fpecified by fingle years; and afterwards, by periods of five or ten years.

IV. LET the BILLS of MORTALITY contain not only a lift of the difeafes of which all die, but alfo exprefs particularly the number dying of each difeafe, in the feveral divifions of life, and different feafons of the year. To accomplifh this, it will be neceffary for the phyficians of the town to confider the prefent lift of diftempers; to reject all fynonymous and obfolete terms; and to give a fhort and eafy explanation of thofe which

(e) Vid: Dr. PRICE's Obfervations on Reverfionary Payments.

are retained. And whenever a perfon dies, who has been attended by any of the faculty, the phyfician, furgeon, or apothecary fhould be defired to certify, in writing, the age and diftemper of the deceafed.

THE following TABLES are conftructed upon this PLAN ; and if the fcale be enlarged, will ferve for the *Church Regifter*, as well as for quarterly or annual publication. It appears to be unneceffary, and in many inftances would be exceptionable, to infert the names of the deceafed: Their *denomination* and *difeafe* therefore may be expreffed, in the columns allotted to each, by dots or units, which are to be fummed up at the end of every three months, and fet down in figures.

The LISTS of *Marriages* and *Chriftenings* may be kept in the common method.

THE additional trouble, which this more comprehenfive and accurate REGISTER will occafion to the Clerks of the feveral churches, &c. may be compenfated by diftributing amongft them, at the difcretion of any judicious clergyman, the money which arifes from the fale of the quarterly BILLS. If a hundred of thefe be fubfcribed for, or fold at the price of one fhilling each, the fum of twenty pounds per annum will thus be raifed, without impofing any new burdens on the town. Every fecond, third, fourth, or fifth year, the bills may be collected into a volume, and publifhed,

lifhed, under the direction of two or more phyficians, with obfervations on the ftate of the weather, the prevalence of epidemic difeafes, their fymptoms and method of cure, and the increafe or decreafe of population during that period. Such a work will afford the moft important inftruction to the public; and from the profits of it, a fund may be eftablifhed for the benefit of the Clerks, and the fupport of the inftitution.

N. B. It is obvious that the plan here propofed is not local, and that it may be executed, with equal facility and advantage, in every town and parifh in the kingdom. BILLS of MORTALITY might be rendered more ufeful in a political view, by taking fometimes the number of houfes and inhabitants, under and above particular ages, wherever fuch regifters are eftablifhed.

TABLE of DEATHS.

January, February, March.

Ages.	Males.	Females.	Ages.	Bachelors.	Married Men.	Widowers.	Maidens.	Married Women.	Widows.
1.			20.						
2.			25.						
3.			30.						
4.			35.						
5.			40.						
10.			45.						
15.			50.						
Total under 15			60.						
			&c. &c.						

TABLE of DISEASES.

January, February, March.

DISEASES.	1.	2.	3.	4.	5.	10.	20.	30.	40.	50.	60.	70.	80.	90.	100.
Casualties.															
Apoplexy.															
Asthma.															
Cancer.															
Chincough.															
Colic.															
Consumption.															
Convulsions.															
&c. &c.															

PROPOSALS

FOR ESTABLISHING MORE COMPREHENSIVE AND ACCURATE

PARISH REGISTERS;

Communicated by the Rev. Mr. DADE, of YORK.

RALPH BIGLAND, Efq. Norroy King at Arms, obferves, in his pamphlet publifhed a few years ago, that " the neceffity of proper " records for afcertaining the marriages, births, " baptifms, deaths and burials of perfons within " their refpective parifhes, is abundantly evident " from a tranfient view of our ancient hiftory, " which, for want of proper names, and real dates, " and family connections occafionally to be re- " ferred to, is oftentimes rendered perplexed and " unintelligible, and fometimes altogether incon- " fiftent even with its own chronology."

To remove this defect, Thomas Cromwell, afterwards Earl of Effex, being the King's Vicar General, in the year 1338 iffued out an order to the clergy throughout England, that in their refpective parifhes a public regifter fhould be kept

for

for the above purpofes. How far the intentions of that Minifter of State are really anfwered, is evident from the incorrect manner in which entries are too generally made. It has been long wifhed that the utility of parifh regifters was thoroughly invefligated, that the defects in making the entries were pointed out, and fuch a plan laid down, as might not only be ufeful, but eafily applied to practice.

Whether the prefent form, with the obfervations upon it, contribute to elucidate any of thefe points, the public will eafily determine.

Each page is divided into fix columns; *the firft,* in the regifter for baptifms, contains in large characters the chriftian name: in the *fecond column* is the furname and feniority of the infant, alfo in large characters. The utility of this difpofition will appear to any perfon who has examined parifh regifters with a degree of accuracy. Left the object of our inquiry fhould efcape us, how frequently are we obliged to undergo the toil of traverfing every line in each page, written perhaps in fmall characters, improperly fpelt, and in a hand fometimes fcarcely legible; whereas according to the prefent form, the reader will be able, with one glance of the eye, to run over the feveral names in each page; and will examine, in a few minutes, what otherwife would take feveral hours to accomplifh.

F f 4

In

In the prefent form it is hoped that care has been taken to identify the perfons: for when we are told that Robert Lutton, James Creyke, and Elizabeth Dealtrey were baptized; or that William Strickland, Mary Strangways and Richard Heblethwayte were buried on fuch a day, in a fucceffion of years, how fhall we inform ourfelves whether the parties were infants, adult, or aged, married or fingle, of what profeffion, or how they ftood related; circumftances we are too apt, at the time of recording thofe particulars, to think of no moment, becaufe their confequences are remote. Nor are our inquiries more gratified in finding John fon of William Fairfax, Mary daughter of Thomas Beckwith, and James fon of Robert Anderfon, baptized; or Mr. John Grimfton, Mrs. Jane Turner, and James fon of William Fountaine were buried on fuch a day. Was there no neceffity for carrying our refearches further than twenty or thirty years, the defect might be fupplied by the teftimony of living witneffes, though perhaps, even then, not without much trouble and inconvenience; but where it happens that the occurrences are not recent, and there are no collateral circumftances to affift us in identifying the parties, we muft naturally be left in the dark. A gentleman in the Weft-Riding of Yorkfhire, fome years ago, felt the full weight of this defect. Being defirous of forming a genealogical

genealogical account of his family, he applied to the regifter of the parifh; and though he col-lected nearly 100 baptifms, and as many burials in the laft century, there was not one circum-ftance that would enable him to digeft them into any form, and to afcertain the refpective branch to which each party belonged. Where families of the fame name refide within the fame parifh, there will arife difficulties in proportion; and after the expiration of half a century, it will be impofli-ble to diftinguifh the defcendants of one houfe from thofe of another. There lived fome years ago, in the neighbourhood of Thirfk, three re-fpectable families, nearly allied, of the name of Kitchingman; and on examining the parifh regi-fter, I find it verifies my affertion.

Mr. Bigland had his eye upon thefe defects, when he obferves, " it is of importance to every " family, not excepting the leaft confiderable, to " pay fome regard to their pedigrees, and con-" fequently that every circumftance, whether of " a public or private nature, that tends to " illuftrate genealogical intelligence, fhould be " attended to with the moft religious exactnefs."

Let us then view the laft mentioned names, regiftered according to the form, at the end of thefe remarks. With the addition of collateral circumftances, we fhall eafily diftinguifh the object of purfuit, whether it may regard the title of our

property,

property, or only the gratification of an inquiry natural to thofe who are defirous of knowing whence they are defcended. We have therefore allotted the *third column* to the name, profeffion, and defcent of the father, and the fourth to the name and defcent of the mother, the particulars of which may eafily be collected when the infant is baptized. Thus fhall we hope, on trials of titles to eftates, and genealogical inquiries, to raife a fund of intelligence to the induftrious antiquary, as well as the gentlemen of the law; and perhaps they may allow this fcheme to bid the faireft for fupplying the place of vifitations or inquifitions *poft mortem*.

The *fifth column* fhews the birth, and the *fixth* the baptifm of the infant; the entry of each being effentially neceffary. When the age bears date from the baptifm only, the child may become fubject to great inconvenience. Let us illuftrate this fuggeftion,

A person leaves £5000 to a diftant relation, in cafe his fon fhould die in his minority. It feems, from the remembrance of creditable neighbours, that the child was certainly born a fortnight before baptifm, that he married in his minority, and died a week under age according to the date of the baptifm, being furvived by his wife and an infant fon. The parents and witneffes of the birth being dead, and no particulars found fufficient

cient to afcertain the precife day of his birth, the entry of the baptifm is admitted as evidence, and the diftant relation poffeffes the fortune, to the great prejudice of a poor relict and her helplefs child.

In parifhes of vaft extent, where families dwell at a great diftance from the church, the winter floods and other accidents frequently delaying the baptifm of the infant, it is not uncommon to fee children brought to the font at three, four, and fix months old; nay upon the moors, and in other remote parts, we have inftances of children receiving baptifm, aged almoft as many years: a moft effential reafon this, why the birth of infants fhould be carefully regiftered, as well as the day of baptifm.   For it fhould be confidered, that under the age of twenty-one years, a perfon cannot marry without confent of parents or guardians, take his freedom in any corporation, vote at an election, be a Reprefentative in Parliament, or, in fhort, fill many important offices in fociety: and may it not happen, from a concurrence of circumftances, that perfons really of that age may be deprived of fuch benefits, and lofe fome great and valuable privileges ?   If then the entry of the birth, as well as baptifm, will be admitted as evidence, and effectually prevent fuch ill confequences, what pity it is that the birth is fo frequently omitted ? It is fomewhat remarkable that a gentleman, who was almoft the firft perfon that did me the favour to infpect the prefent form,

and

and whose family is diftinguished for an ancient refidence upon their property, in the neighbourhood, told me that his baptifm was regiftered at O——, but that after the ftricteft inquiries he never could be informed *when* he was born.

What has been obferved on the page for baptifms, will ferve to illuftrate that for the burials: and as an affection for the memory of thofe we loved prompts us to a defire of mingling our afhes with theirs, I have been particular in afcertaining the place of interment.

I have only to add, that the uniformity of the page has been confulted, and that the *two laft columns*, in the regifter of burials, are intended to diftinguifh places remarkable for longevity, or the reverfe, and to acquaint us what diforders mankind is fubject to under particular feafons and climates; the ufe of which information is fufficiently evinced by Dr. Percival of Manchefter.

Should this form meet with the approbation of the public, I can claim no other merit than having improved upon a hint, given to the community in the year 1715 by Mr. Thorefby, the ingenious author of Ducatus Leodienfis, or the Topography of Leeds, as propofed to him by an eminent Antiquary, Thomas Kirke, Efq. of Cookbridge near to that town.

WILLIAM DADE.

Infant's Chrif-tian Name	Infant's Surname and Seniority.	Father's Name, Profession, and Defcent.	Mother's Name and Defcent.	Born.	Baptized.
JOHN	FAIRFAX, Firft born of	William Fairfax, of Steeton, Efq. 3d. fon of Sir William Fairfax of Denton, Knight. By Mary, eldeft daughter of Hugh Chelmley of Whitby, Efquire.	Mary, only daughter of Sir Walter Bethell, of Ellerton, Knight. By Jane, daughter and coheirefs of William Sotheby, of Birdfall, Efq.	On Monday the 24th of January.	On Sunday the 30th of January.
MARY	BECKWITH. Second daughter of	Thomas Beckwith, counfellor at law, on Friar Wall, only fon of the late Roger Beckwith of Ripon, Gent. By Jane his fecond wife, daughter of John Hungate, of Saxton, Efq.	Margaret, daughter and heirefs of John Darley, of Buttercramb, Efq. By Frances his firft wife, daughter of John Milner, of Tadcafter, Efq.	On Saturday the 22d of January.	On Wednefday the 16th of February.
JAMES	ANDERSON Fourth Son of	John Anderfon, Apothecary, in Caftlegate, youngeft fon of James Anderfon of Brigg com Linc. Gent. By Frances, daughter of William Saltmarfh, of Howden, Gent.	Sarah, late relict of William Ramfden, rector of St. Martin's in the Fields, London, and daughter of Samuel Dixon, Alderman, of Leeds, deceafed.	On Tuefday the 22d of February.	On Saturday the 19th of March.

BAPTISMS at St. MARY's, CASTLEGATE, YORK, for the Year 1774.

BURIALS at St. MARY's, CASTLEGATE, for the Year 1774.

Christian Name.	Surname.	Descent, Profession, and Abode.	When died, and where buried.	Age.	Distemper.
JOHN	GRIMSTON.	Doctor of Physic, a married man, fourth son of John Grimston, of Grimston Garth, in Holderness, Esq. By Charlotte, second daughter of John Wilson, Recorder of Hull.	Died at his house without Monk Bar, on Sunday the second of January, and buried in the vault under the altar on Friday the 7th of January.	56 years.	Apoplexy.
JANE	TURNER.	Relict of Oliver Turner, of Wakefield, Gent. eldest daughter of the late Samuel Palmes of Naburn, Esq. By Isabel, daughter of James Strickland, of Thornton Bridge, Gentleman.	Died at Wakefield on Tuesday the 8th, and buried on Saturday the 12th of February, in the centre of the south aile.	47 years.	Pulmonary Consumption.
JAMES	FOUNTAIN.	Bachelor, and portrait painter in Coppergate, only son of William Fountain of Thirsk, woollen-draper. By Jane Stonehouse, his wife.	Died on Wednesday the 16th, and buried on Sunday the 20th of March, in the church-yard, under the east window of the chancel.	25 years.	Fever,

** This improvement may be extended to the register for marriages, and the form, as established by an Act of Parliament, will in general allow room sufficient for inferring the descent of each party.

OBSERVATIONS

AND

EXPERIMENTS

ON THE

POISON OF LEAD.

ADVERTISEMENT.

THE excellent Treatises of Sir George Baker, on the POISON OF LEAD, first excited the author's attention to the subject; and to him the former edition of this little work was inscribed. The approbation of so able a judge is at once a sufficient motive and apology for offering it again to the public.

OBSERVATIONS and EXPERIMENTS

ON THE

POISON of LEAD.

SECTION I.

THE public has been lately favoured with feveral valuable treatifes on the fubject of Lead, which reflect equal honour on the learning, ingenuity, and benevolence of the author.* His obfervations on its ready admiffion into, and injurious operation on the human body, are highly interefting and important; and clearly evince that many chronic, as well as acute difeafes, proceed from this mineral poifon, when fuch a caufe is unfufpected.

NOR is the action of Lead confined to the human fpecies: It exerts alike its deleterious powers on quadrupeds and birds.

A GENTLEMAN in Staffordfhire ufed to feed his hounds in troughs lined with Lead, and they

---

* Dr. Baker, now Sir George Baker, Bart.

never hunted but three or four of them fell down
during the chace, convulfed, and feemingly in
agonies of pain.   A friend fuggefted to the owner
of the dogs, that thefe convulfions might poffibly
arife from fome portion of Lead diffolved in their
food.   The leaden troughs were, therefore, removed, and the hounds, from that time, were
entirely free from this diforder.   Another inftance,
of a fimilar kind, was related to me by a country
gentleman who refides in Derbyfhire.

An intelligent Plumber in Manchefter affures
me, that he is unable to keep a cat in his houfe
above a month or two.   The animal foon fickens,
becomes rough in its coat, liftlefs, emaciated,
and dies in a fhort time of a *marafmus*.   Thefe
fymptoms he afcribes to the particles of Lead
fcattered upon the floor of his work-fhop, which
adhering to the feet of the cat, and being licked
off, are fwallowed, and exert their virulent powers
immediately on the ftomach and bowels.   A perfon of the fame bufinefs, and of good credit in
Sheffield, has obferved that cats are fond of the
fweet powder with which the furface of Lead is
generally covered; and that they are affected by
it in the manner juft defcribed : But he adds that
they are fometimes driven to the moft outrageous
madnefs ; and that he has cured many of thefe
animals, when labouring under the moft frightful
fymptoms, by pouring fweet oil into them.

At

An ingenious apothecary, whose house is contiguous to a Plumber's shop, has more than once observed appearances of the *colica pictonum* in his cats; and some of them have become quite frantic with pain.

A RED LINNET, very lively and in perfect health, and which had been long used to confinement in a cage, was placed in a parlour, recently painted with white Lead. The bird soon sickened, continually gasped for breath, and died in a few days. Another bird of the same species, and equally healthy, was then purchased to supply its place. This was presently affected in a similar manner, and died in less than a week.

A LADY, who is attentive to the feeding of her poultry, had troughs of Lead made for them, on account of their being more durable and cleanly. After the use of these she observed that her fowls and chickens became sickly, spiritless, and emaciated. The food she gives them consists of bread, potatoes, barley, &c. mixed with butter-milk. The latter ingredient is a powerful solvent of Lead; and thus poison is mingled with their nourishment.

A NUMBER of ducks and geese, the property of a painter, were all killed by being confined, a single night, in a place supplied with the water in which his brushes had been steeped, to prevent their becoming dry.

G g 2   SATURNINE

SATURNINE preparations are now almoft univerfally employed in furgery; and from their
aftringent, antifeptic, and fedative powers, are
juftly claffed in the firft rank of topical remedies.
But Mr. Goulard ftrenuoufly maintains, that the
external ufe of Lead is *never* attended with any of
the pernicious effects of its internal exhibition.
And we have the concurring teftimony of his
very ingenious commentator to thefe facts *(a)*.
The evidence of thefe gentlemen feems to be
further corroborated by the experience of the
faculty at Chefter, on a late melancholy occafion.
November 5, 1772, a large number of people,
affembled at a puppet fhew, were blown up by
the accidental explofion of gun-powder, placed
underneath, in a grocer's warehoufe. The fufferers, admitted into the Infirmary, were in number
fifty-three, not one of whom efcaped without
violent marks of contufion, or large and deep
burns in different parts of the body. They were
all repeatedly wafhed with Goulard's faturnine
water, which in every inftance feemed to produce
the moft falutary effect. And though the circumftances of thefe unhappy patients appear to

(a) Vide Mr. Aikin's Obfervations on Preparations
of Lead, page 10.——My friend Mr. White, who
ufes large quantities of the Extract of Lead both in his
private, and hofpital practice, entertains the fame
opinion with Mr. Aikin, of its innocency, and efficacy.

have

have been peculiarly favourable to the abforption, as well as to the immediate action of this mineral poifon on the nervous fyftem, no fymptoms afterwards occurred, which could reafonably be imputed to its operation.   Three of the fufferers, indeed, died of the locked jaw; but this difeafe, with fufficient probability, was afcribed to the bruifes which they received about the joints. Strong as this evidence may be efteemed of the innocency as well as efficacy of Lead, externally applied, I am ftill inclined, with Dr. Baker, to believe that it *fometimes* produces its fpecific effects upon the body; and the following cafes, though not decifive, will at leaft fhew that my opinion is not entirely without foundation.

THREE years ago a young man had a tumour of the fpine, which had refifted various difcutient remedies.   An emollient cataplafm, mixed with the *extractum faturni* of Goulard, was applied. In a few hours he was feized with violent pains in his bowels, and fevere cramps in the extremities, which ceafed foon after the cataplafm was removed.

A GENTLEWOMAN, in Auguft 1770, was over-turned in a chaife, and thrown on the fide of her head and fhoulder; the mufcles of which were much bruifed and ftrained, but the *humerus* was neither fractured nor diflocated.   She was immediately bled, and the venæfection was re-

peated

peated the next day. A faturnine fomentation
was applied warm to the parts affected, and frequently renewed. Twitchings in the legs enfued,
and afterwards fpafms in the ftomach. The
fomentation was omitted, and thefe fymptoms
ceafed; nor did any other application produce the
like effect. This lady is fubject to the colic;
but as fhe was ignorant of the fpecific action of
Lead, the fpafms in her ftomach cannot be imputed to the force of imagination.

THE governor of the work-houfe in Manchefter, aged upwards of feventy years, had a large
ulcer in his leg, which was wafhed feveral times
in the day with the faturnine water of Goulard,
and then covered with an emollient poultice,
which contained a fmall quantity of the extract of
Lead. After ufing thefe applications four days,
he became affected with the colic, and alfo with
paralytic fymptoms, which though flight in degree, could not fail to be alarming. The preparations of Lead were therefore difcontinued,
a dofe of *oleum ricini* was adminiftered, and he
foon recovered from thefe adventitious complaints.

A LADY of a delicate habit, and the mother
of four children, foon after delivery, to avoid
being a nurfe, rubbed her breafts with oil in
which litharge and red lead had been boiled.
Her milk was by thefe means repreffed; but in
a fhort time fhe began to complain of acute pain
about the ftomach and duodenum, lofs of appetite,

tite, flatulency, and depreffion of fpirits. Opium
and the warm bath were the only remedies that
afforded relief. Whether thefe complaints arofe
from the receffion of the milk, or were occafioned
by the poifonous action of the calces of Lead, I
leave to the decifion of my reader.

IN June 1757, a phyfician of great humanity,
was defired to vifit a woman who had a varicofe
fwelling of the veins of the right foot, attended
with great pain, fwelling, and inflammation. He
directed a folution of *faccharum faturni* and opium,
in elder flower water, to be frequently applied,
by means of linen rags, to the part affected.
The pain was alleviated, the fwelling diminifhed,
and the rednefs foon difappeared. But in a few
days fevere vomitings, a violent colic, and obftinate conftipation of the bowels fupervened; and
the woman was ever afterwards fubject to
frequent returns of thefe complaints. The faturnine folution was ufed only four or five days; nor
was it then difcontinued from any fufpicion of its
injurious effects. For very little attention was
at that time paid to the noxious qualities of Lead.

I HAVE been affured, from undoubted authority,
that Dr. A—— had a flight paralytic affection
of his legs, by the practice of fetting his feet
every evening, on a piece of Lead placed near
the fire. And that a dog, by lying on it, was
entirely deprived of the ufe of his limbs.

ZELLER

ZELLER mentions a remarkable inſtance of the
pernicious effects of litharge, which Dr. Baker
has quoted. *De Lithargyro quoque mihi narra-
vit, matronam quandam nobilem pulverem ejus, in
rubore faciei, poſtquam hic ipſi tanquam ſingulare
et certiſſimum arcanum deprædicatus fuiſſet, in petia
ligatum, axillis bis vel ter die aſperſiſſe cum preſen-
taneo effectu; verum exinde ſubſecuta fuiſſe dyſpnæam,
lipothymiam, dolores vagos in abdomine, vomituri-
tionem, et nauſeam.* This account the doctor has
confirmed by the caſe of a violent and obſtinate
colic, which appeared to be occaſioned by ſome
litharge mixed in a cataplaſm, and applied to
allay a troubleſome itching*(b)*. The teſtimony
of Boerhaave muſt alſo be admitted to have great
weight on this ſubject; and he ſeems to ſpeak
from experience, when he ſays, after deſcribing
the proceſs for making vinegar of Lead, " This
" preparation, if rubbed upon the ſkin, in a ſtate
" of dilution, cures eruptions, redneſs, the eryſi-
" pelas, and inflammations; gives whiteneſs and
" beauty to the ſkin, but proves injurious to the
" body, at length occaſioning a conſumption, as
" appears by many melancholy examples*(c).*"

(b) Medical Tranſactions, vol. I. p. 312.

(c) " SI dilutum corpori affricetur, puſtulas, rube-
" dines, eryſipelas, phlegmonas multum levat; cuti
" candorem, nitoremque conciliat; ſed corpori nocet,
" tandem in phthiſin deducendo, ut triſtiſſimis ſæpe
" conſtitit exemplis." Element. Chemiæ, vol. II.
Proc. 172.   S E C-

SECTION   II.

THE following obfervations concerning the effects of Lead I have collected in Derby-fhire.   There are many mines of this ore, from the working of which no inconvenience enfues *(d)*. But the cafe is otherwife where the vein of ore is narrow, and the lime ftone fides are very hard; for then the fmall particles of the ore, which fly off from the tool by the force employed in digging it, fall upon the faces of the workmen, and are frequently received into their mouths. The fame is true, alfo, of the mines in which the water runs through the ore; for the faces of the men are continually fprinkled with it, by the dafhing of the pick-axes, and they look as if rubbed over with gun-powder.   To render the ore fit for fale it is broken, and carefully wafhed from the impurities which adhere to it. If any cattle drink of the water which has been ufed for this purpofe, they are affected with violent colics, and conftipation of the belly; and they generally die convulfed.   Dogs and cats, from the fame caufe, will fometimes become

(d) THE Earl of Hopetoun informs me that his miners in Scotland are, in general, a very healthy fet of men.

mad,

mad, fall into fits, and often kill themſelves by running headlong againſt a wall.

THE *colica pictonum* is more incident to thoſe employed in the ſmelting of Lead, than to the workers in the mines. But ſince cupolas have been uſed for that operation, it has prevailed much leſs than formerly, even amongſt this claſs of men. For the vapours ariſing from the Lead are thus carried off, by a ſtrong current of air, through a chimney, which is raiſed many yards above the furnace. Theſe vapours deſtroy the verdure of the graſs, which grows in the neigh-bourhood of the ſmelting houſes; and the cattle which feed on it are ſometimes affected with the dry gripes, or, as it is vulgarly termed, the belland. But the moſt frequent cauſe of this diſorder amongſt horſes and cows, is the grazing in paſtures, which have been overflowed by floods from the mines. And it is remarkable that theſe animals, who are generally directed to avoid whatever is injurious to them, by an inſtinct wiſe and unerring in its operation, ſo far from being averſe to this mineral poiſon, are fond and even greedy of it to exceſs. The ſame is true alſo of pidgeons, and other tame fowls, who pick up the ſmall particles of Lead whenever they meet with them. Sheep are ſeldom known, in Derbyſhire, to be affected with the belland.

I AM

I AM indebted to an experienced and judicious practitioner, who resides at Bakewell in Derbyshire, for the following information concerning the usual method of treating the *colica Pictonum*, amongst the workers in Lead. The men first complain of a weight, pain of the stomach, and costivenes, which , are generally relieved, if thy apply early for advice, by a vomit, and pills of soap, rhubarb, and aloes; or by any aperient medicines of the liquid kind, with oil added to them. But if these symptoms be neglected, the patients complain of their saliva becoming sweet, of clammy sweats, lassitude, feebleness of the legs, a total loss of appetite, obstinate costivenes, and a fixed pain in the abdomen, with severe retchings. In this stage of the disorder, oily clysters and gentle purgatives are the most effectual remedies; and are usually repeated at short intervals, till the stools assume a natural appearance. For during the disorder they are hard, dry, and scaly like bran. The *oleum ricini* has of late been used with great success.

I CANNOT omit this opportunity of recommending the trial of alum, both as a prophylactic, and as a remedy in slighter cases of the *colica pictonum*. I have administered it with the happiest effect in various obstinate and painful affections of the bowels. Fifteen grains given every fourth, fifth, or sixth hour, for the most

part

part prove gently aperient; and if the fymptoms
be not very fevere, the fecond or third dofe
feldom fails to mitigate the pain, and fometimes
entirely removes it.   When there is reafon to
apprehend that the alum may be too rough or
auftere in its action, it may be combined with
gum arabic, or fperma ceti; and under this
form it is moft likely to be ferviceable in the
colic arifing from Lead *(e)*.

In Derbyfhire, when the miners or fmelters of
Lead find themfelves affected with the afthma,
they ufually leave their occupation for a while,
and work at the lime kilns, experience having
taught them that the fixed air, or *mephitis*, arifing
from the calcination of lime ftone, is an effectual
and fpeedy remedy in this diforder.   No other
change of employment affords them fo much
relief.   The fame vapour, in a moderate degree,
feems to be falutary to the human conftitution;
for I have been informed by a gentleman of
judgment and veracity, who has the direction
of a confiderable number of lime kilns, that the
men employed in burning lime are remarkable
for their health and longevity.   This obfervation
is the refult of more than thirty year's experience;
and perhaps may corroborate the popular opinion,

(e) See Cafes of Colics, cured by the Ufe of Alum,
p. 461.

that

that in confumptions of the lungs it is good to live near places, where this procefs is carried on.

It is the common practice of the fmelters of Lead, and of others, alfo, who live in the neighbourhood of fmelting mills, to broil mutton, beef, or pork fteaks on the hot pigs of that metal, by which the flefh acquires a peculiarly agreeable flavour. It is probable the flavour depends upon the fweetnefs communicated by the effluvia of the new-caft Lead; but however grateful to the palate, it muft be injurious to the nervous fyftem. A Clergyman, at Bakewell, who was fond of fifhing, and often ufed to broil his fifh in this way, was affected, during feveral years before his death, with colics, frequent retchings, and a total lofs of appetite. His diforder was afcribed to an irregular gout; but the apothecary who attended him is now of opinion, that it was produced by the dangerous practice above mentioned; to the confequences of which he was then a ftranger.

The river Derwent flows through a large tract of Derbyfhire, which abounds with Lead mines; and the ftreams difcharged from many of them, and which are loaded with particles of Lead, fall immediately into it. Yet it is ftored with trout and other fifh, and the water of it is potable, and not efteemed unwholefome. But I have often remarked, that the trout caught in the Derwent

near

near Matlock, are of a fmaller fize, of a fofter texture, paler colour, and of a lefs agreeable flavour than thofe of other rivers. And I am inclined to impute this to the action of Lead; becaufe the fame kind of fifh are found in great perfection in the river Trent, into which the Derwent flows, after a paffage which allows time for the precipitation of the ore which it contains. The following fact alfo, if it be deemed fufficiently authentic, confirms my opinion. It is related in a letter from Dr. Carte, of Manchefter to Dr. Grew, of which I fhall infert a copy in the Appendix, that the reader may determine the degree of credit which is due to it. " I know " a fmall rivulet, on which fome of thefe mills " ftand, wherein trouts have been caught which " have been fuppofed affected with the bellan, by " the irregularity of their growth, their heads " being great and mifhapen, their backs crooked, " their tails very fmall, which I am apt to think " might proceed from their feeding on the " fmitham or duft that is wafhed down at a flood: " For not only the fumes, but alfo the wafhings " of the Lead ore, and the wafte (as they call it) " i. e. the duft that remains after the ore is melted, " is very noxious to moft fort of creatures, and " for this reafon, they that live near the mills " dare not water their horfes at the river upon " a flood."

THE

THE manufacturers of the White and Red Lead Works in Sheffield, are frequently and violently difordered; but they feldom apply to the faculty for affiftance, becaufe they have certain popular remedies amongft themfelves, which are chiefly of the laxative kind. Some of thefe workmen, when labouring under complicated affections of the lungs, ftomach, and bowels, have been fpeedily relieved by a dofe of emetic tartar, fufficient to operate both as a vomit and purgative. And a blifter, applied to the abdomen, has alfo been known to remove a very fevere colic, arifing from the fame poifon.

THE compofition called by braziers pot-metal, becaufe pots for boiling food are made of it, confifts of nearly equal parts of copper and lead, with a fmall proportion of litharge and of antimony. Brafs cocks are, alfo, made of the fame materials. The heat neceffary for fufing this compofition is much greater than what is ufually employed by plumbers, and fufficient to evaporate Lead very copioufly; and this evaporation is much increafed by the flux which is often employed. The workmen, in thefe two articles, ufe few or no precautions excepting chimneys that draw well, but they are unavoidably expofed to the noxious vapours every time they pour the metal into a mould. Yet I have heard, from good authority, that not above one in forty of

thefe

thefe artifts becomes confiderably difeafed, in the manner fuppofed to arife from Lead; although a few of them are fometimes moft violently afflicted with colics and palfies. Indeed there feem to be certain conftitutions very little difpofed to be affected by this mineral poifon, either externally or internally applied. Two cafes have been communicated to me, of the vinegar of Lead being fwallowed in no inconfiderable quantity, without prejudice. It proved in the one inftance powerfully diuretic; in the other it produced no fenfible effect.

A PHYSICIAN, well known to the public by his ufeful and ingenious writings, informs me, that during his refidence in the Weft-Indies, many cafes fell under his obfervation which juftify the utmoft caution in the ufe of Lead, and of its preparations. In one of the fmall Virginia Iflands near Tortola, a Gentleman who poffeffed many flaves, built a fpacious houfe, which was covered with fhingles, or wood cut into the form of tiles, and painted with red Lead. The rain that fell upon this roof, was conveyed by pipes into an open ciftern of Lead, for the ufe of the family; the individuals of which had been peculiarly incident to violent, and fometimes fatal colics. The phyfician very juftly attributed this diforder to the Lead carried off, by the rain, from the fhingles, or corroded by the water in the ciftern.

ciftern.   And he had afterwards the fatisfaction
to find, that thofe who refrained from this water
were no longer liable to attacks of the colic.

A LEARNED friend of mine is of opinion, that
the colic from Lead was more common amongft
the ancients, than is generally fufpected.   Their
drink, he obferves, was chiefly wine of the acefcent kind, which powerfully corrodes this mineral : And pains of the bowels were very general
complaints, as appears from the writings of Celfus.
Oil, alfo, both externally and internally, was the
remedy prefcribed in fuch cafes ; the efficacy of
which is chiefly, if not entirely confined to the
colica pictonum (f).

Two modern books of Cookery contain receipts for recovering wine when four, and preventing it from becoming fo, by means of ceruffe,
and of melted Lead.   From one of thefe books,
I have tranfcribed the receipt, which is as follows.

" To hinder wine from turning."

" *Put a pound of melted Lead, in fair water,*
" *into your cafk pretty warm, and ftop it clofe.*"

The Univerfal Cook, p. 244.

This work was publifhed in 1773, and is written by John Townfhend, late Mafter of the Grey-

(f) Celfus de Morb. Inteft. tenuioris ; Aretæus de Ileo ;
& Cælius Aurelianus.

VOL. I.   H h   hound

hound Tavern, and Cook to his Grace the Duke of Manchefter.

It muft be fuppofed that Mr. Townfhend is ignorant of the poifonous quality of Lead; but he is certainly deferving of cenfure for prefuming to give receipts without better information. And if he, or other vintners have practifed the method which he recommends, they are juftly chargeable with all the mifchiefs fuch deteftable arts muft produce. The adulteration of wine is indeed an evil fo general, and fo dangerous in its confequences, that it is to be hoped the legiflature will interpofe to prevent it.

It may not be unfeafonable here to fuggeft a caution, againft the common practice of cleaning wine bottles with leaden fhot. It frequently happens, I am perfuaded, through inattention, that fome of the fhot are left behind; and when wine or beer is again poured into the bottles, this mineral poifon will flowly diffolve, and impregnate thofe vinous liquors with its deleterious qualities. The fweetnefs (which is fometimes perceived in red port wine) may arife from this caufe, when fuch an adulteration is neither defigned nor fufpected.

The workmen in the fugar-houfe at Manchefter are fupplied with beer, prepared of malt and the refufe of the fugar, which are often fermented together in a large leaden ciftern. The liquor
ferments

ferments fo brifkly, that without the utmoft care it becomes foxed, or inclined to acidity; and the men who drank of it were formerly fubject to the moft fevere and excruciating colics. Of late, proper meafures have been taken to check the progrefs of the fermentation; and the fugar boilers, in confequence of this precaution, have been fince exempt from thofe violent attacks to which they were before incident. Whether thefe colics were owing to a folution of Lead, or to the acidity of the wort, I fhall not prefume to determine.

A LADY of a delicate conftitution, whofe bowels are very irritable, always finds herfelf affected with the colic, if fhe fits half an hour in a room which has been lately painted. And a gentleman and his wife, by fleeping in fuch a chamber, a few years ago, were both violently difordered. The gentleman informs me, that when he firft awaked, he felt a great oppreffion at his breaft, a tremor, naufea, and a fevere pain and great confufion in his head. By changing his apartment, thefe fymptoms were in a fhort time happily removed.

S E C T I O N   I.

EXPERIMENT I. THE very beautiful polifh of the Burflem pottery, commonly called the Queen's ware, inclined me to

fufpect

suspect that Lead, which is easily vitrified with sand and kali, enters into the composition of its glazing. To determine whether my conjectures were well founded, I poured about an ounce and a half of vinegar upon a plate of this ware, that a large surface of the glazing might be exposed to the action of the vegetable acid. In twenty-four hours the vinegar had acquired a deeper colour, and assumed a dusky hue when two drops of the volatile tincture of sulphur were added to it. The same tincture, instilled into fresh vinegar in the like proportion, produced a light cloudiness, which was succeeded by a white sediment; the sulphur being precipitated by the combination of the acid and alkali. From this trial, which was several times repeated, it should seem that Lead is an ingredient in the glazing of the Queen's ware; but the quantity dissolved by the vegetable acid, appears to be very inconsiderable. For two drops of a solution of *saccharum saturni* (which I computed to be equal only to the fiftieth part of a grain of Lead) mixed with half an ounce of vinegar, struck a darker colour with the tincture of sulphur, than the same quantity of vinegar, after its action had been exerted upon the plate forty-eight hours.

THE present experiment, therefore, furnishes no objection to the common use of this beautiful pottery; but it shews that vessels of it are improper for the preserving of acid fruits and pickles.

EXPERI-

EXPERIMENT II. I was a witnefs to the following experiment, when made by my friend Dr. Prieftley, and have fince repeated it. Several pieces of paper, daubed with white lead paint, were put under a receiver, which was then immerfed, about two inches deep, in a veffel of water. In twenty-four hours the air was diminifhed more than one fifth part in quantity, and was become in a high degree noxious. It extinguifhed a candle, did not effervefce with nitrous air *(g)*, and affected a moufe in fuch a manner, as muft quickly have proved fatal, if the animal had not been immediately withdrawn. This air was rendered wholefome by agitation in water; which fhews the propriety of placing veffels of water in rooms recently painted. Perhaps fprinkling water by means of a garden

---

(g) NITROUS air is obtained from all the metals and femimetals, except zinc, by the nitrous acid. When one part of this air is added to two parts of common air, the mixture becomes hot, turbid, and of a red colour, and fuffers a diminution of nearly one third part of its bulk. Thefe effects are obferved to be exactly proportioned to the fitnefs of the air for refpiration. With mephitic, inflammable, or any kind of noxious air, no chemical union is formed, nor any fuch changes produced by it. Hence the nitrous air furnifhes a very accurate teft of the comparative purity of other fpecies of air. Vide Dr. Prieftley's Papers on various Kinds of Air, which will be publifhed in the LXVII. vol. of Philofoph. Tranfactions.

pot, would be ftill more effectual, becaufe the furface is thus increafed, and fome degree of agitation produced.

EXPERIMENT III.   I tried the fame experiment with what the painters term *dead white*, which is a compofition of white Lead, linfeed oil, and fpirit of turpentine.   The refult differed in no other refpect, but in the proportional diminution of air, which was lefs in the prefent than in the former trial.   Surprized at this circumftance, I repeated the experiment feveral times, but the event was uniformly the fame.   It is probable, therefore, that the oil of turpentine, by furnifhing a caufe of addition to the air, diminifhed the apparent deftruction of it by the white Lead. This paint is found to be more injurious to the nervous fyftem than any other, which may be explained by the action of the turpentine, in quickening and increafing the evaporation of the Lead.

EXPERIMENT IV.   I expofed a very large furface of painter's oil to the air contained in a glafs jar, immerfed in water.   In twenty-four hours the air was diminifhed in its bulk one fourth part, and inftantly extinguifhed flame.   Having no nitrous air in readinefs, I could not employ this teft.   Painter's oil is prepared by boiling litharge and a fmall quantity of red lead, in the oil extracted from linfeed.

EXPERIMENT

EXPERIMENT V. I made a fimilar experiment with common linfeed oil, and found that the air was neither diminifhed in quantity, nor rendered noxious in its quality.

EXPERIMENT VI. Having more than once felt myfelf difagreeably affected by the fmell of an oil-cafe hood, I was defirous of trying whether this might arife from any thing injurious, communicated by it to the air. Several flips of frefh oil-cafe were, therefore, put into a receiver, which was then placed in water. The air in twenty-four hours extinguifhed the flame of a candle, and was diminifhed in quantity, but in what proportion I did not afcertain. Various compofitions are employed for making oil cafe: But I believe they all contain Lead, and the moft common one confifts of *faccharum faturni*, gum copal, and other refinous fubftances, which are boiled in oil, to the confumption of two thirds of the original quantity. I am informed by an artift in this branch of bufinefs, that he is never employed in the above preparation, without fuffering a moft violent head-ach. And I have lately had a patient, who laboured under a fevere and obftinate colic, which feemed to be produced by the fame poifonous effluvia. For previous to her diforder, and during the fhort intervals of it, fhe was affiduoufly employed in fhaping and fewing feveral hundred oil-cafe hoods.

H h 4   After

After a variety of remedies had been tried in vain, the cure of this patient was at laſt effected by alum, combined with ſpermaceti.

EXPERIMENT VII.   Red ſealing wafers are made of fine flour, the whites of eggs, iſinglaſs, and a little yeaſt.   They ſhould be coloured with vermilion; but as red lead is much cheaper, I believe it is more frequently uſed.   The common wafers certainly contain a large quantity of it, as any perſon may diſcover, by ſetting fire to a few of them, when ſtuck upon the point of a pin. For the ſurface of the wafers will be covered with an infinite number of the particles of Lead, which running together will fall down into a ſpoon, or whatever is held to receive them. Wafers are pleaſant to the taſte, and they are often held long in the mouth, and ſometimes ſwallowed through inadvertence : I have ſeen children fond of eating them.   It is of importance, therefore, to know that the coarſer or common kinds are poiſonous, and that it is very abſurd œconomy to purchaſe ſuch on account of their cheapneſs.   The poliſhed Iriſh wafers ſeem to contain no Lead.

A LADY in Cheſhire had a favourite bulfinch, which was ſo tame as to be permitted to fly about the room ; a liberty that ſeemed to improve both his health and plumage.   The bird unfortunately picked up ſome ſcraps of wafers, which had been

left

left after fealing a letter.   He foon loft his appetite and fpirits, and in a few days pined away and
died.   Another bulfinch was procured, and when
fufficiently tame, allowed the liberty which the
former had enjoyed; but great care was taken
to keep wafers out of his reach.   However, by
the inadvertence of a ftranger in the family, who
had been ufing them, a piece of one was left
upon the table, which the bird immediately
feized, and like the former fickened and died in
confequence of it.   Dr. Falconer, to whom I
am indebted for thefe facts, adds that fome time
afterwards, a third bulfinch, belonging to the
fame lady, met with a fimilar fate.

Dr. WALL of Worcefter, to whofe friendfhip
I am under many obligations, has lately favoured
me with the following cafe.   " I was fome years
" ago called to the fon of a plumber in this
" town, a child about two years of age, who
" had been remarkably healthy till this illnefs.
" He had been taken, a few days before I faw
" him, with violent pains in the bowels, attended
" with a fever, and convulfive motions in the
" limbs.   Thefe complaints had been attributed
" to worms, and feveral medicines had been
" given unfuccefsfully.   When I vifited him firft,
" I found him paralytic on one fide, and deliri-
" ous.   Upon inquiring into the caufe of his
" diforder, and particularly whether the child had
                                                  been

" been ufed to go into the room where they
" melted the Lead, I was informed that he did
" frequently, and that it was a cuftom with his
" maid to let him run barefooted along the fheets
" of Lead, whilft they were warm, with which he
" appeared to be much delighted. I did not
" then hefitate to attribute his prefent diforder
" to this caufe."

I HAVE fome doubt whether the vapour of
arfenic be fo poifonous, as is commonly fuppofed;
and if the reader will excufe the digreffion, I will
lay before him the facts on which that doubt is
founded. To folder works of filver filigree, and
other delicate manufactures, a compofition is
ufed, of which arfenic is the principal ingredient.
The folder is melted by the flame of a lamp,
directed by a blow pipe; and this operation
cannot be performed with due accuracy, but
in a clofe room. The greateft part of the arfenic
is evaporated by the blaft and flame, and fome
part alfo of the reft of the folder. And the workmen muft conftantly breathe thefe vapours, becaufe there is little or no current of air to carry
them into the chimney. Yet the men appear
to enjoy as good health, and to live as long as
other artifts who purfue their bufinefs in clofe
rooms, and ufe lamps. Amongft other examples
of the truth of this obfervation, I faw one lately
in the manufactory at the Soho, near Birmingham:

ham: A man aged upwards of fifty, who has foldered filver filigree more than five and thirty years; has regularly paffed from eight to twelve hours daily in his occupation; and is at prefent fat, ftrong, active, cheerful, and of a complexion by no means fickly. Neither he, nor his brother artifts, ufe any means to counter-act the effects of their trade.

A N

AN

APPENDIX

TO THE

OBSERVATIONS on LEAD.

EXTRACT OF A LETTER, FROM THE AUTHOR, TO
DR. DUNCAN OF EDINBURGH; ON THE EX-
TERNAL USE OF PREPARATIONS OF LEAD (a).

THOUGH I entertain a very high opinion of
the usefulness of Saturnine preparations,
externally applied, and frequently prescribe them,
yet I am fully convinced that they *sometimes* produce the specific effects of Lead upon the body.
And I could wish that more attention were paid
to the operation of such topical remedies, especially when applied to constitutions to which we are
strangers. There are, indeed, some habits that
appear very little disposed to be affected by this
mineral poison, of which I have given several

(a) Inserted in the Medical Comment. vol. III. p. 199.

examples

examples in my *Obfervations and Experiments on Lead,* and can now add two others. The firft was communicated to me by Mr. Barker, furgeon in Bakewell; the fecond, by the late Dr. Small, an excellent philofopher, and a phyfician of great eminence at Birmingham.

Two fmelters, who have worked *nineteen years* at the fmelting mills, have conftantly, during that time, toafted the cheefe, and broiled the bacon, and other provifions which they ufed, on the hot pigs of lead, without the leaft apparent inconvenience. They are ftout, healthy men, and have never experienced any pains in their bowels. And, as this method of dreffing meat renders it remarkably fweet and palatable, Mr. Barker could not prevail upon them to difcontinue it.

A GENTLEMAN, who had been long troubled with the heart-burn, difcovered, from repeated trials, that his malady was relieved by fwallowing a large quantity of faliva. To increafe this fecretion, he chewed, many hours every day, a piece of Lead, which being neither hard, friable, nor offenfive to the palate, fuited his purpofe better than any other fubftance. This practice he continued many years, with great advantage, and without injury, in any refpect, to his health.

But the fame learned phyfician informed me, that he had feen three inftances of the

fatal

fatal effects of Goulard's Extract of Lead externally applied. Two of the cases were incipient White swellings; the third was a tumour of a more uncommon kind. Each of the patients became paralytic, and two of them were convulsed several days before death. I lament that Dr. Small did not favour me, in his letter, with a more circumstantial relation of these cases; but his judgment and accuracy may be relied on with confidence.

From the present universal use of the Saturnine Water of Goulard, it may be thought surprizing that such melancholy examples, as these, do not more frequently occur. But this preparation happily contains so small a portion of Lead, that it is capable, in the most irritable habits only, of producing its peculiar effects. An ounce phial, filled to the brim with the *Extractum Saturni*, weighed sixty-five grains and a half heavier than the same quantity of the vinegar with which it was prepared. A hundred drops of this Extract, the quantity usually mixed with a quart of rain-water, are about the fifth part of an ounce, and may be supposed to suspend thirteen grains of Lead, if no change be produced, by combination, in the specific gravity of the compound. Each ounce, therefore, of the vegeto-mineral

mineral water contains only four tenths of a grain of this metal.

The *Aqua Saturnina*, employed in the following cafe, was ftrongly impregnated with Lead, having an ounce of the Extract in every quart of water. On Thurfday February 16, 1775, Mr. P——, a young man of a delicate habit of body, had a tea-kettle full of boiling water thrown upon his leg, by which the cuticle was feparated from the knee to the toes. Oily applications were immediately ufed; but the pain and inflammation were fo great, the following day, as to require the affiftance of the ingenious furgeon *(b)*, to whom I am indebted for this account. A gentle laxative was directed; the patient's leg and foot were well wafhed, every three hours, with Goulard's Saturnine Water; and afterwards covered with linen foaked in the fame lotion, and wetted with it from time to time. The relief obtained, by thefe means, encouraged the young man's friends to ufe the lotion in an immoderate quantity; for, in fix days, no lefs than feven quarts of water were confumed. On Wednefday night, the fixth from the firft application of this remedy, the furgeon was called to his patient, and found him violently af-

(b) Mr. Starkie, of Manchefter.

flicted

flicted with colic, trembling of the limbs, continual naufea, and frequent vomitings. He had been coftive three days, and had neglected to take a purgative medicine prefcribed for him. It may be proper to point out the progrefs of thefe fymptoms, as they feem to mark the gradual operation of the Lead. On Monday the conftipation commenced, and a flight tremor was perceived in the fcalded limb: The tremor continued on Tuefday: On Wednefday the colic fupervened, which grew extremely fevere and alarming in the evening, and was aggravated by the ficknefs and retchings which accompanied it. Directions were given to difcontinue the lotion; the *Ceratum Sambucinum*, fpread upon linen, was applied to the parts affected; and the following draught was adminiftered every four hours.

> R. *Ol. Ricini V. O. fubact. ʒſs.*
> *Aq. Menth. Pip. fimp.* ʒ i.
> *Tinct. Thebaicae gutt. vii.*
> *Syr. e Meconio* ʒ i. m. f. *hauftus.*

SEVERAL motions were procured by the repetition of this draught; the complaints of the patient became more moderate; and the colic entirely ceafed before the next evening. But a forenefs of the *abdomen* remained, and the body was left in a very irritable ftate.

The

The fcalded leg and foot, in eight days, were more healed than is ufual, after fuch accidents, in three weeks, when unctuous remedies are employed.

I have feen and examined the patient, whofe cafe is here related; and can atteft the faithfulnefs and accuracy of this account.

The facts which I have now adduced, in conjunction with thofe contained in my Treatife on the Poifon of Lead, afford a ftrong prefumption, that Saturnine preparations, externally applied, are not fo perfectly innocent as they are too generally afferted and believed to be. One pofitive proof, well authenticated, out-weighs a thoufand negative ones; efpecially when fuch pofitive evidence is acknowledged but rarely to occur. And I fhall be happy in the idea of having done fome fervice to the community, if I can excite more attention to the operation, and more caution in the ufe of thefe topical remedies, which are defervedly efteemed, and univerfally employed. My defign is not to difparage them, but only to recommend a juft difcrimination of their effects. Whenever tremors of the limbs, paralytic affections, coftivenefs, yellownefs of the countenance, or pains in the bowels fucceed the application of any Saturnine compofition, the ufe of it fhould be for a while fufpended, or entirely difcontinued;

and the proper antidotes to the poison of Lead should be sedulously administered. Thus will the danger be obviated on its first approach; and we shall not be reduced to the sorrow and disgrace of having cured an ulcer, a burn, or a contusion, by inflicting the most excruciating tortures, or perhaps at the expence of life.

It has been observed in the Medical Essays, published by a Society at Edinburgh, " that " though opium produces such certain effects in " the stomach, yet it is not clear, that it has any " operation externally, even when applied to the " bare nerves, in a part excoriated by a blister." This has been urged as an argument against the topically poisonous action of Lead. But the observation is not founded in truth, and is contradicted by facts which daily occur in medical practice. For what physician is a stranger to the powers of opium when applied to the nerve of of an aching tooth, or to the eyes in an *ophthalmia* ?

Dr. Heberden remarks, in his very ingenious lectures on poisons, that Lead affords a singular instance of a poison which only affects the nerves of motion : " Tremblings, strong spasms, " and palsies, are its usual consequences; but " I apprehend it has been seldom or never found " to injure the understanding, or to make the " patient delirious, till he becomes so, as is
" common

" common in moſt diſtempers, by the near ap-
" proach of death." I believe this curious obſervation, with reſpect to the human ſpecies,
may be juſt; but cats become frantic by ſwallowing Lead.

I HAVE obſerved, that peſtles and mortars, for
the uſe of apothecaries and others, are made of
the *glazed* Burſlem pottery. This muſt be attended with pernicious conſequences; becauſe the
vitrified Lead will be diſſolved by the acids,
which are frequently employed in medicine; and
the particles of it will be abraded by conſtant
friction. Perhaps theſe particles may, alſo, be of
ſuch a ſize and ſharpneſs, as to injure, by their
mechanical action, the coats of the ſtomach; for
the glazing is very unequally diffuſed over the
ſurface of the coarſer ware.

COPY OF A LETTER FROM DR. HAYGARTH, TO
　THE AUTHOR, CONTAINING A PARTICULAR
　ACCOUNT OF THE EFFECTS OF GOULARD'S
　SATURNINE WATER ON THE SUFFERERS BY
　THE EXPLOSION OF GUN-POWDER, AT CHESTER,
　NOVEMBER 5, 1772.

CHESTER, May 31, 1773.

I SHOULD fooner, my dear friend, have
anfwered your benevolent inquiries concerning the effects of Goulard's faturnine water upon
the patients who fuffered by the explofion of
gun-powder in this city, on the fifth of November
laft; but the horrors of that tremendous fcene,
even at this diftance of time, are fo painful, that
I feel a peculiar reluctance in recollecting their
anguifh and variety of wretchednefs.　Happy
fhould I be, if this dreadful calamity could afford
any ufeful inftruction how, in future, to alleviate
the miferies of mankind.

　FROM the neighbouring coal-pits there are
frequently fent to our Infirmary, patients, who,
by the explofion of the inflammable vapour they
contain,

contain, have been burnt on their faces, hands, and often a great part of their bodies which happened to be uncovered. Oil, in the usual method, had been generally applied to these burns. But the integuments were often so deeply affected, and to so large an extent, and the patients continued for many days in such exquisite pain, that their groans and lamentations were heard over the whole house. On this account, a trial was made in these cases of the saturnine water, and with the most happy event; the excruciating pains were immediately relieved, and the burns soon healed. The striking similarity of the cases afforded the most convincing argument, that the same remedy should be used in the burns from gun-powder.

On the night of the fatal accident, thirty-three patients were admitted into the Infirmary; the hands and faces of all, with the arms and thighs of the women, were, in general, severely burnt. A considerable number of old patients, with other assistants, were most assiduously employed in washing all the burnt and bruised parts with the saturnine water, many times over, that night. The next morning I examined very attentively the appearance of the burns; they were very moderately inflamed, and upon their being asked, none of the patients complained of that painful burning vulgarly attributed to fire in the part,

except

except one young man whose legs were so deeply affected, that all the integuments sloughed off, and the sores could not be healed in less than six months.

I COMPARED very attentively the state of the burns, which had been thus treated, with those of twenty patients, who were admitted into the Infirmary the next and following days. Though the latter in general had received incomparably much slighter injuries, yet their burns appeared red, tense, and highly inflamed; and they complained of a severely painful burning in the parts affected. When the saturnine water had been plentifully applied to these burns, the pain and inflammation very soon abated.

As preparations of Lead, when taken internally, are known to produce such pernicious effects, the faculty have, with reason, doubted whether their external application were universally safe. On this account, I was particularly attentive in watching every symptom that might possibly arise from the poison of Lead, and can assure you, that, of these fifty-three patients, whose burns and contusions were very plentifully and frequently washed with the saturnine water, not one had the slightest symptom of colic or palsy, during the whole time of their recovery, though so many nerves were exposed to the immediate contact of the Lead.

THE

The only cafes that proved fatal were three young girls, who were feized with the locked jaw, and died convulfed. Though this difeafe has never, that I know, been attributed to the poifon of Lead, yet as this is a purely nervous affeftion, I will mention fuch particulars of each cafe, as will entirely remove all fufpicion of this caufe, by fhewing that the injuries they received were fully adequate to fuch an effeft. The poor girl, who was firft feized with a locked jaw, had been fo much hurt by the explofion, as to be unable to fpeak for twenty hours after the accident; and befides many fevere contufions and burns, the *tendons* on the back of her hand were all laid bare by a deep burn. The fecond, befides large burns on her face, arms, and thighs, with a bad contufion on her head, had the *tendons* of her ham feverely lacerated and burned. This patient complained to me, particularly, that a pain alter-nated between this wound, and the mufcles of her neck and jaw, that were fpafmodically af-feéted. The third had a broken arm, large burns and contufions, but was not feized with a locked jaw, till the integuments on her *facrum* were deeply mortified.

It is of importance to obferve on the whole, that of one hundred and fix perfons, who were blown up by eight hundred pounds of gun-powder, twenty-three died almoft inftantly by the ex-

plofion;

plofion'; that among fo large a number of the
remainder as eighty-three, who had received fuch
fevere burns, contufions, fractures, and dif-
locations, fo fmall a proportion as three only
terminated fatally : fifty-three, who of this
number had received the worft injuries, were
admitted into the Infirmary. This very uncommon fuccefs I would chiefly attribute to a
plentiful application of the faturnine water,
together with copious evacuations, acid and
acefcent drinks, and fupplying the wards both
day and night fo freely with frefh air, as entirely to clear away all the putrid effluvia, produced by fo great a number of very large
fores.

I am ever,

DEAR SIR,

With the fincereft Regard,

Your moft faithful, and affectionate,

J. HAYGARTH.

COPY

COPY OF A LETTER FROM DR. ROTHERAM, OF
NEWCASTLE-UPON-TYNE, TO THE AUTHOR.

S I R,

I AM much obliged to you for the specimen
of your Experiments and Observations upon
the Poison of Lead. The subject is truly
interesting; and I am very glad that you
have taken it in hand, as I am sure the public
will reap both pleasure and benefit from your
inquiries.

WHILST I practised at Hexham, I was frequently consulted for the workmen in the Lead
mines, Smelting mills, and Refineries, of which
there are many in that neighbourhood; and I
most sincerely repent my negligence in not
taking proper minutes of those cases; had I done
that, I might have now been able to have sent
you an hundred of them; but alas! I have nothing but my memory to trust to, and therefore
must speak chiefly in generals.

I HAVE ever looked upon Lead to be highly
poisonous, when its particles are so minutely divided by heat, corrosion, solution, &c. as to

enter

enter the pores or abforbents of any part of the body, but more particularly thofe of the lungs and ftomach; though I have fometimes fufpected them to reach the brain itfelf; for as thefe very minute parts are rendered extremely volatile, efpecially by a ftrong heat, it is no wonder that they pervade fome of the fmalleft pores, and penetrate into the inmoft receffes.

THE people who work in the mines here are generally pretty healthy; and I believe your obfervation with regard to this point will commonly hold: Their diforders may moftly arife from the fmall broken pieces, duft, or wafhings: but I dare not affert this as an univerfal maxim, becaufe I have fome reafon to believe that noxious effluvia are fometimes mixed with the air in old workings, and where they have not a proper number of air-fhafts; and the people affected by this kind of foul air, fhew very different fymptoms from thofe who work in our coal mines. Afthmas, and thofe very obftinate ones, are a frequent confequence, and I believe almoft univerfally attended with a blue expectoration, which lafts for feveral months, often attended with a *conftipatio alvi*, and fometimes with fpafmodic contractions of the mufcles. I think I remember fome of them paralytic; but, as I lamented before, for want of proper minutes I dare not be pofitive.

YOUR

Your obfervation of the cupolas is a very juft one, and confirmed by plentiful experience in this neighbourhood; which leads me to make fome remarks on the three branches of fmelting, refining, and reducing; though they may not be new to you, yet as I have had frequent opportunities of attending to them, I fhall trouble you with a few hints in each.

The effluvia rifing from all thefe works are foon condenfed and concreted when they come into the cool air, and form a great deal of white fubftance, which lines the chimney of flues, and what rifes out falls perceptibly on the ground, fometimes in fmall duft, at other times in little flakes, deftroying a great part of the herbage; what remains gives the cattle the belland, and neither dogs, cats, nor poultry will thrive near any of thefe mills. The fmelting bufinefs has generally been reckoned lefs noxious than the refining, and the reducing or running the litharge into Lead the worft of all; for they ufed always to reduce the litharge upon hearths, and indeed they ftill purfue this fenfelefs method in fome of our works; but the more provident ones have erected proper furnaces for this procefs, which convey the fmoke to a greater diftance; whilft the refiner ftands at the mouth of the teft conftantly fupplying it with Lead, regulating the fire and taking away the litharge, whilft the bel-

lows

lows behind, which are conftantly fkimming off the litharge, blow the effluvia full in his face. The quantity of thefe effluvia may be in fome meafure computed from the lofs of Lead in refining, which generally amounts to at leaft one ton in thirteen, though I am apt to believe that more of this evaporates in the reducing than the refining; for the litharge like minium always exceeds the weight of the Lead from which it is produced; whereas probably twelve tons of litharge when it is run down will fcarce produce eleven of Lead.   To illuftrate this a little farther, I took, the other day, five grains of litharge, and the like quantity of lead, and laid them upon feparate pieces of charcoal which I held in my hand, and threw the flame of a lamp very ftrong upon them with a blow pipe.   The litharge in a very few feconds run down into a clear piece of lead which weighed four grains and a half, the half grain evaporating almoft inftantly, and the vapour covered the charcoal for about an inch round, where it lay with a thin yellow, or rather greenifh cruft.   The Lead was near half an hour in evaporating, but threw off the fame kind of vapour; I obferved from this that the litharge is much more volatile than lead, and the firft fumes are probably more fubtile and eafier raifed.

THE workmen in this country call the diforder by the name of the Mill-reek, and in general it

anfwers

anfwers to the fhort defcription you have given of it in Derbyfhire. The moft particular cafe which I remember was that of Thomas Wallace, a refiner, and who had formerly wrought in the mines; he confulted me about fixteen years ago; he had then violent pains and gripings, with coftivenefs and a numbnefs in his limbs. The medicine with which he was chiefly relieved was the gum pill with a third part of aloes, taken morning and evening. He went to work again, when his diforder foon returned, and brought a *gutta ferena* upon one eye, and rather hurt the fight of the other; his left hand, if I remember aright, turned paralytic; which complaints baffled every effort which I made for his relief by purgatives, blifters, and nervous medicines. He then went recommended to the Bath Hofpital; but, after ufing the waters, and fuch medicines as the phyficians there prefcribed for fome time, he returned in the fame paralytic ftate. I heard of him about two years ago, and I do not know but he may be yet living, and in the fame condition; but as he is forty miles from hence, I have not frequent opportunities.

I KNOW not whether the following experiment may lead to any conclufion in your way, but you may perhaps not be difpleafed with a trial, which you may eafily make at your leifure. Some time ago I made feveral unfuccefsful attempts to cor-

rode

rode or diffolve Lead in the vitriolic acid: I knew
full well that infufing, boiling, or digefting would
not do it; but I digefted ground litharge for
fome time in oil of vitriol ftill without effect. At
laft an ingenious acquaintance, to whom I had
communicated my thoughts, moiftened fome
powdered litharge with diftilled vinegar, and a
day or two afterwards poured fome water and oil
of vitriol upon it, which inftantly turned the
whole mafs into the moft beautiful white Lead I
ever faw; the vinegar doubtlefs acting as a medium of attraction betwixt the litharge and the
vitriol. But the acid of vitriol feparates the parts
of the Lead too far, fo that the fubftance, though it
exceeds the beft white Lead of the fhops in colour,
is greatly deficient in fpecific gravity; and no
art which we have yet ufed can remedy this fault,
and here I am afraid it muft reft. For after feveral trials, it wants body to be of any ufe in
painting; nor does it flux or vitrify eafily enough
to be of ufe in glazing the white earthen ware.
But may not the minerals in fome waters meet
with fome proportion of a fimilar medium, by
which they may attract particles from leaden
pipes, cifterns, &c. and thus carry off with them
many noxious particles.

I HAVE long thought, and am lately more certain, that not only the generality of Lead Ores
in this country, but often the Lead itfelf is more
heterogeneous,

heterogeneous, than has been imagined. I even doubt whether some of our Lead mines may not produce every known metal. Silver is well known to be contained in them all, though in widely different proportions; Mr. Cox, if I am not much misinformed, has lately produced a great quantity of copper from the slags or refuse of some of our smelting mills, and for this purpose has purchased large quantities; zinc we are sure is in some parts of the ore, and zaffre I have produced from other specimens, though I have not yet brought this last to such a certainty as I could wish. The copper sometimes unites with the Lead in smelting, and greatly injures it for the market, as it renders it harder and more brittle.

I MUST trouble you a little farther with expressing my doubts about your last paragraph. How far the fluxes used in soldering the filigree may fix the parts of the arsenic, or from what other cause those workmen might escape, I dare not say; but I should notwithstanding strongly suspect the fumes of this very volatile and caustic mineral to be very prejudicial. Hildanus gives us several instances of bad effects from its external application in small quantities. Hoffman, in his *Metallurgia Morbifera*, sect. xvii. says, *Tristis casus memini, qui Lipsiæ contigit, dum in domo Stanniarii, qui arsenicum cum cupro admisceret, ab haustis ejus venenatis fumis, plures in eadem domo habitantes,*

habitantes, maligno morbo adfecti et mortui funt.
Hoffman likewife tells us, in the fame fection,
that the men employed in both digging and manufacturing the cobalt at Kuttenberg in Bohemia,
are fo affected with vomitings, fyncoptic anxieties,
cardialgias, difficulties of breathing, fuffocations,
tremors, &c. that they appear like living fkeletons.

I FEAR I have too long trefpaffed upon your
patience, and I doubt to little purpofe; as you
will have fo much better and more pertinent information. I moft heartily wifh you all the fuccefs which you can defire: I hope you will com-
mand a great deal, but am fure you will merit
more.

I AM, with thanks for the honour of your laft
correfpondence,

Your much obliged,

and very humble fervant,

J. ROTHERAM.

NEWCASTLE,
JULY 8, 1773.

A LETTER

A Letter from Dr. Saunders, of London to the Author, on Preparations of Lead.

Jeffries-square, *February* 1, 1776.

DEAR SIR.

BEING informed that you are preparing for the prefs a volume of Effays on philofophical and medical fubjeĉts, on the fame plan with thofe already publifhed, I am happy in this opportunity of communicating to you a few ftriking faĉts and experiments on fome of the preparations of Lead, a fubjeĉt which has already engaged your attention. Much has been written on the efficacy of the preparations of Lead, on external application; and their operation and effeĉts are fo well underftood by furgeons, that little remains to be faid upon this fubjeĉt. It being however generally admitted, that the *Acetum Lithargyrites* or Goulard's extraĉt is in its operation and powers the fame as the *Saccharum Saturni*; I am defirous of correĉting this popular error, by ex-

Vol. I. K k plaining

plaining the difference between thefe two preparations.

METALLIC BODIES acquire their caufticity by
an union with acids, with which they enter into
a ftate of mixture; the activity is proportioned
to the quantity of acid and the degree of folubility in the metallic falt. The variety in this refpect in fome metallic falts is fo great, even
where the acid in combination is the fame, that
the caufticity acquired by a moderate proportion
of metal is almoft deftroyed, when a larger proportion is added: This is illuftrated by attending
to the difference between corrofive fublimate and
calomel, which are both preparations of mercury
with the fame acid. This reafoning will apply
to the fubject of Lead.

IN the preparation of the *Acetum Lithargyrites*,
the acid is fully faturated with Lead; in the preparation of the faccharum faturni, the acid is in
a much larger proportion to the Lead. The *Acetum Lithargyrites*, when diluted by the pureft
diftilled water, gives out a copious precipitation
which, from experiment, I find to be Ceruffe.
The *Saccharum Saturni* remains diffolved in diftilled water, and is therefore applied topically in
a ftate more immediately active, both from its
greater proportion of acid, and its preferving its
folubility under high degrees of dilution. I find
                                    from

from experiment that, by adding a very fmall proportion of diftilled vinegar to the *Aqua Satur-nina* of Goulard, the white precipitate is re-diffolved, and that the folution procured in this manner is more active, but lefs adapted to remove inflammation, and abate irritation, as a fedative, than the *Aqua Saturnina* itfelf. I was firft led to apply to this fubject from an averfion to the ufe of turbid liquors, efpecially when the preci-pitation is produced by the pharmaceutical treat-ment of chemical mixtures. I am, however, perfectly convinced, that no degree of dilution of *Saccharum Saturni* will anfwer the many valu-able purpofes to be obtained from the ufe of the *Acetum Lithargyrites*. In the operation of medi-cines on the human body, a flow and gradual action is often to be defired, in preference to a more immediate operation from the fame remedy, applied in a more foluble form. It is upon the fame principle that the *Flores Zinci,* when diffufed in water, in many cafes, produce a better effect than a folution of the *Vitriolum Album* in any ftate of dilution; and that the *Kermes Mineral,* and fome other preparations of antimony of a flow folubility, produce a more lafting opera-tion, and poffefs more powers than even the *Tartar Emetic*, except in fuch cafes where imme-diate and active evacuations are required, as in

K k 2   the

the beginning of fevers and acute difeafes. Water alone therefore, in the cafe of the *Aqua Saturnina*, proves a precipitant of Lead by attracting the acid, and reducing the preparation to a ftate of Ceruffe, an intermediate ftate between Lead and the *Saccharum Saturni*; fo that Ceruffe diffufed in water more nearly refembles the *Aqua Saturnina* of Goulard, than a folution of the *Saccharum Saturni* does. There is however an advantage in external application from the ufe of powdery bodies, in their ftate of precipitation, becaufe they are in a more fubtle form than any body can be rendered by mechanical triture. I have fometimes been of opinion, that various chemical mixtures are formed by the union of the fame metal in its application to different proportions of the fame acid, and that *Calomel* may be confidered as the union of Mercury with *Corrofive Sublimate*, in which the acid was fo much attracted and engaged, that it entered into a very imperfect union with the additional quantity of Mercury in *Calomel*; and that therefore the Mercury employed which produces Calomel, diminifhes the activity of Corrofive Sublimate without acquiring folubility itfelf, and without lofing much of its own phlogifton; hence the precipitates from Calomel and Corrofive Sublimate, by alkaline fubftances, differ fo effentially

in

in their nature. In the fame manner the *Saccharum Saturni* may be confidered as an union of Ceruffe with Vinegar, whereas Goulard's *Acetum Lithargyrites* is an union of Lead with Vinegar.

To the fame principle may be referred the power of fixed air in re-diffolving calcareous matter, after it had proved, in a fmaller proportion, a precipitant for quicklime: So that although chalk may be confidered as a combination of quick-lime and fixed air; calcareous matter diffolved in water by fixed air is an union of chalk and fixed air. We even find that though quicklime attracts fixed air ftronger than the cauftic fixed alkali; yet the cauftic fixed alkali attracts fixed air more ftrongly than chalk does, and therefore precipitates chalk held in a ftate of folution by fixed air. This will probably beft explain why the cauftic alkali fhould prove a precipitant of calculous matter diffolved in the mephitic acid. I have mentioned thefe facts with a view to illuftrate that it is a principle in chemiftry, that various mixts are formed from the combination of two bodies, in different proportions to one another. It is upon a fimilar principle that metallic falts are rendered lefs active by abftracting their acid, either by attraction or calcination. An attention to thefe circumftances, derived from a knowledge of the chemical hiftory

of

of bodies, may lead to some future improvements in the pharmaceutical treatment of many valuable remedies, and enable us to render chemical preparations more or less active, or more or less soluble, as the indications of cure may seem to require.

A LETTER

A Letter from Dr. John Carte to Dr. Grew, concerning the Belland, caused by the fumes of Lead; extracted from Dr. Hooke's philosophical experiments, published by Mr. Derham, f. r. s.

Manchester, *October* 27, 1678.

I THOUGHT it might be worth while to give you a short account of a distemper in Derbyshire, very common among those, who are employed in the smelting-mills, *i. e.* the houses where they melt the Lead down from the ore; it is by the country people called the *belland,* but for what reason I cannot learn; it is hard to give a concise definition of it, because it seldom appears but under the disguise of another disease.

This *belland* frequently imitates the *tormina ventris scorbutica,* but in a most exquisite manner, which is usually accompanied with extreme costiveness, and a continued suppression of urine; sometimes appears like an *asthma convulsivum,* sometimes a continued and obstinate *dyspnœa,* and often seizes the *genus nervosum,* either in a paralytic resolution of the parts, or in spasms.

It

It has a different effect upon men, according to their age; if they come not to the work of the mills, till they are full grown, or of a middle age, they suffer mostly the aforementioned pains of the belly, or difficult breathing. But if taken in while young, and growing, they are subject to the palsy; their limbs (especially their fingers) being often irrecoverably resolved: Or sometimes have their fingers so contracted, as to render them, perhaps for ever, incapable of working: Both which I have seen.

I could not be informed of any specifics, they had for this disease; but that a decoction of *coloquintida*, in ale, was very common among them. I remember once an old man complained to me of the *belland*; it oppressed him in the nature of an *asthma*; I advised him to sulphurate medicines, which did relieve him. The contraction of the fingers I have known cured, by often putting the arms into hot grains after brewing.

I have not observed, whether any of those, that are paralytic by the *belland*, die hectic, as Dr. *Pope* relates of them, at the *mercurial* mines in *Firmly*, but it seems not improbable that they may.

This distemper is not only incident to men, but other creatures, as horses, cows, dogs, cats, hens, geese, &c. but, especially, cats are subject

to

to it: Indeed few creatures that are young, will live near these mills without the *belland*.

Dogs do in their fits howl and tumble up and down, foaming like *epileptics*; this the people impute to the pain of their bellies.

I know a small rivulet, on which some of these mills stand, wherein trouts have been caught, which have been supposed affected with the *belland*, by the irregularity of their growth, their heads being great and mishapen, their backs crooked, their tails very small, which I am apt to think might proceed from their feeding on the *smitham* or *dust* that is washed down at a flood: For not only the fumes, but also the washings of lead ore, and the *waste* (as they call it) *i. e.* the dust that remains, after the ore is melted, is very noxious to most sorts of creatures, and for this reason, they that live near the mills, dare not water their horses at the river, upon a flood.

These poisonous fumes are not only hurtful to animals, but also injurious to vegetables; for if the smoke be driven much upon any one place, it destroys all the grass of it.

Now that the *belland* in men, or other creatures, proceeds mostly from the smoke, will be easily granted; but what these fumes are impregnated with, is the question. Some fancy them to be antimonial; but then, methinks, they

Vol. I.   L l   should

should have the same effect with the flowers of that mineral, and I never heard that any of them were inclined to vomit. I am much more apt to think, that the *mercury* in the ore is the cause, both because they that work in the *mercurial* mines, are subject to the like symptoms, especially the palsy; and also I am told, that this *belland* often begins with a swelling of the glands about the throat, which, perhaps, if not prevented, might terminate in salivation. But why *mercury* should operate so variously upon bodies, differing in age, is a question will hardly be solved, till it appear more plainly, whether it be nearer akin to alcalies or acids: Its effect is easily foretold in bodies that abound with acids, whether scorbutic or venereal; but in younger persons whose humours are more insipid, and their blood freer from both fixed salts and acids, it may, perhaps, fix itself upon the nerves, as the coolest parts, and impede the motion of the spirits; but I had rather hear other's reasons about the cause of these things, than trouble you with my own.

SOME other things I have been informed of by the workmen, as that a little spar mixed with the lead ore, promotes its fusion, I suppose, as the yellow marchasite, that's found with silver, makes that metal flow the sooner: That if there be any hollywood in the fire, it hinders the flux-

ing

ing of the ore, which is certainly caufed by the glutinous fap of that wood.

THAT the fmoke is obferved to follow the water very much: I fuppofe the coldnefs of the water does condenfe the fumes, as is feen in reviving *mercury* from *cinnabar*. A blue film is obferved on the furface of thofe waters, where the fmoke falls.

THAT a man may, by wetting his finger in his mouth, or common water, draw it through melted lead or iron, without any prejudice.

SIR, thefe obfervations will feem barren, yet as good as I could make among thefe people of the *Peak*, few of which can give a rational account of either what they do, or fuffer, in fuch matters.

I am,

SIR,

Yours, &c.

END OF VOLUME FIRST.

Printed in the United States
By Bookmasters